MEDICARE

A Strategy for Quality Assurance

Volume I

Committee to Design a Strategy for
Quality Review and Assurance in Medicare

Division of Health Care Services

INSTITUTE OF MEDICINE

Kathleen N. Lohr, editor

NATIONAL ACADEMY PRESS
Washington D.C.   1990

National Academy Press • 2101 Constitution Avenue, N.W. • Washington, D.C. 20418

NOTICE: The project that is the subject of this report was approved by the Governing Board of the National Research Council, whose members are drawn from the councils of the National Academy of Sciences, the National Academy of Engineering, and the Institute of Medicine. The members of the committee responsible for this report were chosen for their special competencies and with regard for appropriate balance.

Volume I of this report has been reviewed by a group other than the authors according to procedures approved by a Report Review Committee consisting of members of the National Academy of Sciences, the National Academy of Engineering, and the Institute of Medicine.

The Institute of Medicine was chartered in 1970 by the National Academy of Sciences to enlist distinguished members of the appropriate professions in the examination of policy matters pertaining to the health of the public. In this, the Institute acts under both the Academy's 1863 congressional charter responsibility to be an adviser to the federal government and its own initiative in identifying issues of medical care, research, and education.

This study was supported by the Health Care Financing Administration, U.S. Department of Health and Human Services, under Cooperative Agreement No. 17-C-99170/3.

Library of Congress Cataloging-in-Publication Data

Institute of Medicine (U.S.). Division of Health Care Services.
    Medicare : a strategy for quality assurance : a report of a study
by a committee of the Institute of Medicine, Division of Health Care
Services / Kathleen N. Lohr, editor.
       p. cm. — (Publication IOM ; 90-02)
    "Committee to Design a Strategy for Quality Review and Assurance
in Medicare"—P. following t.p. verso.
    "This study was supported by the Health Care Financing
Administration, U.S. Dept. of Health and Human Services, under
cooperative agreement no. 17-C-991/3"—T.p. verso.
    Includes bibliographical references.
    ISBN 0-309-04230-5 (v. 1)
    1. Medical care—United States—Quality control. 2. Medicare.
I. Lohr, Kathleen N., 1941- . II. Institute of Medicine (U.S.).
Committee to Design a Strategy for Quality Review and Assurance in
Medicare. III. United States. Health Care Financing
Administration. IV. Title. V. Series: IOM publication ; 90-02.
    [DNLM: 1. Health Insurance for Aged and Disabled, Title 18.
2. Quality Assurance, Health Care—United States. WT 30 I591m]
RA395.A3I56 1990
362.1'0973—dc20
DNLM/DLC
for Library of Congress   90-5787
                                                          CIP

Printed in the United States of America

Committee to Design a Strategy for Quality Review and Assurance in Medicare

STEVEN A. SCHROEDER,* *Chair,* Division of General Internal Medicine, University of California at San Francisco, San Francisco, California

MARK R. CHASSIN, Value Health Sciences, Santa Monica, California (formerly of The RAND Corporation)

LEO M. COONEY, Yale University School of Medicine and Yale-New Haven Hospital, New Haven, Connecticut

ROBERT B. COPELAND,* Georgia Heart Clinic, LaGrange, Georgia

CHARLES J. FAHEY,* Third Age Center, Fordham University, New York, New York

PAUL F. GRINER,* University of Rochester Medical Center and Strong Memorial Hospital, Rochester, New York

WILLIAM S. HOFFMAN, Social Security Department, International Union, United Auto Workers, Detroit, Michigan

ROBERT L. KANE, School of Public Health, University of Minnesota, Minneapolis, Minnesota

HAROLD S. LUFT,* Institute for Health Policy Studies, University of California at San Francisco, San Francisco, California

MAXWELL MEHLMAN, The Law-Medicine Center, Case Western Reserve University School of Law, Cleveland, Ohio

MARIE MICHNICH, American College of Cardiology, Bethesda, Maryland

MARILYN MOON, Public Policy Institute, American Association of Retired Persons, Washington, DC (until October 1989); The Urban Institute, Washington, DC

JAMES D. MORTIMER, Midwest Business Group on Health, Chicago, Illinois

ALBERT G. MULLEY, Jr., General Internal Medicine Unit, Massachusetts General Hospital, Boston, Massachusetts

EDWARD B. PERRIN,* Department of Health Services, University of Washington, Seattle, Washington

MARGARET D. SOVIE,* Hospital of the University of Pennsylvania, Philadelphia, Pennsylvania

LORING W. WOOD, NYNEX Corporation, White Plains, New York

---

*Institute of Medicine Member

STUDY STAFF

Division of Health Care Services

KARL D. YORDY, *Director*
KATHLEEN N. LOHR, *Study Director*
MOLLA S. DONALDSON, *Associate Study Director*
JO HARRIS-WEHLING, *Staff Officer*
ALLISON J. WALKER, *Research Associate*
MICHAEL G. H. McGEARY, *Senior Staff Officer*
DONALD TILLER, *Administrative Assistant*
THELMA COX, *Secretary*
DENISE GRADY, *Secretary*
THERESA NALLY, *Secretary*

Contents

PREFACE . . . . *ix*

INTRODUCTION TO THE STUDY AND THIS REPORT . . . . *xiii*

SUMMARY 1

1 HEALTH, HEALTH CARE, AND QUALITY OF CARE 19
   Defining Quality of Health Care, 20
   Health and Health Care in the United States, 25
   Quality of Health Care as a Public Policy Issue, 31
   Summary, 37

2 CONCEPTS OF ASSESSING, ASSURING, AND IMPROVING
   QUALITY 45
   Quality Assessment, Quality Assurance, and Quality Improvement, 45
   Criteria for Judging an Effective Quality Assurance Program, 49
   Quality Assurance Conceptual Models, 52
   Traditional and Continuous Improvement Models Compared, 62
   Summary, 64

3 THE ELDERLY POPULATION 69
   Size and Growth of the Elderly Population, 69
   Sociodemographic Characteristics, 71
   Economics of Aging, 75
   Use of the Health Care System, 79
   Health Status, 85
   Summary, 91

v

4 THE MEDICARE PROGRAM 96
Structure, Eligibility, and Benefit Coverage of the Medicare
  Program, 97
Administration and Financing of the Medicare Program, 102
Expenditures of the Medicare Program, 104
The Prospective Payment System (PPS), 108
Quality Assurance in Medicare, 110
Summary, 111
Appendix A The Medicare Catastrophic Coverage Act of 1988, 114
Appendix B The Medicare Decision Support System, 117

**5 HOSPITAL CONDITIONS OF PARTICIPATION IN
MEDICARE** 119
Standards and Conditions, 120
Inspection and Enforcement, 128
Federal Government's Roles and Responsibilities, 131
Conclusions, 132
Summary, 134

**6 FEDERAL QUALITY ASSURANCE PROGRAMS FOR
MEDICARE** 138
Experimental Medical Care Review Organizations, 139
Professional Standards Review Organizations, 139
Utilization and Quality Control Peer Review Organizations
  (PROs), 147
Controversial or Problematic Aspects of the PRO Program, 182
Conclusions About the PRO Program, 195
Summary, 199

7 QUALITY PROBLEMS AND THE BURDENS OF HARM 207
Introduction, 207
Evidence of Problems in Technical Quality of Care, 211
Evidence of Overuse, 220
Evidence of Underuse, 225
Summary, 230

**8 SETTINGS OF CARE AND PAYMENT SYSTEM ISSUES
FOR QUALITY ASSURANCE** 238
Settings, 238
Payment Systems, 254
Other Setting and System Factors, 258
Summary, 259

9   METHODS OF QUALITY ASSESSMENT AND
    ASSURANCE 265
    Introduction, 265
    Prevention of Problems, 267
    Detection of Problems, 274
    Factors that Impede or Enhance the Effectiveness of Quality
        Interventions to Correct Problems, 289
    Summary, 297

10 CRITICAL ATTRIBUTES OF QUALITY-OF-CARE
    CRITERIA AND STANDARDS 303
    Types of Criteria Sets, 304
    Effect of the Type and Use of Criteria on Specification of
        Desirable Attributes, 309
    General Attributes of Criteria Sets, 310
    Differences Among Key Attributes for Different Criteria Sets, 319
    Methods and Strategies for Developing Quality-of-Care Criteria, 323
    Other Issues, 325
    Summary, 328
    Appendix A   Criteria-Setting Expert Panel Activity, 334

11 NEEDS FOR FUTURE RESEARCH AND CAPACITY
    BUILDING... 343
    Research Needs, 344
    Capacity Building, 360
    Funding Issues, 363
    Summary, 363

12 RECOMMENDATIONS AND A STRATEGY FOR QUALITY
    REVIEW AND ASSURANCE IN MEDICARE 368
    Findings and Conclusions, 369
    Recommendations, 375
    Organizational and Operational Features of the Medicare
        Program to Assure Quality, 387
    Responsibilities and Tasks of the MPAQ, 394
    Responsibilities and Tasks of the MQROs, 400
    Implementation Strategy and Phases, 412
    Summary, 419

    ACKNOWLEDGMENTS 422

    INDEX 427

Preface

Medical care in the United States presents a paradox. At its best, U.S. medicine is a marvel, featuring state-of-the-art diagnostic and surgical technology augmented by sophisticated pharmaceutical agents. Most citizens report that they are happy with their medical care. Yet, at the same time our health care system merits serious criticism: it is by far the most expensive in the world, consuming almost 12 percent of the nation's gross national product; its health status, as measured by such standard indices as life expectancy from birth or infant mortality rates, lags that of most developed countries; its organization and distribution of health care resources are unbalanced, with a serious skew toward technology-intensive services, sometimes at the expense of primary care, preventive services (especially for the poor), home care, and long term care; and more than 30 million persons lack any form of health insurance, thereby posing severe problems of access and equity.

By contrast, the elderly enjoy comprehensive coverage and usually excellent access to hospital and acute care facilities under the Medicare program. Coverage for ambulatory care is also good, although benefits for home and long term care are limited. By international standards, the U.S. elderly enjoy excellent health status. As judged by life expectancy from age 65, and especially from age 75, the U.S. ranks among the countries with the best longevity in the world.

Driven largely by concerns about relentlessly rising expenditures for medical care, many health policy analysts now believe that explicit rationing of health services is the appropriate strategy for medical cost containment. The prospect of rationing, however, must be viewed in the context that, for the elderly in the United States, utilization of services such as coronary artery bypass surgery, prosthetic replacements of diseased hips, and treatments for end-stage renal disease already greatly exceed levels occurring in any other country.

As a result of these conflicting trends and forces, the current health care system in the United States presents a confusing picture:

- Despite the comparatively high use of medical services, there are strong pressures to increase access and use of virtually every type of health care, including organ system transplants, treatment for AIDS, and long term care.
- At the same time, employers, employees, federal and state government, and the elderly are increasingly vocal in their opposition to paying more for medical care for themselves and others.
- Governmental and industrial efforts at medical cost containment have been persistent, incremental, and largely ineffective in their overall effect on the costs of medical care. Previous and current efforts include incentives for health maintenance organizations, hospital prospective payment, utilization review, limitations on benefits and eligibility, imposition of co-payments and deductibles, mandated local entities to ensure planning of new facilities and technologies, and limits on medical malpractice awards. These cost containment strategies have had, at best, marginal effects on the ever-increasing costs of medical care, and essentially no impact of the quality of care. It is not unreasonable to expect that the current "hot prospects" for medical cost containment, such as physician payment reform and the promulgation of practice guidelines, will be equally ineffective.
- An unintended but increasingly intrusive result of the cumulative efforts at medical cost containment has been the establishment of an administrative bureaucracy to review medical care delivered in all sites—hospital, office, home, and nursing home. Although it is unclear that the procedures that have resulted from this effort have reduced the cost of medical care, it is clear that they have introduced a layer of complexity for patients and providers and have contributed to a mounting sense of frustration among physicians.
- The advent of sophisticated data collection and analytic techniques, made possible by computer technology, offers the opportunity to measure and compare the outcomes of medical care for certain conditions across comparable settings. In addition, newer ways of conceptualizing the approach to quality measurement and improvement provide the stimulus to reassess our goals and efforts.

Emerging from this tangle has come an increasing concern about the quality of medical care, particularly focused on the question of whether cost containment efforts (both successful and unsuccessful) will harm quality. To address that question it is necessary to define quality of medical care, to measure it, to assess its current state, and to understand how it can be improved and how it might be jeopardized. From concerns and questions such as these comes this report. Requested by the Congress, the authorizing legislation called for an ambitious and far-reaching strategic plan for assessing and assuring the quality of medical care for the elderly during the next decade. Emboldened by the scope of this charge, the Institute of Medicine study took a broad and comprehensive view. Its deliberations and fact-finding included commissioned papers, public hearings, panel meetings, site visits, focus groups, and many meetings.

The resulting report indicates that although the current quality of medical care for Medicare enrollees is not bad, it could be improved; that the current system in place to assess and assure quality is in general not very effective and may have serious unintended consequences; and that exciting opportunities—still to be tested in the field—are now emerging to set in place a comprehensive system of quality assurance that can address itself to improving the health of the elderly population.

STEVEN A. SCHROEDER
Chairman, Committee to Design a Strategy
for Quality Review and Assurance in Medicare

Introduction to the Study and This Report

CONGRESSIONAL CHARGE

The commission from the Congress of the United States to "design a strategy for quality review and assurance in Medicare" was contained in Section 9313 of the Omnibus Budget Reconciliation Act of 1986 (OBRA 1986). It called for the Secretary of the U.S. Department of Health and Human Services (DHHS) to solicit a proposal from the National Academy of Sciences (NAS) to conduct the study that would address eight legislative charges, namely "among other items," to:

(A) identify the appropriate considerations which should be used in defining "quality of care";

(B) evaluate the relative roles of structure, process, and outcome standards in assuring quality of care;

(C) develop prototype criteria and standards for defining and measuring quality of care;

(D) evaluate the adequacy and focus of the current methods for measuring, reviewing, and assuring quality of care;

(E) evaluate the current research on methodologies for measuring quality of care, and suggest areas of research needed for further progress;

(F) evaluate the adequacy and range of methods available to correct or prevent identified problems with quality of care;

(G) review mechanisms available for promoting, coordinating, and supervising at the national level quality review and assurance activities;

(H) develop general criteria which may be used in establishing priorities in the allocation of funds and personnel in reviewing and assuring quality of care.

STUDY METHODS

Studies undertaken by the NAS and the Institute of Medicine (IOM) are conducted by expert committees. These committees comprise individuals selected for their expertise who can provide information and insights from all disciplines and social sectors that are important to the topic of the study. The 17-member IOM committee for this study included experts in medicine, nursing, home health and social services, law, economics, epidemiology and statistics, decision analysis, and quality assessment and assurance. Committee members also represented major consumer, purchaser, and business interests. The committee had a broad representation by age, sex, and geographic location.

The OBRA legislation required consultation with specific organizations and representatives of major groups with an interest in this issue. To this end, a 14-member Technical Advisory Panel (TAP) was appointed; it met twice during the study, and IOM staff maintained regular contact with TAP members.

Review of the congressional charges reveals that the scope of this study could have been extraordinarily, and possibly unmanageably, broad. The committee thus decided to constrain the breadth of the work in several ways. First, it considered quality issues only as they relate to elderly Medicare beneficiaries. Second, it focused on three major settings of care: inpatient hospital care, outpatient physician-office-based care, and home health care. Collectively, those locales and types of care provide important insights in problems of and opportunities for quality review and assurance not only in their own right but for other settings (such as ambulatory surgery) that could not be studied in depth. Third, the study included both fee-for-service and prepaid group practice but did not look in detail at different types of prepaid, capitated, or managed care arrangements.

Another decision was to emphasize long-range issues, that is, specifically to respond to the congressional call to ". . . design a strategy . . . ." The committee elected to consider the elements of a strategy that might be put in place over the decade of the 1990s; the aim was to articulate a goal for the year 2000 and the major steps that need to be taken to reach that goal. Thus, the emphasis of this study is on strategy, not immediate tactics, although some recommendations deal with nearer-term changes and activities.

The study was conducted in three phases: planning (summer 1987 through January 1988); data collection and report preparation (February 1988 through February 1990), and dissemination (through May 1990). The work was financed by two grants from the Health Care Financing Administration (HCFA), one for the planning phase and one for the remainder of the study. HCFA also asked that the IOM undertake a second effort, mandated in Section

9305 of OBRA 1986, to examine the capacity of standards used for hospitals to meet the Conditions of Participation for Medicare to assure the quality of hospital care. The IOM included this work in the larger effort.

The committee and IOM staff carried out several major activities during this study; they fall into the general categories of convening, gathering background information, consulting broadly with groups across the country, and acquiring or producing technical documents (some of which are in Volume II). The committee met nine times for two-to-three-day meetings. A total of 10 background papers was commissioned; in addition, several papers and reports were produced by IOM staff or consultants on various specific activities of the study.

Early in the study two sets of focus groups were conducted. Eight focus groups were carried out among elderly Medicare beneficiaries in four cities (New York City, Miami, Minneapolis, and San Francisco); an additional eight groups were done among practicing physicians in five cities (Philadelphia, Chicago, New Orleans, Los Angeles, and Albuquerque). A public hearing process was also carried out in the early months of the study. It featured two formal public hearings, one in San Francisco and the other in Washington, D.C., at which a total of 42 groups gave oral testimony before the entire committee; in addition, written testimony only was received from nearly 100 groups (of nearly 575 contacted).

The most extensive study task was a series of site visits across the country. In the major site visits (two-to-three-day trips to the states of California, Georgia, Illinois, Iowa, Minnesota, New York, Pennsylvania, Texas, Virginia, and Washington), committee and staff visited Medicare Peer Review Organizations (PROs), hospitals and hospital associations, home health agencies and aging groups, health maintenance organizations (HMOs), state departments of health, and other organizations; in addition, meetings with practicing physicians, hospital administrators, and other individuals were organized. The shorter site visits were to specific organizations (e.g., multispecialty clinics or HMOs) that appeared to offer particular insights into approaches for quality assurance. Altogether, site visitors spoke with more than 650 individuals.

To address the congressional charge of prototypical criteria and standards, a special expert panel was convened late in the study to develop recommendations concerning the criteria by which quality-of-care criteria and appropriateness or practice guidelines might be evaluated. Other consultants were used to advise on different study topics, such as legal and regulatory issues. For instance, we acquired data on staffing and costs of quality assurance programs from a survey that was being conducted at the same time by a large multihospital system. Additionally, at several of its meetings, the committee heard from a range of experts in quality assurance and related topics. Finally, committee and staff consulted with staff at

HCFA and at several federal and congressional agencies with interests in the Medicare quality assurance program.

ORGANIZATION OF THIS REPORT

This report first examines concepts of quality of care and of assessing, assuring, and improving quality of care. Chapter 1 presents the committee's definition of quality of care and examines the topic of the quality of health care as a public policy issue. Chapter 2 focuses on a conceptual framework and models for implementing quality assurance and continuous improvement programs and explores the key attributes of a quality assurance program.

The report then turns to a description of the context and environment for quality assessment and assurance in Medicare. Chapter 3 discusses aspects of the elderly population. Chapters 4, 5, and 6 examine the Medicare program and its quality assurance efforts (hospital conditions of participation in Chapter 5 and the peer review programs, particularly the PRO program, in Chapter 6).

Chapter 7 examines quality problems and the burdens of harm they pose to the elderly; these include poor technical or interpersonal performance of practitioners, overuse of services, and underuse of services. Conceptual and practical issues posed by setting and payment systems are dealt with in Chapter 8, and Chapter 9 discusses certain strengths and limitations of key quality measurement and assurance approaches. Chapter 10 deals with the special topic of desirable characteristics of quality-of-care criteria sets, practice guidelines, and case-finding tools. Chapter 11 presents the committee's views about long-range needs for research and for capacity building for quality assurance.

Finally, Chapter 12 presents the committee's quality assurance strategy for Medicare. It highlights the committee's conclusions about the current program, states the committee's recommendations about new directions for a Medicare quality assurance program, and suggests the steps and the timetable by which such a new program might be put into place. Volume II of this report contains major background documents.

We expect this report to be of interest to a wide audience. Its principal purpose is to address the strategic concerns of Congress about a viable approach to maintaining and improving the quality of care for the elderly. We believe it will be useful for those who lead the development of quality assurance programs at the local level, by documenting the wide array of tools and the rich store of quality assurance experience in the country today. The considerable research agenda called for by remaining unanswered questions about the measurement and assurance of quality should be of value for investigators in health policy, health services research, and education. Finally, we believe it will provide guidance for policymakers responsible for designing a farsighted yet pragmatic quality assurance program for Medicare.

KATHLEEN N. LOHR
Study Director, Study to Design a
Strategy for Quality Review and
Assurance in Medicare

MEDICARE

Summary

Good health is a highly valued attribute of life. It is also difficult to define; it means different things to different people. In general, however, Americans would cite similar goals for their health and principles for health care. The nation has long held a common concept of what constitutes desirable health services.

What is different today is a broad concern among the health professions about the quality of health care. This is coupled with rising dissatisfaction about the health care system on the part of the public and policymakers, unremitting pressures for cost containment, and uncertainty about the effect of future cost containment on quality of care.

Focusing these concerns on the elderly, the Congress of the United States, through the Omnibus Budget Reconciliation Act of 1986, called on the Secretary of the Department of Health and Human Services (DHHS) to request the National Academy of Sciences to conduct a study "to design a strategy for quality review and assurance in Medicare." The Academy's Institute of Medicine (IOM) appointed a 17-member committee to undertake the study. In response to the congressional mandate this committee report covers four main themes:

- appropriate definitions of quality of care and quality assurance;
- the range and adequacy of methods for measuring quality and for preventing, detecting, and correcting quality problems;
- needed research and building of a professional cadre; and
- a strategy for implementing a program to assure the quality of health care for Medicare beneficiaries.

1

The remainder of this summary first describes the methods of the study and summarizes the committee's findings and conclusions. It then gives the committee's 10 major recommendations and describes the main operational features of a Medicare Program to Assure Quality (MPAQ), as the committee denotes the new program it recommends be established. Finally, it outlines a three-phase, 10-year implementation strategy, during which time many details of the program will evolve.

FINDINGS AND CONCLUSIONS

The nation is generally perceived to have a solid, admirable base of good quality health care, and the elderly are usually satisfied with the quality of care they themselves receive. Contrasting with this positive perception of the overall quality of care in the nation is a large literature that documents areas of deficiencies in all parts of the health sector. Some of these relate to the overuse of unnecessary and inappropriate services, some to underuse of needed services, and some to poor technical skills, interpersonal care, or judgment in the delivery of appropriate services.

Significant problems exist in quality of care and in the nation's present approaches to quality assurance. These problems are sufficient to justify a major redirection for quality assurance in this country and, in particular, a more comprehensive strategy for quality assurance in Medicare.

Our major findings and conclusions include the following:

• A quality assurance program should be guided by a clear definition of quality of care.

• No single approach or conceptual framework to quality assurance is likely to suit all purposes.

• Regarding the elderly,
    —their population continues to grow, both in absolute numbers and as a proportion of the entire population,
    —the average number of years lived after age 65 continues to increase, and
    —an increasing number of the elderly live with chronic illness and disabling conditions.

• Regarding Medicare and the elderly,
    —health care costs continue to rise,
    —pressures for cost containment increase, and
    —use of sites of care other than inpatient (i.e., outpatient, long-term-care, and home) continues to expand.

• Near universal coverage of the elderly population by the Medicare program gives them better access to health care than any other age group; nevertheless, gaps in coverage and financial barriers do exist and adversely affect quality.

- Regarding the burden of poor quality,
  —evidence of overuse of health services is substantial,
  —underuse is hard to detect under existing surveillance systems, but we suspect it is considerable, and
  —numerous examples of poor performance have been documented.
- Different approaches to quality assurance may be necessary for different sites of care (e.g., hospital, home care, and ambulatory settings) and for different organizational structures such as health maintenance organizations (HMOs) and fee-for-service practices.
- Criteria by which quality of care can be reviewed or assured
  —can be classified into three main groups—appropriateness (or clinical practice) guidelines, patient management and evaluation criteria, and case-finding screens, and
  —vary considerably in internal and external validity.
- Those groups of quality-of-care criteria can be described in terms of substantive (or structural) attributes, such as scientific grounding, latitude for clinical and patient judgment, design, and efficiency and implementation (or process) attributes such as feasibility of use, ease of use, ability for special cases to be appealed, and dynamic aspects of review and updating.
- Currently available methods of quality assurance
  —suggest that a small number of outliers account for a large number of serious quality problems,
  —are inadequate in coping successfully with outlier providers,
  —tend to focus on single events and single settings,
  —may not identify underuse and overuse of services,
  —are constrained (sometimes in counterproductive ways) by regulatory and legal systems, and
  —are of questionable value in improving average provider behavior.
- Medicare Utilization and Quality Review Peer Review Organizations (PROs) constitute a potentially valuable infrastructure for quality assurance. Nevertheless, it is the perception of the committee that Medicare PROs
  —give primary attention to utilization rather than quality,
  —focus on outliers rather than the average provider,
  —concentrate on inpatient care,
  —impose excessive burdens on providers,
  —do not use positive incentives to alter performance,
  —are perceived as adversarial and punitive,
  —use a sanctioning process that is largely ineffective,
  —are rendered relatively inflexible by program funding arrangements,
  —use methods that are redundant with other public and internal quality assurance programs, and
  —have not been evaluated with respect to their effect on quality.

• Mechanisms for ensuring that hospitals meet the Medicare Conditions of Participation are generally sound in terms of the concept of "deemed status" but warrant strengthening in several aspects, especially the survey and certification procedures for hospitals that are not accredited.

• The present structure does not have the capacity to achieve a comprehensive and maximally effective quality assurance system. Required research and capacity building include basic methodological research, applications research, research on methods of diffusion, training of professionals in research and quality assurance, and methods to improve patient decision making.

A MODEL OF QUALITY ASSURANCE FOR MEDICARE

On the basis of these findings and conclusions, the committee outlined its vision of a quality assurance system for Medicare. It focuses on health care decision making and health outcomes of Medicare beneficiaries, enhances professional responsibility and capacity for improving care, uses clinical practice as a source of information to improve quality of care, and can be shown to improve the health of the elderly population. This "ideal" system stands in sharp contrast to the existing quality assurance system; the latter relies too heavily on provider-oriented process measures, regulation, and external monitoring, contributes little new clinical knowledge to improve the quality of care, and has not been evaluated in terms of impact on the health of the elderly. We believe that any future quality assurance program requires a better balance than exists today between regulation and professionalism, provider orientation and patient orientation, and processes of care and desired health outcomes.

DEFINING QUALITY OF CARE

The committee identified critical dimensions of quality of care and adopted the following definition:

Quality of care is the degree to which health services for individuals and populations increase the likelihood of desired health outcomes and are consistent with current professional knowledge.

According to this definition, the health care services provided are expected to have a net benefit (to do more good than harm, given the known risk when compared to the next-best alternative care). That benefit is expected to reflect considerations of patient satisfaction and well-being, broad health status and quality-of-life outcomes, and the processes of patient-provider interaction and decision making. The values of both individuals and society are explicitly to be considered. How care is provided should reflect appropriate use of the most current knowledge about scientific, clinical, technical, interpersonal, manual, cognitive, and organizational and management elements of health care.

RECOMMENDATIONS

In responding to the congressional charge to design a strategy for quality review and assurance in Medicare, the committee has three aims. The first is to have in place a fully functioning program by the year 2000. The second is to have many of its parts operating well before that time. The third is to create a system that itself can grow and mature well into the next century, when health care needs, health care delivery systems and financing mechanisms, and social realities may be vastly different from those we encounter today. In furtherance of these aims, the committee agreed on 10 recommendations, which are based on its findings and conclusions and its vision for a new quality assurance program for Medicare.

Medicare Mission and Quality Assurance

RECOMMENDATION NO. 1. **Congress should expand the mission of Medicare to include an explicit responsibility for assuring the quality of care for Medicare enrollees, where quality of care is defined as the degree to which health services for individuals and populations increase the likelihood of desired health outcomes and are consistent with current professional knowledge.**

A critical requirement of a quality assurance program is that it respond conceptually to an accepted definition of quality of care. For this report we have adopted the definition offered above, which implies a markedly stronger and broader mission statement for the Medicare quality assurance than appears in the legislation that presently guides the Medicare peer review program. A more explicit commitment to quality is needed to counter the perception that monitoring efforts in Medicare are primarily concerned with cost containment.

By focusing on health services, desired health outcomes, and levels of professional knowledge, our definition of quality calls for broad action by provider organizations and by the Medicare program in the collection, analysis, feedback, and dissemination of data and in the initiation of creative quality interventions. This definition implies a considerably expanded and richer conceptualization of the outcomes about which data will be acquired than has been evident heretofore in any (external or internal) quality assurance efforts. It also implies greater attention to the scientific knowledge base, to health care technology assessment, and to the actual processes of everyday practice. It requires that better use be made of what is known about the effectiveness of health care services and about the links between process and outcome. Finally, by highlighting the need for attention to both individuals and populations, this definition underscores the importance of requiring the Medicare program to take responsibility for understanding the health outcomes of the populations for which they are accountable, not just for the persons actually served.

Quality Assurance Goals of the Medicare Program

RECOMMENDATION No. 2. **Congress should adopt the following three goals for the quality assurance activities of the Medicare program:**

• **Continuously improve the quality of health care for Medicare enrollees, where quality is as defined in our first recommendation;**
• **Strengthen the ability of health care organizations and practitioners to assess and improve their performance; and**
• **Identify system and policy barriers to achieving quality of care and generate options to overcome such barriers.**

We recommend below an ongoing evaluation of the quality assurance program and its impact. The goals for which that program should be held accountable are improved health, enhanced capabilities of providers in quality assurance, and better understanding of broad system obstacles to high quality of care. These goals are at once more explicit and more comprehensive than the status quo.

Medicare Program to Assure Quality (MPAQ)

RECOMMENDATION No. 3. **Congress should restructure the PRO program, rename it the Medicare Program to Assure Quality (MPAQ), and redefine its functions.**

To discharge the responsibilities implied by earlier recommendations, Medicare will need a revised and expanded quality assurance program at the federal level. To underscore this point, Congress should deliberately shift the focus and responsibility of this new program—the MPAQ—to functions more explicitly oriented to quality of care. In addition, Congress should authorize the Secretary of DHHS to support new local entities— Medicare Quality Review Organizations (MQROs)—in the performance of the MPAQ activities. To build on the personnel and skills already available, these local entities would in many instances be (or be similar to) the organizations with which the Health Care Financing Administration (HCFA) presently contracts through the PRO program. Responsibilities and functions of these organizations are discussed below.

Public Accountability and Evaluation

RECOMMENDATION No. 4. **Congress should establish a Quality Program Advisory Commission (QualPAC) to oversee activities of the MPAQ and to report to Congress on these activities.**

RECOMMENDATION No. 5. **Congress should establish within DHHS a National Council on Medicare Quality Assurance to assist in the implementation, operation, and evaluation of the MPAQ.**

RECOMMENDATION No. 6. **Congress should direct the Secretary of DHHS to report to Congress, no less frequently than every two years, on the quality of care for Medicare beneficiaries and on the effectiveness of MPAQ in meeting the goals outlined in recommendation no. 2.**

In addition to the MPAQ and its MQROs, we have recommended that two other entities be created to form a comprehensive structure to promote, coordinate, and supervise quality review and assurance activities at the national level. Because of the importance of these public accountability and oversight activities, we also suggest that the Secretary of DHHS establish a Technical Advisory Panel to assist in the evaluation efforts. These bodies will have four major purposes, namely to bring a greater degree of public and scientific oversight and input into the quality assurance program, provide a way for both the MPAQ and the MQROs to avail themselves of the most advanced techniques available through the private sector, provide a basis by which the program itself can be more effectively evaluated, and assist the program in management and operations.

Hospital Conditions of Participation

RECOMMENDATION No. 7. **Congress should direct the Secretary of DHHS to initiate a program to make the Medicare Conditions of Participation consistent with and supportive of the overall federal quality assurance effort.**

This report emphasizes the use of process-of-care information and especially patient outcomes data in evaluating quality of care. Nevertheless, all conceptual frameworks of quality assurance emphasize the importance of the *capacity* of an organization to render high quality care—essentially a structural measure. Indirectly, such capacity is measured through mechanisms such as accreditation. For the hospital sector and Medicare, this translates into "deemed status" for those facilities accredited mainly through the Joint Commission for Accreditation of Healthcare Organizations and certification through state survey and certification agencies for those not so accredited.

Our recommendation is intended to prompt HCFA to strengthen its current program for survey and certification of hospitals and for delegating certification of unaccredited hospitals to state agencies. Four aspects of this program deserve attention. First, HCFA should update the Conditions of Participation, and their related standards and elements, within the next two years and continually thereafter (no more infrequently, say, than every three years). Second, HCFA should continue to support the concept of deemed status for hospitals. The agency should encourage the Joint Commission in its efforts to develop a state-of-the-art quality assurance program and in its program to disclose information to the agency about conditionally accredited and nonaccredited hospitals in a timely fashion. Third, HCFA should increase the capacity of the survey and certification system to encourage and enforce compliance with the conditions (i.e., for those hospitals not meeting them by virtue of deemed status). Finally, HCFA should improve the coordination of federal quality assurance efforts by developing criteria and procedures for referring cases involving serious quality problems from the MQROs to the Office of Survey and Certification (and vice versa).

Research and Capacity Building

RECOMMENDATION No. 8. **Congress should direct the Secretary of DHHS to support, expand, and improve research in and the knowldge base on efficacy, effectiveness, and outcomes of care and to support a systematic effort to develop clinical practice guidelines and standards of care.**

RECOMMENDATION No. 9. **Congress should direct the Secretary of DHHS to establish and fund educational activities designed to enhance the nation's capacity to improve quality of care.**

We applaud recent developments in the attention and support that Congress and DHHS have given to effectiveness and outcomes research and to efforts to stimulate the development of clinical practice guidelines. We endorse expanded funding for all of these efforts. DHHS should also undertake broad efforts to improve coordination of data systems and data collection efforts within the Department.

Long-term financial and other support for research and special projects is needed in many areas:

• variations, effectiveness, and appropriateness of medical care interventions;

• practice guidelines and the mechanisms by which they can be developed, refined, disseminated, and updated;

• better measures of the technical and interpersonal aspects of the process of care;

- more and improved measures of health status and health-related quality of life;
- effectiveness of methods for changing provider and practitioner habits, behaviors, and performance;
- data and information management systems (computer hardware and software); and
- improved methods of program evaluation.

Capacity building is that set of activities that will enhance the ability of professionals and patients to assess and improve quality of care. If quality assurance is to move forward aggressively, it will require a corps of professionals prepared to provide both technical skills and leadership. At present we lack such a group in anything like adequate numbers to staff a national set of organizations for this purpose. An early priority must be, therefore, to establish training programs to prepare these health professionals, taking account of the following circumstances and needs:

- Educational programs would likely require an extended period of study (e.g., a year);
- They can be built on existing programs in epidemiology, health services research, and biostatistics;
- Education for the existing staffs of facilities and those senior professionals already in, or just about to enter, this work will have to use techniques of intensive continuing education and technical assistance;
- More organized programs of training with field experience will be needed to prepare a new cadre of health workers with the tools needed to collect and apply information based on outcomes in quality assurance;
- Resources will be needed to underwrite the curriculum development and to support the education of these professionals; and
- Ways to make quality assurance more of a profession with a clear career path should be developed.

In addition, it will be important to educate patients and consumers about how best they can contribute to evaluating and improving the care they receive and participate in informed decision making about their health care.

FUNDING

RECOMMENDATION NO. 10. **Congress should authorize and appropriate such funds as are needed to implement these recommendations.**

The MPAQ must be adequately funded from the start, if it is to be successfully implemented and operated. We propose a considerably expanded data collection and evaluation effort in the new MPAQ and assume that Congress and HCFA will continue to expect the MPAQ to do much, although not all, of what the PRO program now does. For those reasons, we concluded that an increase in the MPAQ budget over present PRO levels is necessary. In addition, we advised that the MPAQ shift from a purely competitive contracting mechanism for MQROs to a funding mechanism that relies more heavily, if not exclusively, on grants or cooperative agreements.

This recommendation is potentially costly, but an underfunded quality assurance program cannot discharge its responsibilities effectively and thus wastes the funds it is provided. It earns little respect from providers, and it cannot demonstrate any meaningful impact on either quality of care or health of the beneficiary population.

The program we are proposing is intended to avoid some of those pitfalls. It is also intended to provide a considerably enhanced body of knowledge about the health and well-being of the elderly and to improve the mechanics of quality review and assurance in all major settings of care. Furthermore, we have built into our proposals a rigorous evaluation component, so that society can know what it is getting for its investment. In our view, the MPAQ simply will not be able to accomplish its objectives with funding that remains at customary levels, and we thus advocate an appreciable increase in support.

We have not specified a target amount, however. Implementation of this proposed program will take time, and many details will emerge only with time. Moreover, internal and external quality assurance efforts have an element of joint production, and not all the activities envisioned in this plan may involve new federal costs. Nevertheless, a reasonable estimate of the costs of this program might be that it would eventually double the investment in the present PRO program, but it should be recognized that this is an order-of-magnitude estimate, not a detailed point estimate.

ORGANIZATIONAL AND OPERATIONAL FEATURES OF THE MEDICARE PROGRAM TO ASSURE QUALITY

Starting Points

The conceptual foundation of the MPAQ approach is the classic triad of structure, process, and outcome. We also draw on five constructs of the continuous improvement model: (1) differentiate external quality monitoring from internal quality improvement and assurance efforts; (2) emphasize increased use by internal programs of data on outcomes, systems, and processes of care; (3) reward providers that implement successful internal quality improvement programs; (4) focus on a broad range of "customer" outcomes that include those of patients, practitioners, and the broader community; and (5) foster cooperative communication and negotiation between many different pairs of actors in the health care delivery setting.

The practical starting point for the MPAQ is the existing Medicare program and the private, local, peer review organizations that presently do (or could) carry out the current PRO agenda. We emphasize transition, not starting over, and we believe that many elements of the PRO program can and should be retained. At the same time, we have renamed the program to emphasize the substantial changes in concept and function that we have recommended.

Structure

The Federal and Local Levels

MPAQ. The first level of our model of quality assurance is that of the federal program, the MPAQ. It might also embrace other organizations that operate nationally and that might be considered complementary to this effort, such as the accreditation programs of the Joint Commission.

Briefly, the MPAQ would be responsible for the planning and administration of the quality assurance program for Medicare. It would have three major responsibilities: (1) to engage in long- and short-term program planning for MQROs (e.g., to define the program guidelines for the MQROs, to review applications and make awards to MQROs, and to provide or arrange for technical assistance to MQROs); (2) to monitor and evaluate MQRO operations and performance; and (3) to aggregate, analyze, and report data.

MQROs. The middle level is that of local or regional entities, the MQROs. They would have several primary responsibilities: (1) to obtain information on patient and population-based outcomes and practitioner and provider processes of care; (2) to analyze these data, making appropriate adjustments for case mix, patient characteristics, and other pertinent information by various types of providers; (3) to use these data to make judgments about practitioner or provider performance; (4) to feed such information back to the internal quality assurance programs of practitioners and providers (as well as report it to the MPAQ); and (5) to carry out quality interventions and technical assistance to internal organization-based quality assurance programs.

The Internal Organization-Based Level

We have given considerable recognition to the emerging concepts of continuous quality improvement and organization-based, internal quality assurance efforts. Self-review and self-regulation remain the hallmark of the healing professions. Therefore, our third level is one based on internal, organization-based quality assurance.

We do not prescribe the approach to quality assurance that such institutions, agencies, or practices might take. Some internal programs may pursue traditional efforts; others may implement advanced continuous quality improvement models; still others may experiment with novel review and assurance efforts tailored to their particular needs and circumstances. The MQROs should encourage and assist in the development of all such internal efforts. Internal programs will no doubt use outcome data for their own purposes, but they will also need to emphasize the actual systems and processes of care as a means of knowing where to act when problems arise or to improve care more generally. Finally, these internal programs will have to document that their surveillance systems identify and attempt to solve important quality problems.

If internal programs cannot document their quality assurance procedures and impact, or if the results of the external MQRO monitoring suggest that these activities are not being done well, then the MQRO will have to become more actively involved. Such MQRO interventions might involve abstracting process-of-care information on-site, consulting in the planning of quality assurance activities, imposing corrective actions of the sort now available to PROs, and pursuing new intervention strategies developed during the implementation of the MPAQ.

Operational Overview of the Proposed Model

An Emphasis on Outcomes

A central theme of our recommendations and the proposed MPAQ is a greater emphasis on the outcomes of care. Attention to outcomes offers several advantages. It allows monitoring of the system while leaving providers able to undertake their own quality improvement efforts. It collects systematic data that can be used to inform the field about how process components are related to outcomes. It provides a means to look across time and to appreciate the temporal and service linkages within episodes of care. It emphasizes aspects of care that are most relevant to patients and to society.

The MPAQ and MQROs must choose outcomes that are easily and reproducibly defined, can be practically obtained, and are important to Medicare beneficiaries. These outcomes should include mortality and medical complications; relevant physiologic measures; functional outcomes such as patients' mental and emotional status, physical functioning (for instance, ability to walk), and social interaction; activities of daily living; placement of the patient at home or in a long-term-care facility; and the patients' and their families' satisfaction with care.

A difficult aspect of outcome-directed quality assurance efforts will be to adjust outcomes for the risk factors present in the population being studied (e.g., case mix, severity of illness, and demographic factors). The choice of conditions to be monitored in this new program must reflect the availability of information about known risk factors. Furthermore, the size of this undertaking means that not all discharges could be monitored for outcomes. At least some conditions would be studied nationally for periods of time to acquire adequate comparative data. In other cases, local or regional topics (perhaps based in part on variations in performance) might be used as the basis for selecting conditions.

Adjusted, comparative information would be returned to the appropriate providers. In addition, providers in a region can be evaluated according to the relative outcomes of their patients. Those whose performance was significantly poorer than the mean would be asked to examine their activities carefully—to identify the specific systems or processes of care that contributed to these results and to make appropriate corrections. Follow-up studies should be performed to assess the impact of these corrections. Failure to improve would result in closer monitoring and potentially more stringent actions, including public disclosure of their status.

Aggregate information would be shared with provider groups to serve as a basis for better understanding of the processes of care. This information would form part of a national data base to be used to improve clinical decision making.

The Importance of the Process of Care

This attention to outcomes is not intended to slight the importance of process-of-care measurement. Process measures have strengths missing in an outcome focus, including the lack of sensitivity of outcome measures for detecting certain rare but catastrophic events. Process measures may need to be used as proxies for outcomes for patients with complex medical conditions, when the many variables that influence outcomes of care cannot be controlled. Further, the long lead time required for some adverse outcomes is such that process surrogates are needed.

Identifying key processes of care and responding to them are best done by internal quality assurance programs of these institutions, organizations, or provider groups. Related activities, such as the development of clinical practice standards and appropriateness criteria, will be best done by national groups drawing on data generated by this quality assurance program as well as the increased interest and research in effectiveness and outcomes of care. The MPAQ and MQROs should encourage, stimulate, and participate in this work as much as possible.

Continuity of Quality Assessment

The emphasis on care beyond a single setting is a new direction in quality assurance. It is essential if ultimate outcomes are to be understood and affected. Superb inpatient care followed by poor post-hospital care, for instance, cannot be acceptable. Each care provider and institution is part of a system of care. Each must recognize a responsibility to ensure that the continuum of the process of care results in a good outcome for the patient.

Potential Problems

It is appropriate here to acknowledge real or potential drawbacks with this model. This ambitious design will be more difficult to develop in the ambulatory and home care setting than in the institutional one. The data and methods to implement such a system today are inadequate or not easily transferable from other research applications; furthermore, assessment techniques to identify problems are more advanced than techniques to intervene successfully once problems are identified. It is this dearth of off-the-shelf methods that necessitates the research agenda and the proposed 10-year implementation strategy. Any system has the potential for "gaming" by providers; a program as invested in promoting internal quality improvement efforts as this one is more at risk for such gaming. There is little experience to draw on to evaluate a program as complex and ambitious as this one, and it therefore may run a considerable risk of seeming to be ineffective, inefficient, and wasteful of the public's dollars. Relying on self-review, delegated review, and self-regulation are problematic approaches, and they deserve careful study.

IMPLEMENTATION STRATEGY AND PHASES

Our 10-year implementation strategy is divided into three phases from 1991 to 2000. The major activities that should be undertaken are outlined below. Activities beginning in one phase need not end in that phase; for instance, special studies begun in Phase II may well continue into Phase III, and certain efforts to be started in Phase I (such as public oversight or capacity building) are expressly intended to continue throughout implementation and beyond.

Phase I: Years 1 and 2

Congress or DHHS, or both, should take the basic steps to establish the MPAQ. These include establishing the program and the entities in the first five committee recommendations and providing the appropriate authorizations and appropriations, and beginning operations of QualPAC and the National Council. PRO program activities, financing instruments, survey and certification procedures for Conditions of Participation for hospitals, and other aspects of existing programs should be reviewed and revamped as necessary to meet MPAQ goals. MPAQ public oversight and evaluation activities (e.g., articulating specific goals for the MPAQ, appointing the

TAP) should be begun and the first program evaluation report should be submitted. Research and capacity building efforts should be started.

Phase II: Years 2 through 8

The middle phase of implementation entails data collection, data analysis, information dissemination, and four areas of special projects. These activities focus on the design, testing, and implementation of major components of the MPAQ model. We assume that these activities would be started in the second or third year of the MPAQ and generally would take anywhere from three to six years to complete. We assume further that the best of the approaches would then be incorporated into the full MPAQ in Phase III, taking into explicit account the advice and consent of QualPAC, the National Council, or both.

Data Collection

We have consistently emphasized the importance to this Medicare quality assurance program (and to the Medicare program more broadly) of a greatly enhanced data base on use of services, patient outcomes, and the process of care. To create and maintain such an information base—only the foundations of which are in place—and to make it useful for assuring the quality of health care for the elderly over the long run is a massive undertaking. We expect that getting this data collection effort underway will take the middle part of this 10-year strategy because the development and testing of such a system is necessarily evolutionary and must be responsive to environmental and technical factors.

Data Analysis Capabilities

The data analysis capabilities that would be needed in a program with the level of information gathering just described exceed those available in contemporary quality assurance programs, both public and private. Thus, HCFA will need to begin early in implementation to expand and improve its internal data analysis capacity and, more importantly, the data analysis capacity of the MQROs. Specific attention should be given to strengthening several key elements, especially analytic personnel and computer capability, and initiating a technical assistance effort (use of outside expert consultants on an advisory or contracting basis).

Information Dissemination

Our proposed program calls for a sophisticated approach to feeding useful clinical-practice and quality-related information back to practitioners and provider institutions of all types. Few good models of such feedback loops exist, so a considerable effort will be needed to design, test, and refine such models. Also, formal, external studies of issues relating to public release of information and data sharing might be undertaken, with a focus on their legal, regulatory, and policy ramifications.

Special Projects

Distinguishing providers on the basis of quality and outcomes. If the MQROs are to be able to respond differently to providers according to their capacity to render superior, acceptable, or only poor care, they have to be able to create "quality distributions" of providers, so that performance along that distribution can be acknowledged and acted upon. To overcome the enormous conceptual, practical, and political difficulties of this, we recommend studies to test different methods for creating such quality distributions for the major types of Medicare providers.

Improving the average level of performance. Improving average performance ("shifting the curve") is, in our view, a critical aspect of the MPAQ; so is fostering better internal, organization-based quality assurance programs. Because this is such a new area, various research and demonstration studies (including current PRO pilot projects as appropriate) will be needed during this phase. These projects might be done through joint efforts of the MQROs and individual providers, focus on geriatric-specific quality concerns, be community-wide, and/or involve several providers in either similar or different care settings.

Incentives for good and exemplary performance. Early in Phase II, the MPAQ should study ways to identify and reward both good and exemplary (or superior) providers. These might include lowering the amount of intrusive external review to which they might be subjected, publishing superior rankings, giving special recognition for performance and innovation, selective contracting, and sharing information on exemplary providers with private third-party purchasers.

Dealing with outliers. Providers not meeting the criteria of satisfactory performance on the quality indicators will be subjected to more intensive review and other quality interventions; we have noted in the report that more innovative approaches to these quality interventions will need to be developed. Better mechanisms also need to be devised for real-time intervention in the event of catastrophic malfeasance or poor performance.

Phase III: Years 9 and 10

Our aim is a functioning quality assurance program at the end of a 10-year period, one that can respond creatively to changing environmental circumstances. Some of these circumstances can be foreseen (even if their particulars cannot be specified), such as a larger and older elderly population and different Medicare payment systems. Others are a matter of speculation, such as the strength of the nation's economy. Most of the reforms suggested for the first two phases of this implementation strategy are intended to provide a firm foundation for this program, and we expect them to continue into Phase III.

Thus, in Phase III, we expect to see a shift from demonstrations to full-scale implementation, continued improvement in quality of care and in the conduct of quality assurance, and a major reassessment to determine if the MPAQ is on target. The report highlights four other sets of activities in this third phase because of their very broad and long-range public policy implications: research, capacity building (both discussed earlier), public oversight of the Medicare quality assurance effort, and program evaluation.

A consistent theme of the report is engagement of patients and consumers in quality assurance. A corollary is that the public is entitled to know and have some voice about public monies spent on quality assurance programs. The public also needs a way to bring quality-related problems to the policymaker's attention. The report suggests that efforts be coordinated among all the Medicare commissions (especially ProPAC, PPRC, and QualPAC), so as to avoid duplication of effort and forestall major policy difficulties. Among the issues that might be monitored is the likelihood and severity of quality problems confronting the MPAQ as reimbursement mechanisms and Medicare benefits change over the 1990s, but other issues may well arise.

We clearly put very strong emphasis on rigorous evaluation (of the program itself, not only its agents). We have suggested that HCFA devise and test various program evaluation techniques, including ways to assess the cost-effectiveness of a quality assurance program. We suggest that a formal, operational program evaluation effort (outside the MPAQ) be in place by the time the MPAQ itself is fully operational.

CONCLUDING REMARKS

This report presents a strategy for a quality review and assurance program for Medicare.

It envisions an evolution from the present Medicare PRO program but with several different emphases that present extraordinary challenges. It looks more to professionalism and internal quality improvement than to regulation and external inspection. It gives more attention to patient and consumer concerns and decision making, and it adopts an aggressive regard for outcomes. It seeks to generate new knowledge from clinical practice and to return that information to providers in a timely way that improves clinical decision making. It places stronger emphasis on systems of care, the joint production of services by many different providers, and continuity and episodes of care. Related to this, it moves more forcefully into settings not traditionally subjected to formal quality assurance, such as physician office-based care and home health care. It becomes far more publicly accountable through an extensive program oversight and evaluation effort. It intends to be responsive to a changing environment, with principles that will stand the tests of time and change. Finally, it is grounded in a clear definition of quality of care.

The Medicare program has a large responsibility to assure the quality of care for the elderly population. By no means does it have the sole responsibility. Patients, providers, and societal agents must work together if we are to meet the challenges inherent in this strategy for quality review and assurance.

1

Health, Health Care, and Quality of Care

Good health may be the most valued attribute of life. Daily, we express our concern for others by inquiring about their health and wishing them well. Material concerns are overshadowed when our own health is threatened; good health is recognized as essential for the pursuit of happiness.

Good health is as difficult to define as it is important. It means different things to different people. Health is influenced by many factors, including the genes we inherit, the environment into which we are born, and our own behavior.

The influence of health care is variable. In some cases, it is essential and its effect in preserving or restoring health is dramatic. In others, it has a marginal impact, at least on those attributes of life and health that can be objectively measured. Although health cannot be bought and sold, health care can be and is, with expenditures that are far greater in the United States than in other industrialized nations.

Personally, people in the United States want health care that will maximize their health potential and meet their health goals. Collectively, they want to ensure equitable access to essential health services. These wants, together with the uncertainty about the effectiveness of component health services in preserving or improving health, provide the context for rapidly increasing health care costs and unexplained variations in use of services by different providers for seemingly similar patients.

New policies and programs, implemented to contain costs and manage care, have exacerbated concerns about potential deficiencies in our ability to assure quality (Ellwood, 1988; *Health Affairs*, 1988; *Inquiry*, 1988; Roper and Hackbarth, 1988; Berwick, 1989; *Generations*, 1989). As individuals and as a society we are now challenged to develop and implement an effective and broad-based strategy to assure the quality of the health care provided in this nation. This report of a committee of the Institute of Medicine (IOM) presents such a strategy to assure the quality of care provided to Medicare beneficiaries.

Congress has evidenced concern for quality of care in the Medicare program since its inception in 1965.[1] For instance, legislation in the early 1970s, which created Experimental Medical Care Review Organizations and later Professional Standards Review Organizations (PSROs), dealt directly with ensuring that care met professional standards of quality. This concern continued with the passage in 1982 of legislation that created the Utilization and Quality Control Peer Review Organizations program (commonly called the PRO program). Despite these efforts, Medicare quality assurance to date has been insufficient, in large measure because the programs were also heavily charged to control utilization and costs. The congressional mandate for this study reflects both an appreciation of the shortcomings of the current Medicare quality assurance program and apprehension that past and future efforts to curb Medicare expenditures, control use of services, and reform payment mechanisms will have negative effects on the quality of care rendered to the elderly.

Defining health is difficult because of differences in what may be valued and attainable and because of the sometimes tenuous relationship between health services and health outcomes. These are not theoretical issues for those responsible for operating a program to assure quality health care. The process involves eliciting and balancing value judgments, often when legitimate interests are in conflict. Responsibilities are often shared and are therefore ambiguous. Even when the decisions are sound and the appropriate services are delivered with technical proficiency, poor outcomes can occur. Conversely, bad decisions or inept care will not always be followed by poor outcomes. The quality of care cannot necessarily be judged by the outcome for an individual, so accountability is further diffused. These issues must be understood in defining quality health care and designing programs and systems to assure it.

A pragmatic strategy also requires an understanding of the problem to be solved and the potential barriers. How does one define quality of care? What is the health status of the United States citizenry, and what can we infer about the quality of care from that information? Why is quality of health care a public policy issue? This chapter provides a foundation for the committee's strategy by addressing these questions.

DEFINING QUALITY OF HEALTH CARE

In 1974 the IOM published the following statement about quality assurance: "The primary goal of a quality assurance system should be to make health care more effective in bettering the health status and satisfaction of a population, within the resources which society and individuals have chosen to spend for that care" (IOM, 1974, pp. 1-2). Despite the continuing appeal of this statement, it does not define quality of care. Furthermore, some experts assert that strategies for reviewing and assuring quality depend on how quality is defined (Palmer and Adams, 1988).

Through the activities of this study, over 100 definitions of (or sets of parameters to consider in defining) quality of care were collected from the relevant literature. An analysis of existing definitions is beyond the scope of this chapter but is included in Volume II, Chapter 5. We reviewed each definition for the presence or absence of 18 dimensions (Table 1.1). This analysis enabled the committee to develop a sense of the key terms used in a definition by others (such as use of the term "patient"), the more common variations of terms applicable to a given dimension (such as patient versus consumer or client), and the specific combinations of dimensions used in a given definition. From this information and with considerable debate, the committee developed a consensus definition of quality of care.

As defined by the committee, **quality of care is the degree to which health services for individuals and populations increase the likelihood of desired health outcomes and are consistent with current professional knowledge.** This definition has the following properties. It

- includes a measure of scale (. . . degree to which . . .);
- encompasses a wide range of elements of care (. . . health services . . .);
- identifies both individuals and populations as proper targets for quality assurance efforts;
- is goal-oriented (. . . increase...desired health outcomes . . .);
- recognizes a stochastic (random or probability) attribute of outcome but values the expected net benefit (. . . increase the likelihood of . . .);
- underscores the importance of outcomes and links the process of health care with outcomes (health services . . . increase . . . outcomes);
- highlights the importance of individual patients' and society's preferences and values and implies that those have been elicited (or acknowledged) and taken into account in health care decision making and policymaking (. . . desired health outcomes . . .); and
- underscores the constraints placed on professional performance by the state of technical, medical, and scientific knowledge, implies that that state is dynamic, and implies that the health care provider is responsible for using the best knowledge base available (. . . consistent with current professional knowledge).

In this definition, the care provided is expected to have a net benefit (to do more good than harm, given the known risk when compared to the next best alternative care). In turn, that benefit is expected to reflect considera-

TABLE 1.1 Dimensions in Definitions of Quality

 1. Scale of quality
 2. Nature of entity being evaluated
 3. Goal-oriented
 4. Aspects of outcomes specified
 5. Acceptability

 6. Type of recipient identified
 7. Role and responsibility of recipient asserted
 8. Continuity, management, coordination
 9. Professional standards
10. Technical competency of provider

11. Interpersonal skills of provider
12. Acceptability
13. Statements about use
14. Constrained by resources
15. Constrained by consumer and patient circumstances

16. Constrained by technology and state of scientific knowledge
17. Risk versus benefit tradeoffs
18. Documentation required

NOTE: The first eight dimensions are explicitly incorporated in the committee's definition.

tions of patient satisfaction and well-being, broad health status or quality-of-life measures, and the processes of patient-provider interaction and decision making. The values of both individuals and society are explicitly to be considered in the goal-setting process. How care is provided should reflect appropriate use of the most current knowledge about scientific, clinical, technical, interpersonal, manual, cognitive, organizational, and management elements of health care.

Elements of the Committee's Definition

In contrast to other common definitions that refer to medical or patient care our definition of quality refers to health services. Health care implies a broad set of services, including acute, chronic, preventive, restorative, and rehabilitative care, which are delivered in many different settings by many different health care providers. This broad dimension is particularly important for the elderly, who often receive a wide range of services from different sources. There is great potential for fragmentation of care unless programs and resources are available and dedicated to assure coordination and continuity. The need for attention to continuity has been greatly heightened by the shifts in settings of care resulting from the Prospective Payment System (PPS) and other cost-containment policies.

Our definition identifies both individuals (but not just "patients") and populations for three reasons. First, even though traditionally quality assurance has focused on the technical care rendered to individuals (for instance, in medical record review), we believe advances must be made in population-based measures. This is particularly important for assessments of overuse of certain services and of underuse that results from lack of access to the health care system or from less than adequate care for those who do have access to the system. Second, we believe that only by emphasizing both individuals and populations can we underscore the importance of identifying determinants of health and illness. Third, we have described some strategies for assessing and assuring quality of care that can be used more widely than in a single public program.

The committee adopted a broad set of outcome measures to encompass health-related quality-of-life variables, which include physical and social functioning, mental health, and physiologic measures (Lohr, 1988; Kane and Kane, 1989). We also intend to include both patient and provider satisfaction as important elements of the process and the outcomes of care. Provider-patient trust and the art of care emphasize the humaneness with which health care is delivered and contribute to the level of patient satisfaction experienced in the health care encounter; they are thus critical to quality assurance (Davies and Ware, 1988; Cleary and McNeil, 1988).

Although our definition emphasizes outcome measures, it links the processes of health care to outcomes. Interpersonal and technical skills used in health care are important in increasing the likelihood of desired outcomes and decreasing the likelihood of undesired outcomes. In contrast, several definitions reviewed by the committee focused only on process or only on outcomes. Because chance and other factors such as the environment also influence outcomes, our definition focuses on the selection of treatment courses (processes) believed to provide the best possible desired outcome rather than on the frequency of outcomes. In this manner, the committee's definition is consistent with that proposed by Avedis Donabedian (1980), which also emphasizes the expected net benefit attendant on the process of care.

Health care goals may differ for the government, administrators, patients, health care providers, or other parties such as payers. The decision-making process frequently must consider the values of multiple parties before the desired goal is defined.

The lack of professional knowledge of the effectiveness of many technologies and the vast dimensions of medical science yet unexplored limit the achievable level of quality (Brook, 1988; Greenfield, 1988; Roper et al., 1988). Our definition accepts this reality but acknowledges that the information base is dynamic. It also implies that professionals have a responsibility to stay informed about current advances in the technical and scientific knowledge pertinent to their profession (Farber, 1988) rather than adopting an average standard of practice that may fall short of the best wisdom.

Implications of the Committee's Definition

The committee acknowledges limitations in the scope and level of benefits covered in the Medicare program; we also acknowledge that use of the term "health services" in our quality definition could be interpreted as broadening the mission of the Medicare program. This clearly poses a challenge to Medicare and to society. Issues of financing, access, and health care delivery can restrict the capacity for achieving quality care.

After deliberating whether its definition should explicitly incorporate resource constraints, the committee agreed that it should not. (Several existing definitions of quality do reflect considerations of resource availability; a few explicitly state that resource considerations should not be included in defining quality.) The committee decided that quality should not be defined on a sliding scale and that judgments of quality should not fluctuate just because resources are constrained or unavailable. Excluding resource constraints in the definition of quality should enable quality assurance efforts to identify situations in the health care system where quality would be improved if additional resources were available. Responsible parties (individuals, public and private payers, and societal agents) should be able to distinquish quality problems from those arising from resource availability and subsequently be able to make informed decisions about the level of quality that is desired and affordable.

The committee recognizes the implications of excluding explicit consideration of the theoretical and real constraints on what our society can spend on health care. Efficiency in the delivery of services necessary to produce health benefits is important. Equity, too, is important. Delivery of all health services including those that provide only the smallest of benefits to everyone would divert resources from education, housing, or other services that could provide greater benefits to individuals and society. The highest level of quality, as defined by the committee, may not be attainable for everyone; it may not be a societal goal to attempt to achieve the highest level. Such conflicts between individual and societal goals challenge our capacity for collective decision making and action.[2]

Most of society perceives health care to be different from other goods and services. Many health problems occur beyond the control of individuals, and the consequent need for health care is distributed very unevenly among people. In addition, health care has a symbolic aspect beyond the technical and practical elements; it signifies not only mutual empathy and caring, but mysterious and awesome aspects of curing and healing (President's Commission, 1983).

Health care is frequently delivered in a personal and intimate manner that reflects the social, religious, and ethical values of individuals and society (Fuchs, 1988); thus, health care decision making is not taken lightly. Although health care is typically purchased, a relationship based on mutual trust and confidence between the health care provider and patient (rather than an adversarial attitude of caveat emptor) is believed to contribute greatly to a better "product" or "outcome," that is, improved health status (Fuchs, 1988).

A quality assurance program has ethical obligations paralleling those of the health care professional: to prevent harms (nonmaleficence), to promote good care (beneficence), and to consider first its clients (fidelity to patients).[3] Increasingly, experts point out that physicians in both fee-for-service and prepaid settings are in positions of inherent conflict of interest when their incomes depend on how they execute the duty to beneficence (Povar, 1989). Similar conflicts of interest are perceived to exist in situations when third-party payers, including Medicare, exercise their multiple and perhaps incompatible responsibilities as both prudent purchasers and agents for assuring quality of care. Countervailing forces or conflicts in delivering quality health care exist for other reasons as well: differences among competing values for goods and services (such as health, privacy, financial resources, and assets) held by the same individual or agent, and differences among competing individuals or agents (such as payer, patient, physician, and society) in values held in common as well as disagreed upon (President's Commission, 1983).

As the field of health care advances and the knowledge bases improve on all fronts (scientific, interpersonal, and clinical), the frequency with which ethical and moral dilemmas occur may diminish. Our abilities to identify issues having ethical dimensions will be heightened, and our responses can be more timely. The art of care, the fiduciary relationship between the patient and clinician, their mutual respect for dignity and freedom, and the practice of humanism in health care are important dimensions of quality. Few quality assurance programs acknowledge or address these elements of health care (Nelson, 1989); we believe they should.

HEALTH AND HEALTH CARE IN THE UNITED STATES

Neither a definition of quality of care nor a strategy for quality assurance is particularly useful outside a context. We take the appropriate context to have three major components: (1) the health status of the citizenry, both individually and collectively; (2) the health care system that attempts to meet the needs of that citizenry; and (3) the major policy issues that must be taken into account as one attempts to put a quality assurance program into place.

Health and Illness

In the early nineteenth century, the primary causes of death in this country were infectious diseases (e.g., smallpox, diphtheria, tuberculosis, and pneumonia). With improved nutrition and identification and control of the responsible infectious agents, death rates began to drop, with a corresponding increase in life expectancy. Since that time, disease patterns here (as in all industrial countries) have changed markedly. Today, the leading causes of death are chronic processes, the effects of which occur mainly in older age groups,[4] and the trends of declining death rates and increases in life expectancy continue (NCHS, 1988, 1989).

Many observers, however, regard these trends with a mixture of pride and dismay when viewed in a more global context. In 1985, the U.S. infant mortality rate was higher than that of 21 other countries, including several (e.g., Singapore, Spain, Italy, and the German Democratic Republic) that are not as economically developed as the United States (NCHS, 1989). In 1986, the United States ranked nineteenth in life expectancy at birth for males and fourteenth for females, behind such countries as Japan, Sweden, Canada, and Spain (NCHS, forthcoming, Table 20). Life expectancy at age 65 could be seen to be at least partly indicative of the contribution of health care for the elderly. Life expectancy for both males and females ranks considerably higher in international comparisons than rankings at birth. Males rank tenth, and females share the rank of seventh with Australia and the Netherlands, behind such countries as Japan, Switzerland, Canada and Sweden (NCHS, forthcoming, Table 20).

For the elderly population in particular, little is known about the direct relationship of health status to the level of quality of care it receives or the relationship of health status to the burden of harm attributable to quality problems (i.e., frequency and severity of quality problems).[5] The traditional measures of patient health and the effectiveness of medical treatments have long been confined to rates of life expectancy, mortality, and morbidity. These measures do not meet today's needs for characterizing the health of the Medicare population in a comprehensive manner because they do not reflect the impact of chronic disease on daily functioning.

Structure of the U.S. Health Care System

The modern American health care system has evolved through several important periods (Torrens, 1978). Beginning with the period of development of the first hospitals and followed with the period establishing the introduction of the scientific method into medicine, the evolution has continued into a current period that is characterized by acknowledgment of limited resources, reorganization of methods for financing and delivery of care, and a greater examination of the respective roles and responsibilities of patients, providers, and society in the protection of health and well-being.

The composition of the U.S. health care delivery system is presently in flux. For example, although the country's acute general hospitals differ dramatically in size and type of services offered, the growth rate in the overall number of facilities and the proportionate profit status of ownership (mainly not-for-profit) were fairly stable over the last two and one-half decades. In the mid-1980s the growth of not-for-profit hospitals and beds began to level off and then decline, whereas the growth of proprietary hospitals and beds continued (NCHS, 1989). More recently, the rate of hospital closures has increased, particularly in rural areas. In addition, an economic environment that now encourages competition for financial resources and patients has led hospitals to become more involved in both vertical and horizontal integration of services. Free-standing surgical and urgent care facilities have multiplied.

The number and size of nursing homes and the number of persons served and visits per person by home health agencies are also increasing (Ruther and Helbing, 1988; NCHS, 1989) although the rate of growth in the use of Medicare home health services has decreased since 1983. The reasons for these increases include the growth and aging of the elderly population and the need for alternatives to inpatient hospital care. The desire to enhance independent functioning and quality of life for the elderly is another factor in the increased use of home care.

Arguably the most important component of the health care system is the training, supply, and distribution of health care personnel. Even though the number of persons employed in the health care industry has grown dramatically, the shortage of personnel in many areas continues to be severe. For example, the shortage of registered nurses is widespread and of a magnitude sufficient to affect quality of care (Aiken and Mullinix, 1987; Iglehart, 1987; Secretary's Commission on Nursing, 1988; Aiken, 1989; Hinshaw, 1989; Minnick, 1989; Wilensky, 1989). The implications of the nursing shortage and shortages of other types of allied health professionals (IOM, 1988a) are considered ominous for the nation's ability to preserve high quality care in general and for the elderly in particular, since the elderly are the major consumers of care rendered in hospitals, nursing homes, and the home.

Growth in physician manpower has been uneven over at least the last two decades as a result partly of shifting levels of financing for undergraduate medical education and partly of inconsistent projections of the country's need for physicians. On the surface the number of physicians available to serve the elderly appears to be adequate. However, the relative proportions of primary care physicians and specialists is markedly skewed toward specialists, and some experts believe that many physicians lack an adequate appreciation of the complexities of caring for elderly patients. In addition, some observers fear that present (or at least future) levels of Medicare reimbursement will induce some physicians to restrict their Medicare practices and thus reduce the pool of physicians available to provide care to the growing elderly population. Finally, some experts argue that greater numbers of physicians (by themselves) may not improve quality; instead, more benefit might be expected from improving the services that physicians supply (Perrin and Valvona, 1986).

If the past predicts the future, the U.S. health care system is certain to be characterized by continual and occasionally unpredictable patterns of change. Severe economic constraints, the aging of the population, and the appearance of serious sociomedical problems such as substance abuse (Harwood et al., 1984; Blendon and Donelan, 1989) and AIDS (IOM, 1986a, 1988b; Nichols, 1989) will all drastically affect both supply and demand for services. The system is likely to move into a period of retrenchment and unstable developments in financing, structure, and manpower. All these factors will generate health policy issues even beyond those most salient today for the quality of health care.

Major Health Policy Issues with Implications for Quality of Care

Health Care Expenditures

The dominant health policy issue of the past 15 years has been the upward spiral of health care expenditures, both in the nation as a whole and in the Medicare program. In 1965, national health care expenditures were $41.9 billion, or 5.9 percent of the U.S. Gross National Product (GNP). In 1987, health care expenditures stood at $500.3 billion, or 11.1 percent of GNP (Division of National Cost Estimates, 1987). Health care spending will be an estimated $647 billion in 1990. Although a variety of payment and financing systems exists in the nation, none seems protected from the upward spiral of expenditures.

Medicare expenditures have also risen dramatically over the last several decades. In 1970, Medicare spending amounted to $7.3 billion, rising to $35 billion in 1980 and to $81.6 billion in 1987 (Long and Welch, 1988). It is estimated to reach $114 billion in 1990. The United States spends a higher percentage of its Gross Domestic Product (GDP) on health care than most other countries in the Organization for Economic Cooperation and Development (OECD). For example, in 1986, the United States spent 11.1

percent of its GDP on health care, which was almost 52 percent higher than the OECD mean of 7.3 percent (Schieber and Poullier, 1988).

Past efforts to control rising expenditures have taken many forms, such as price controls and Medicare's PPS. Their effect on the quality of care is generally unknown. Most evidence to date suggests that the fears about potential impacts of Medicare PPS on quality (Lohr et al., 1985) have not been borne out (ProPAC, 1988, 1989; Kahn et al., 1989), but some signs about excessively shortened hospital stays are disturbing (Fitzgerald et al., 1987, 1988).

The interest in quality of care must be viewed in a larger social and economic context. On the one hand are the staggering reality of a federal budget deficit created during the 1980s (now conservatively estimated at over $135 billion), a growing desire to protect the 35 million persons who are uninsured for health care (most of whom are not elderly), and much discontent about numerous other components of the social fabric (housing and the homeless, education and literacy, and the pervasiveness of illegal drugs). On the other hand are the increasing need for care by a growing elderly population and the concomitant pressure to broaden the benefits within the Medicare program, as seen most recently in the debates about the Medicare Catastrophic Coverage Act of 1988 and about expanded coverage for long term care.

Access to Services

Germane to any discussion of health policy are the twin issues of geographic and financial access to services. Persons in need of care are forced on occasion to forgo treatment because they live in areas that are underserved by medical practitioners or otherwise face limited access to health care institutions and technologies; this is particularly evident in rural areas and inner cities. Gaps in coverage, restrictions on the use of needed services, inconsistencies in the application of reimbursement policies, and cost-sharing can all be obstacles to the receipt of appropriate levels of care.

Settings of Care

Changes in the settings of care, such as the shift of some types of surgery to the ambulatory setting and the growth of home care, produce uncertainty about quality and continuity of care. These changes complicate quality assurance efforts because needed data systems may be lacking for these nontraditional settings. Ensuring high quality in the diagnosis and treatment of mental health problems, conditions recognized as important health issues for the elderly, is difficult because they, too, often fall outside the usual practice domains (Brook et al., 1982).

Integration of Financing and Delivery of Services

The strong trends toward the integration of financing and delivery of services and the growth of for-profit enterprise in health care (IOM, 1986b) have serious implications for quality of care. Prospective payment systems, capitated programs, and many other payment methodologies put providers at financial risk. Price competition among providers and insurers is vigorous, and competition for market share is being pursued through overt marketing to consumers and employees to an unprecedented degree. These developments, it is feared, lead to conflicts within, or erosion of, the traditional physician-patient relationship. Others perceive these trends as obstacles to providing continuity of care; instead of increasing the choices, these developments limit the choices of providers available to consumers.

Utilization Management and Utilization Review

Utilization management encompasses efforts to monitor the appropriateness of treatment and treatment sites to control unnecessary utilization[6] without jeopardizing individuals' equitable access to needed medical care. Integrating utilization management with other strategies for balancing cost, quality, and access should improve the effectiveness and efficiency of the health care system (Gray and Field, 1989), but overly aggressive, poorly understood, or badly administered efforts may prove detrimental by imposing harmful confusion or delay on patients and by taking practitioner time away from patient care. Because the private sector has been much more aggressive about installing utilization management requirements in health care plans for the nonelderly than has the government for Medicare (Brown et al., 1989; MBGH, 1989), the potential net impact of greater utilization management efforts on the elderly remains to be determined.

Growing use of utilization management techniques by third-party payers to reduce costs of health care by decreasing (presumably) unnecessary or inappropriate services places pressure on quality assurance programs to ensure that decisions resulting from such techniques do not affect quality negatively. Quality assurance programs frequently are jointly responsible for utilization management and utilization review, and they often view their efforts as one branch of the overall responsibility to balance concerns about cost, access, and quality (Gray and Field, 1989).[7] Utilization management and utilization review increasingly evaluate the need for a health care service in addition to the more traditional review of the appropriateness of setting and length of stay. The very recent push to develop practice guidelines, which would then be used in utilization management programs, is evidence of the concern about overuse of inappropriate and unnecessary services and hence about quality of care.

Operational links between the structures of quality assurance and utilization management and review need to be more clearly defined in a number of areas. These include consistency in clinical guidelines and criteria for making prospective decisions about care; consistency in guidelines and criteria in retrospective review of care; methods (both informal and formal) for resolving disagreements about the level of quality of care in those situations when the utilization and the quality programs yield conflicting findings; and procedures for sharing information between the two efforts.

Medicare's Physician Payment System

Reform of the physician payment system for Medicare has emerged recently as a contentious issue (PPRC, 1988, 1989). Expenditures for physician services have grown significantly over the years, increasing the financial burden on both beneficiaries and the taxpayers. In addition, increases in physician charges, the unwillingness of some physicians to accept Medicare assignment, and the impact on beneficiary out-of-pocket expenditures (in terms of copayments and extra billing) raise concern about diminished access to quality care for Medicare beneficiaries who, under the constraints of limited financial resources, avoid seeking services that may not be reimbursed.

Summary

The current revolution in the organization and financing of health services is unprecedented in this country and without parallel elsewhere. It calls for imaginative and carefully constructed approaches to quality review and assurance. These should cover a comprehensive range of services; evaluate complex health care organizations involving widely varying institutions and providers; be sensitive to the availability of appropriate health services; monitor the appropriate use of services and counter both underuse and overuse; and be reasonable in the resource use they entail. With that goal in mind, we examine the question of quality of health care as a public policy issue.

QUALITY OF HEALTH CARE AS A PUBLIC POLICY ISSUE

Burden of Harm of Poor Quality

The elderly are usually quite satisfied with their own medical care and the health care providers with whom they interact, although they may express dissatisfaction about access or financial barriers to care. Despite this positive view, a large body of literature documents specific areas of deficiencies in quality in all parts of the health sector—what we have called the burden of harm of quality problems. Some of these deficiencies relate to poor technical and interpersonal skills or judgment in the delivery of appropriate services, some to the overuse of unnecessary and inappropriate services, and some to underuse of needed services by those receiving some care and by those having difficulty obtaining access to the health care system.

Both the types of quality problems and the level of quality may vary considerably across geographic areas, among beneficiaries, and among individual and institutional health care providers. The use of health care services varies greatly even across small geographic areas of the country in ways for which we cannot fully account. The effectiveness and the outcomes of that care may also vary greatly. Chapter 7 provides a more detailed discussion on quality problems and the burden of harm.

Assuring Quality: A Professional and a Public Responsibility

As we increase our knowledge and understanding of the complexities of good health care, we also increase the quantity of factors that apparently impinge on the quality of health care. Furthermore, advances in health care are accompanied by a corresponding increase in our expectations for even better quality of care.

No single party or individual can be held accountable for all that happens in health care; the factors are too diverse and diffuse. Patients have different preferences, needs, and capacities. Numerous providers render care in thousands of delivery settings. Interventions of vast number occur over both short and long time frames. Finally, a multiplicity of outcomes can occur with only fuzzy and wavering lines to distinguish causal relationships from chance occurrences.

The lack of a single point of accountability can be perceived as both a blessing and a misfortune. The opportunities for improving health care singly and through cooperative ventures are almost unlimited. Conversely, lack of a single point of accountability creates an environment conducive to shifting or shirking responsibility. Helping to focus on the appropriate points of accountability in the system should be the aim of a successful quality assurance program.

Professional Responsibilities

Through the activities of the study (public hearing testimony, the focus groups, and the site visits), we heard almost without exception that the single party most responsible for quality care is the party closest to the point of delivery of care, that is, the professional care provider. Historically professionalism has been relied on as the primary quality assurance mechanism (Donabedian, 1988a, 1988b). It is realized in numerous ways: explicit professional codes of ethics; the unstated contract between patients (or society) and health care professionals sealed with the practitioner's obligations to competence, integrity, and humaneness;[8] and even the impetus behind the several federal peer-review programs. Quality assurance is imbedded in what is referred to as the most fundamental safeguard of quality, that of self-governance and virtuous behavior on the part of individuals and organizations (Pellegrino, 1977; Farber, 1988; Vladeck, 1988).

Regulatory efforts have attempted to take advantage of and support the drive for professionalism, but at times regulatory agents have been perceived as being hostile and even actively detrimental to professionalism. The idea of professionalism clashes fundamentally with those of competition and market forces and with the adversarial atmosphere entailed in malpractice litigation. Some professionals perceive that the foundation of the provider-patient relationship is eroding as a result of these other forces (Blendon, 1988; Eisenberg and Kabcenell, 1988; Goldsmith, 1988; Nelson, 1989).

Nevertheless, professional self-examination has facilitated the development of standards and criteria and of efforts at continuing professional growth. In the broader institutional or corporate provider sense, professionalism supports participation in voluntary accreditation programs such as those of the Joint Commission for Accreditation of Healthcare Organizations. It also fosters implementation of internal quality assurance programs, in particular those based upon the continuous quality improvement model.[9]

Public Sector Responsibilities and Regulation

Because several factors and parties contribute to health care, it is not surprising to find countervailing forces at work within the environment in which health care is delivered. The health of individuals has important implications for the health of the community; in some circumstances the natural balancing of these countervailing forces has not brought the level of health care desired. Thus, government bodies have assumed some responsibility to monitor the quality of health care and to direct or control some of the forces thought to influence the quality of health care.[10]

For almost a century, quality of health care has been a public concern. Only recently have private market forces and competition been seen to have a valid role in ensuring the quality of health care, and many health care providers remain skeptical about any positive impact on quality within a heavily emphasized cost competitive environment. Traditionally, public policy has used regulations and legislation to exert external controls on the health care industry. These range from licensing professionals and certifying facilities (mainly with the intent of assuring at least a minimal level of quality) to controlling expansion of providers and services through health planning and certificate of need, invoking explicit cost and utilization controls, and mandating quality assurance efforts in the publicly financed health programs. Other public policy efforts directed toward improving access to quality care include programs such as educational assistance for residency training programs and the National Health Service Corps to improve the distribution of providers. The responsibility of the Health Care Financing Administration (HCFA) for the quality of care rendered to Medicare beneficiaries is fundamentally a regulatory issue, although in recent years quality assurance activities have taken on a competitive marketplace orientation.

The health care industry is among the most regulated industries in this country. According to Vladeck (1988, p. 100), "Concern...for the quality of health care services has led to external controls in the United States that are more extensive, more intrusive, and more complex than they are elsewhere in the world." None of these regulatory controls has provided a completely satisfactory approach to assuring the quality of health care in this country, yet none has ever been completely abandoned, for reasons partly related to the "public good" aspects of health care.

Health Care as a Public Good

Perhaps more important than the actual (and extensive) involvement of governmental bodies in health care is the perception of health care as a public responsibility, indeed, a public good.[11] Members of our society widely believe that an adequate level of medical care should be available to the poor and elderly, if not all citizens (Enthoven, 1988; Estes, 1988; Fuchs, 1988; Goldsmith, 1988; Arnold, 1989; Leader and Moon, 1989).

One simple aspect of health care as a public good is the gathering and dissemination of information. In the case of quality assurance, this includes information about the effectiveness and appropriateness of medical practices. As stated by Roper et al. (1988, p. 1197), "the benefit of better information accrues to the public at large, not just to those collecting it, [and] the market system may not ensure adequate investment in the necessary research and data collection."

The rationale of viewing health care as a public good, although not a Constitution-backed entitlement or right, is similar to the thinking behind any other public good. The health of individuals affects the health of the community at large; clear distinctions are not easily made between public health and private medicine. Changes in the health status of the community have a domino effect on various sectors of our society and economy.

Other Forces for Quality Assurance

Market Forces and Competition

The last decade or two has seen growing support for the notion that the untrammeled exercise of market forces and competition would serve patients' interests more fully than does health care regulation. The movement toward release of provider-specific information, such as HCFA's publications of hospital-specific mortality rates, is a manifestation of this idea (Brinkley, 1986; Bowen and Roper, 1987).

In an ideal market,[12] competition among health care providers in response to the consumer demand will work to improve the quality of health care, largely by eliminating so-called outliers but possibly also by rewarding good performers by, say, increasing their volume of patients. This tenet is viable only to the extent that someone—patients, outside evaluators, the clinician community itself—can recognize good and bad care. A competitive environment should support good information flow and should value personal choices and preferences. When competitive markets fail, as is often held to be the case in health care, consumers may be at risk of both overuse and underuse. An ideal environment should also permit relatively easy movement of providers (i.e., suppliers) into and out of the market. All these characteristics of a market are assumed to lead to better levels of quality than do purely regulatory mechanisms;[13] none has yet been shown to do so.

Malpractice and Risk Management

Ours is a society that values individual choice, rests its economy on capitalistic principles of competition, uses regulatory methods to place basic (or entry) controls on the health care industry, supports a health delivery system that is decentralized, pluralistic, and fragmented, and uses the courts to resolve both the most trivial and the most complex of social and political issues. It is thus not surprising that patients resort to private legal means, largely that of malpractice suits, when they believe that quality of care has fallen demonstrably below acceptable levels.

The malpractice issue presents very difficult problems for society and for the medical and provider community (Schwartz and Komesar, 1978; OTA, 1988; Hatlie, 1989; Hiatt et al., 1989).[14] At the level of individual practitioners, physicians are widely believed to practice defensive medicine (erring in favor of doing more, rather than less) as a protection against possible malpractice claims should anything go amiss in the care of patients.

Some institutions have incorporated risk management programs into their quality assurance structure in an effort to harness the forces of professional-ism, competition, and malpractice in a more mutually supportive way.[15] Some malpractice insurers also offer incentives in the form of lower premi-ums for organizations that have an effective risk management program in place (GAO, 1989).

Value Purchasing

Perhaps more a hybrid than a separate and unique force are the joint efforts of purchasers, providers, and consumers to promote the idea of value or quality within the context of cost.[16] As the environment for health care delivery has become more competitive, the call for accountability in both the economic and quality spheres is dispersed among many more parties than was true a decade or two ago. Providers see the responsibility for quality assurance shifting away from them and a growing involvement by purchasers and consumers. By contrast, providers and consumers (frequently through unions) are assuming some of the responsibility for cost contain-ment heretofore assumed by private third-party payers, by employers, and, in the case of Medicare, by the federal government. Coalitions developing between payers and capitated prepayment health care systems are attempt-ing to promote quality and contain cost. The need for large corporations and self-insured groups to reduce their health care expenditures while re-taining some confidence that quality of care will not be harmed may pro-duce an impetus for quality assurance that will far exceed the pressures already discussed.

Successful value purchasing depends on access to useful information; inability to judge the reliability, validity, or relevance of available informa-tion on quality of care limits the potential of value purchasing. The move-ment toward population-based outcome measurements may help address some of these problems.

Decision Making and Population-Based Outcomes

Utilization management, practice guidelines, more competition, more regulation in health care, and so forth can all be seen as manifestations of a perceived need for better decision making on the part of purchasers, provid-ers, and patients. Interest and research in population-based outcomes and the potential use of such measures in improving decision making have in-creased (Tarlov et al., 1989). One very significant dimension to current research into patient outcomes is patient preferences and values (sometimes denoted "utilities"); this links the patient-provider decision-making process with outcome measures (Greenfield, 1988).

Informed decision making involves numerous parties with different capacities for using different types of information. Accountability must be accompanied by access to information; such information must be in the public domain. Meaningful information must provide insight to those parties struggling with the cost-related issues of health care; decision makers need to know the value of health care rather than keep separate "balance sheets" on cost and quality. A focus on decision making promotes the strategy of using information to improve quality overall rather than simply to isolate and punish outliers. Finally, as a unifying factor such a focus on decision making helps bridge the conflicting elements of professionalism, regulation, competition, malpractice, and value purchasing.

SUMMARY

The committee identified critical dimensions of quality of care and adopted the following definition: quality of care is "the degree to which health services for individuals and populations increase the likelihood of desired health outcomes and are consistent with current professional knowledge."

We briefly reviewed the United States health care system and the health status of the population to provide a broader context for the recommendations made in this report. We also discussed several factors that affect the quality of care and promote or retard effective quality assurance, such as rising health care expenditures, geographic and financial access, changes and shifts in settings of care, integration of financing and delivery of services, cost-control and utilization management efforts, and Medicare payment systems. Quality of health care is a transcendent public policy issue. The availability and use of meaningful information for decision making by purchasers, providers, and patients will affect the success in balancing the forces of professionalism, regulation, market forces and competition, malpractice and risk management, and value purchasing in a manner that improves quality overall.

NOTES

1. Chapter 4 describes the Medicare program in more detail, and Chapter 6 covers Medicare's peer review and quality assurance efforts.
2. The situation characterized by unlimited access to common constrained resources with decreasing nontransferable marginal benefits to individual consumers has been called the "tragedy of the commons." Pursuit of individual interests will impoverish all in the absence of collective decision making and action (Hardin, 1968; Hiatt, 1975).
3. The independent literatures on bioethics and on quality of care are extensive; the literature on the intersection of the two fields is sparse. Three recent works in this area are McCullough, 1988; Whiteneck, 1988; and Povar, 1989.
4. Other conditions are much more important for specific population groups other

than the elderly. For instance, acquired immune deficiency syndrome (AIDS) affects young to middle-aged adults and, increasingly, infants born to affected mothers; homicides, suicides, and accidents affect young males more than persons in other age or sex groups. These epidemiologic and medical developments are beyond the scope of this study.

5. We return to a more complete description of the health status of the elderly in Chapter 3, and Chapter 7 discusses quality problems and the burden of harm.

6. The IOM defines utilization management as techniques used by or on behalf of purchasers of health benefits to manage health care costs by influencing patient care decision making through case-by-case assessments of the appropriateness of care before it is given (Gray and Field, 1989). Prior review techniques used include pre-admission review, admission review, continued-stay review, discharge planning, and second opinion programs; the other major effort of utilization management is to conduct focused high-cost case management. Both of these efforts rely on case-by-case assessments of care. Generally, utilization management is distinguished from utilization review, which is conducted after care has been rendered (although sometimes before it is reimbursed).

7. In hospitals at least, no clear pattern emerges for lumping or splitting quality assurance and utilization review, utilization management, or risk management. In data obtained through a survey of several hospital systems, we observed many different combinations of these activities, from separate offices responsible for each task to a single unit responsible for all of them. At one hospital included in our site visits, the quality assurance activity was subsumed in the utilization review unit; the notion that it should engage in direct actions intended to assess and improve quality of care was not an important part of that unit's responsibilities. Thus, although in theory utilization review and management can be viewed as an integral part of quality assurance, the provider community in practice does not necessarily see it that way.

8. This is sometimes termed a fiduciary responsibility of professionals to their patients, in explicit contradistinction to a contractual relationship. Hence, the term contract here is not meant to be taken literally.

9. Chapter 2 discusses the quality improvement model. Chapters 5 and 10 provide more detailed discussion of voluntary accreditation through the Joint Commission and quality-of-care criteria, respectively.

10. The use of external regulatory efforts as one of the mechanisms for assuring quality is discussed more fully in Chapters 5, 6, and 9.

11. Public good can be taken as synonymous with public welfare, common good, social good, public interest, and similar ideas. It has a more specific meaning drawn from the field of economics (Eckaus, 1972; Musgrave and Musgrave, 1976)—namely, goods consumed collectively with a joint or societal use or where one person's use does not in theory prevent any other person's use, in contrast to a private good where consumption is exclusive and benefits are internalized. The arguments put forth in this section can be understood in either the broader or the narrower context.

12. A complete discussion of the topics of competition and market economies is beyond the scope of this study. The simple assumptions of an ideal market include notions of perfect information, homogeneous products, large numbers

of suppliers and customers (here, professionals and patients), and free entry of competitors into the marketplace. None of these assumptions holds for health care (Weisbrod, 1983; Lohr, 1986). Information in health is never perfect or complete, and patients do not and cannot learn quickly or at low cost what they may need to know about providers. The products—the processes and the outcomes—cannot be totally homogeneous, because they apply to unique individuals. Although the numbers of suppliers and customers may be large (except in situations of scarcity, such as rural areas), the free entry of competing suppliers is not a sustainable notion because of professional (guild), regulatory, and cost barriers.

13. The debates about the relative merits of regulation and competition are sharp and likely to continue. For key discussions of these issues, see Dallek, 1986; Blendon, 1988; Brook and Kosecoff, 1988; Enthoven, 1988; Enthoven and Kronick, 1988; Estes, 1988; Fuchs, 1988; Ginsburg and Hammons, 1988; Goldsmith, 1988; Iglehart, 1988; McEachern, 1988; Shortell and Hughes, 1988; Rubin and Blehart, 1989; and Smith, 1989.

14. Chapters 7 and 9 briefly discuss malpractice issues in a quality assurance context.

15. Generic or occurrence screens, which are now widely used in quality assurance programs in hospitals and which are discussed more fully in Chapters 6, 9, and 10, are a product of a large study of malpractice cases, the California Medical Insurance Feasibility Study (Mills, 1977).

16. A number of innovative projects are underway through the value purchasing efforts of business, health, and consumer coalitions. These include the "Buy Right" effort of the Center for Policy Studies (Iglehart, 1988), efforts of the Health Care Purchasers Association of Seattle (Castell, 1988), and a recent project of the Midwest Business Group on Health (MBGH, 1989). A large body of literature is emerging on value purchasing and the shifting and sharing of responsibilities and risks, including New York Business Group on Health, Inc., 1987; Ellwood, 1988; Enthoven, 1988; Fuchs, 1988; Iglehart, 1988; Eisenberg, 1989; and McLaughlin et al., 1989.

REFERENCES

Aiken, L.H. The Nursing Shortage: Is it Real? Paper presented at The Sixth Annual Meeting of the Association for Health Services Research and the Foundation for Health Services Research, June 1989.

Aiken, L.H. and Mullinix, C.F. The Nurse Shortage: Myth or Reality? *New England Journal of Medicine* 317:641-646, 1987.

Arnold, M.D. The Politics of Assuring Quality of Care for Elders. *Generations* 13:34-37, Winter 1989.

Berwick, D.M. Sounding Board. Continuous Improvement as an Ideal in Health Care. *New England Journal of Medicine* 320:53-56, 1989.

Blendon, R.J. The Public's View of the Future of Health Care. *Journal of the American Medical Association* 259:3587-3593, 1988.

Blendon, R.J. and Donelan, K. The 1988 Election: How Important was Health? *Health Affairs* 8:6-15, Fall 1989.

Bowen, O.R. and Roper, W.L. *Medicare Hospital Mortality Information 1986.* Washington, D.C.: U.S. Government Printing Office, 1987.

Brinkley, J. U.S. Releasing Lists of Hospitals with Abnormal Mortality Rates. *The New York Times* March 12, 1986, pp. A1, A22.

Brook, R.H. Quality Assessment and Technology Assessment: Critical Linkages. Pp. 21-28 in *Quality of Care and Technology Assessment.* Report of a Forum of the Council on Health Care Technology. Lohr, K.N. and Rettig, R.A., eds. Washington, D.C.: National Academy Press, 1988.

Brook, R.H. and Kosecoff, J.B. Competition and Quality. *Health Affairs* 7:160-161, Summer 1988.

Brook, R.H., Kamberg, C.J., and Lohr, K.N. Quality Assessment in Mental Health. *Professional Psychology* 13(1): Special Issue, February 1982.

Brown, R.E., Sheingold, S.H., and Luce, B.R. *Options for Using Practice Guidelines in Reducing the Volume of Medically Unnecessary Services.* BHARC-013/89/027. Washington, D.C.: Battelle Human Affairs Research Centers, June 1989.

Castell, A.B. Gateway to Better Health. *Business and Health* 5:16-17, November 1988.

Cleary, P.D. and McNeil, B.J. The Measurement of Quality. *Inquiry* 25:25-36, 1988.

Dallek, G. Commentary: Politics of Privatization. *Case Western Reserve Law Review* 36:969-984, 1986.

Davies, A.R. and Ware, J.E., Jr. Involving Consumers in Quality Assessment. *Health Affairs* 7:33-48, Spring 1988.

Division of National Cost Estimates, Office of the Actuary, Health Care Financing Administration. National Health Expenditures, 1986-2000. *Health Care Financing Review* 8(4):1-36, Summer 1987.

Donabedian, A. *Explorations in Quality Assessment and Monitoring: The Definition of Quality and Approaches to Its Assessment.* Vol. 1. Ann Arbor, Mich.: Health Administration Press, 1980.

Donabedian, A. Quality Assessment and Assurance: Unity of Purpose, Diversity of Means. *Inquiry* 25:173-192, 1988a.

Donabedian, A. Monitoring: The Eyes and Ears of Healthcare. *Health Progress* 69:38-43, November 1988b.

Eckaus, R.S. *Basic Economics.* Boston, Mass.: Little, Brown and Company, 1972.

Eisenberg, J. Economics. *Journal of the American Medical Association* 261:2840-2841, 1989.

Eisenberg, J.M. and Kabcenell, A. Organized Practice and the Quality of Medical Care. *Inquiry* 25:78-89, 1988.

Ellwood, P.M. The Shattuck Lecture: Outcomes Management. *New England Journal of Medicine* 318:1549-1556, 1988.

Enthoven, A. Managed Competition: An Agenda for Action. *Health Affairs* 7:25-47, Summer 1988.

Enthoven, A. and Kronick, R. Competition 101: Managing Demand to Get Quality Care. *Business and Health* 5:38-40, March 1988.

Estes, C. Healthcare Policy in the Later Twentieth Century. *Generations* 7:44-47, Spring 1988.

Farber, S.J. Perspectives in Quality Assurance and Technology Assessment. Pp. 11-20 in *Quality of Care and Technology Assessment.* Report of a Forum of the Council on Health Care Technology. Lohr, K.N. and Rettig, R.A., eds. Washington, D.C.: National Academy Press, 1988.

Fitzgerald, J.F., Fagan, L.F., Tierney, W.M., et al. Changing Patterns of Hip Fracture Care Before and After Implementation of the Prospective Payment System. *Journal of the American Medical Association* 258:218-221, 1987.

Fitzgerald, J.F., Moore, P.S., and Dittus, R.S. The Care of Elderly Patients with Hip Fracture. *New England Journal of Medicine* 319:1392-1397, 1988.

Fuchs, V.R. The Competition Revolution in Health Care. *Health Affairs* 7:5-24, Summer 1988.

GAO (General Accounting Office). *Health Care Initiatives in Hospital Risk Management.* Washington, D.C.: General Accounting Office, July 1989.

Generations 13:4-68, Winter 1989 (Special Topic: Assuring Quality of Care).

Ginsburg, P. and Hammons, G. Competition and the Quality of Care: The Importance of Information. *Inquiry* 25:108-114, 1988.

Goldsmith, J.C. Commentary: Competition's Impact: A Report from the Front. *Health Affairs* 7:162-173, Summer 1988.

Gray, B.H. and Field, M.J., eds. *Controlling Costs and Changing Patient Care? The Role of Utilization Management.* Washington, D.C.: National Academy Press, 1989.

Greenfield, S. The Challenges and Opportunities That Quality Assurance Raises for Technology Assessment. Pp. 134-141 in *Quality of Care and Technology Assessment.* Report of a Forum of the Council on Health Care Technology. Lohr, K.N. and Rettig. R.A., eds. Washington, D.C.: National Academy Press, 1988.

Hardin, G. The Tragedy of the Commons. *Science* 162:1243-1248, 1968.

Harwood, H.J., Napolitano, D.M., Kristiansen, P.L., et al. *Economic Costs to Society of Alcohol and Drug Abuse and Mental Illness: 1980.* RTI/2734/00-01FR. Research Triangle Park, N.C.: Research Triangle Institute, June 1984.

Hatlie, M.J. Professional Liability. *Journal of the American Medical Association* 261:2881-2882, 1989.

Health Affairs 7:1-113, Spring 1988. (Special Issue. The Pursuit of Quality.)

Hiatt, H.H. Protecting the Medical Commons: Who Is Responsible? *New England Journal of Medicine* 293:235-241, 1975.

Hiatt, H.H., Barnes, B.B., Brennan, T.A., et al. Special Report. A Study of Medical Injury and Medical Malpractice. *New England Journal of Medicine* 321:480-484, 1989.

Hinshaw, A.S. Determinants of Nurse Retention, Job Satisfaction, and Turnover. Paper presented at The Sixth Annual Meeting of the Association for Health Services Research and the Foundation for Health Services Research, June 1989.

Iglehart, J.K. Health Policy Report: Problems Facing the Nursing Profession. *New England Journal of Medicine* 317:646-651, 1987.

Iglehart, J.K. Competition and the Pursuit of Quality: A Conversation with Walter McClure. *Health Affairs* 7:79-90, Spring 1988.

Inquiry 25:1-192, Spring 1988. (Special Issue. The Challenge of Quality.)

IOM (Institute of Medicine). *Advancing the Quality of Health Care.* A Policy Statement by a Committee of the Institute of Medicine. Washington, D.C.: National Academy of Sciences, 1974.

IOM. *Confronting Aids. Directions for Public Health, Health Care, and Research.* Washington, D.C.: National Academy Press, 1986a.

IOM. *For-Profit Enterprise in Health Care.* Washington, D.C.: National Academy Press, 1986b.

IOM. *Allied Health Services: Avoiding Crises.* Washington, D.C.: National Academy Press, 1988a.

IOM. *Confronting AIDS: Update 1988.* Washington, D.C.: National Academy Press, 1988b.

Kahn, K.L., Rubenstein, L.V., Kosecoff, J., et al. DRG-Based Prospective Payment System and Quality of Care. *AFCR Clinical Epidemiology and Health Care, Clinical Research.* Vol. 37, No. 2, 1989.

Kane, R.A. and Kane, R.L. Reflections on Quality Control. *Generations* 13:63-68, Winter 1989.

Leader, S. and Moon, M. Forging the Agenda. Pp. 111-123 in *Changing America's Health Care System.* Leader, S. and Moon, M., eds. American Association of Retired Persons. Glenview, Ill.: Scott, Foresman and Company, 1989.

Lohr, K.N. Commentary: Professional Peer Review in a "Competitive" Medical Market. *Case Western Reserve Law Review* 36(4):1175-1189, 1986.

Lohr, K.N. Outcome Measurement: Concepts and Questions. *Inquiry* 25:37-50, 1988.

Lohr, K.N., Brook, R.H., Goldberg, G.A., et al. *Impact of Medicare Prospective Payment on the Quality of Medical Care. A Research Agenda.* R-3242-HCFA. Santa Monica, Calif.: The RAND Corporation, March 1985.

Long, S.H. and Welch, W.P. Are We Containing Costs or Pushing on a Balloon? *Health Affairs* 7:113-117, Fall 1988.

McCullough, L.B. An Ethical Model for Improving the Patient-Physician Relationship. *Inquiry* 25:454-468, 1988.

McEachern, J.E. Comment. John Mannix Quality of Care Symposium. *Health Matrix* VI:11-14, Summer 1988.

McLaughlin, C.G., Zellers, W.K., and Brown, L.D. Health Care Coalitions: Characteristics, Activities, and Prospects. *Inquiry* 26:72-83, 1989.

MBGH (Midwest Business Group on Health). *Value-Managed Health Care Purchasing Project.* Vols. I-IV. Chicago, Ill.: Midwest Business Group on Health, 1989.

Mills, D.H., ed. *Report on the Medical Insurance Feasibility Study.* San Francisco, Calif.: California Medical Association, 1977.

Minnick, A. The Nursing Shortage: A Study of Nursing in Six Urban Areas. Paper presented at The Sixth Annual Meeting of the Association for Health Services Research and the Foundation for Health Services Research, June 1989.

Musgrave, R.A. and Musgrave, P.B. *Public Finance in Theory and Practice.* Second Edition. New York, N.Y.: McGraw-Hill, 1976.

Nelson, A.R. Humanism and the Art of Medicine. *Journal of the American Medical Association* 262:1228-1230, 1989.

NCHS (National Center for Health Statistics). Prevalence of Selected Chronic Conditions, United States, 1983-85. *Advancedata.* No. 155. DHHS Publ. No. (PHS) 88-1250. Public Health Service. Hyattsville, Md.: National Center for Health Statistics, May 1988.

NCHS. *Health, United States, 1988.* DHHS Publ. No. (PHS) 89-1232. Public Health Service. Washington, D.C.: U.S. Government Printing Office, March 1989.

NCHS. *Health, United States, 1989.* Public Health Service. Washington, D.C.: U.S. Government Printing Office, forthcoming.

New York Business Group on Health, Inc. *Quality of Care Discussion Paper* 7:(Supplement No.4), 1987.

Nichols, E. *Mobilizing Against AIDS.* Cambridge, Mass.: Harvard University Press, 1989.

OTA (Office of Technology Assessment). *The Quality of Medical Care: Information for Consumers.* OTA-H-386. Washington, D.C.: U.S. Government Printing Office, 1988.

Palmer, R.H. and Adams, M.E. Considerations in Defining Quality in Health Care. Paper prepared for Institute of Medicine Study to Design a Strategy for Quality Review and Assurance in Medicare, 1988.

Pellegrino, E.D. A Humanistic Base for Professional Ethics in Medicine. *New York State Journal of Medicine* 77:1456-1462, August 1977.

Perrin, J.M. and Valvona, J. Does Increased Physician Supply Affect Quality of Care? *Health Affairs* 4:64-71, Winter 1986.

Povar, G. Quality Assurance: Ethical Considerations. Paper prepared for the Institute of Medicine Study to Design a Strategy for Quality Review and Assurance in Medicare, 1989.

President's Commission. *Summing Up. The Ethical and Legal Problems in Medicine and Biomedical and Behavioral Research.* Washington, D.C.: President's Commission for the Study of Ethical Problems in Medicine and Biomedical and Behavioral Research, 1983.

PPRC (Physician Payment Review Commission). *Annual Report to Congress.* Washington, D.C.: Physician Payment Review Commission, 1988.

PPRC. *Annual Report to Congress.* Washington, D.C.: Physician Payment Review Commission, 1989.

ProPAC (Prospective Payment Assessment Commission). *Medicare Prospective Payment and the American Health Care System. Report to the Congress.* Washington, D.C.: Prospective Payment Assessment Commission, 1988.

ProPAC. *Medicare Prospective Payment and the American Health Care System. Report to the Congress.* Washington, D.C.: Prospective Payment Assessment Commission, 1989.

Roper, W.L. and Hackbarth, G.M. HCFA's Agenda for Promoting High-Quality Care. *Health Affairs* 7:91-98, Spring 1988.

Roper, W.L., Winkenwerder, W., Hackbarth, G.M., et al. Effectiveness in Health Care, An Initiative to Evaluate and Improve Medical Practice. *New England Journal of Medicine* 319:1197-1202, 1988.

Rubin, R.N. and Blehart, B.D. Government. *Journal of the American Medical Association* 261:2849-2851, 1989.

Ruther, M. and Helbing, C. Use and Cost of Home Health Agency Services under Medicare. *Health Care Financing Review* 10:105-108, Fall 1988.

Schieber, G.J. and Poullier, J.P. International Health Spending and Utilization Trends. *Health Affairs* 7:105-112, Fall 1988.

Schwartz, W.B. and Komesar, N.K. Doctors, Damages and Deterrence: An Economic View of Medical Malpractice. *New England Journal of Medicine* 298:1282-1289, 1978.

Secretary's Commission on Nursing. *Final Report.* Vol. I. Washington, D.C.: Department of Health and Human Services, 1988.

Shortell, S. and Hughes, E. The Effects of Regulation, Competition, and Ownership on Mortality Rates Among Hospital Inpatients. *New England Journal of Medicine* 318:1100-1107, 1988.

Smith, N.H. The Struggle for Lawmakers. *Generations* 13:42-44, Winter 1989.

Tarlov, A.R., Ware, J.E., Jr., Greenfield, S., et al. The Medical Outcomes Study. *Journal of the American Medical Association* 262:925-930, 1989.

Torrens, P.R. *The American Health Care System: Issues and Problems.* St. Louis, Mo.: Mosby, 1978.

Vladeck, B.C. Quality Assurance Through External Controls. *Inquiry* 25:100-107, 1988.

Weisbrod, B. Competition in Health Care: A Cautionary View. Pp. 61-71 in *Market Reforms in Health Care: Current Issues, New Directions, Strategic Decisions.* Meyer, J.A., ed. Washington, D.C.: American Enterprise Institute, 1983.

Whiteneck, M.R. Integrating Ethics with Quality Assurance in Long Term Care. *Quality Review Bulletin* 14:138-143, 1988.

Wilensky, G. An Economic Analysis of the Nursing Shortage. Paper presented at The Sixth Annual Meeting of the Association for Health Services Research and the Foundation for Health Services Research, June 1989.

2

Concepts of Assessing, Assuring, and Improving Quality

In this chapter we describe quality assurance concepts and models as a context in which to understand where our proposed quality assurance program for Medicare fits in the long tradition of quality assurance in this country. We attempt to answer these questions: What do quality assessment, quality assurance, and quality improvement mean? What are the roles of structure, process, and outcome in these concepts? What are the key properties of a quality assurance program?

The final section of this chapter examines two quality assurance conceptual models, that is, the traditional structure-process-outcome model and the continuous quality improvement model. During this study the health care industry became increasingly interested in the potential application of the continuous improvement model for health care. The committee took advantage of numerous opportunities to explore its concepts and practices, and it thoroughly debated how this relatively new model might be incorporated into a strategy for quality assurance in Medicare.

QUALITY ASSESSMENT, QUALITY ASSURANCE, AND QUALITY IMPROVEMENT

Definitions

The concepts of quality assessment and assurance in the health sector are not new; the literature documents efforts over the last 80 years or so to place them into operational frameworks.[1] Quality assessment is the measurement of the technical and interpersonal aspects of health care and the outcomes of that care. Assessment is expressly a measurement activity;

although it is the first step in quality assurance, it does not imply a solution to problems that may be uncovered.

Classically, quality assurance encompasses a full cycle of activities and systems for maintaining the quality of patient care. One definition has it as "a formal and systematic exercise in identifying problems in medical care delivery, designing activities to overcome the problems, and carrying out follow-up monitoring to ensure that no new problems have been introduced and that corrective steps have been effective" (Lohr and Brook, 1984, p. 585). Generally, that cycle involves a set of steps proceeding from identification and verification of quality-related problems and their causes to the implementation of solutions to the problems with the specific intent that the solution be long-lasting or preventive; these activities are followed by a timely review to determine if the problem has been solved and no new ones generated in the process. If the last two conditions are met (one problem solved and no new ones generated), attention turns away from that aspect of patient care to other areas or topics.

Quality improvement is a set of techniques for continuous study and improvement of the processes of delivering health care services and products to meet the needs and expectations of the customers of those services and products. It has three basic elements: customer knowledge, a focus on processes of health care delivery, and statistical approaches that aim to reduce variations in those processes. In understanding the place of continuous quality improvement it is helpful to think in terms of a bell-shaped curve that distributes numbers of providers or volume of care against quality. The leading tail is the province of research, the lagging tail is the focus of regulation; and the middle is the focus of continuous improvement. The design of a quality assurance system (for Medicare or for any other health care program) should attend to all three parts of the distribution.

Purposes of Quality Assurance

Quality assurance neither promises nor guarantees error-free health care. Its ultimate goal is to build confidence and faith in the quality of the health care being rendered. Achieving error-free health care at all times is impossible; trying to do so ultimately discourages quality assurance efforts. The ultimate goal, however, is achievable and thus encourages continuous effort. An effective quality assurance program is not an end in itself; rather, it is a means of maintaining and improving health care (O'Leary, 1988).

Quality assurance programs vary widely in their purposes, targets, and methods. Four major purposes can be identified.[2] First, in some circumstances the main goal is to identify providers whose delivery of care is so far below an acceptable level that immediate actions are needed to ensure that they no longer deliver care or that responsible third-party payers, such as Medicare, no longer reimburse for any care delivered. Second, quality assurance programs, on identifying providers whose delivery practices are determined to be unacceptable, may concentrate on working with those providers to correct the problems and bring care up to an acceptable level. Both these examples reflect an orientation to "outliers,"[3] although the remedies (and hence the underlying philosophies) differ.

A third purpose focuses on improving the average level of quality of care delivered by a community of providers. Improving average performance, sometimes referred to as "shifting the curve," by moving a large number of providers forward on the quality scale usually occurs only gradually. It implies, among other things, a considerable educational effort. From a statistical point of view however, one can shift the curve by removing outliers from the professional community when their abnormal practices are truly extreme and constitute a significant percentage of the community's practices. Implicit in this process of shifting the curve is the understanding that acceptable levels of quality are protected from erosion.

Fourth, quality assurance may also motivate and assist providers to achieve high levels of quality. Programs may identify excellent providers who serve as models or mentors. They may explicitly recognize and reward exemplary performance or underwrite incentives for practitioners and organizations to reach and surpass desirable levels of quality. This approach supplements direct efforts at improving average practice by highlighting and rewarding superior performance.

Internal and External Programs

This report often distinguishes "internal" and "external" quality assurance. Internal quality assurance programs are those implemented by organizations or systems, for example by hospitals, HMOs, home health agencies, or similar groups of practitioners. Internal programs have (or could be brought to have) several key features. They can be integrated into ongoing patient care and adapted to the local environment and the degree of sophistication and interest of the practitioners. They can emphasize professionalism and the desire on the part of most practitioners to do better. They can minimize the adversarial "we-they" attitude that can and does provoke mistrust of the outside reviewer (Weiss, 1972). To the extent that internal programs involve their entire staffs in quality-of-care matters, they can reinforce the concept of the "virtuous" organization. Theoretically, they can serve all four purposes of a quality assurance program outlined above, although they may find it difficult to identify or, more importantly, remove the true outlier provider. Further, they are not likely to identify systemic problems that exist within the organization.

Internal programs face several problems. Conflict over authority, lack of commitment or expertise, and concern about financial repercussions for individuals or of financial stress in the organization may result in inaction despite well-known and well-documented problems. When individual organizations develop idiosyncratic methods, collect data without an external reference for comparison, or fail to follow through when internal data suggest problems, valuable resources and opportunities for improvement are wasted. The time-honored principle of peer review may be difficult to implement in a small organization.

External quality assurance programs typically serve a broader social purpose and clientele. Examples include the accrediting activities of the Joint Commission on Accreditation of Healthcare Organizations and the National League for Nursing, the Medicare Utilization and Quality Control Peer Review Organization (PRO) program, and state medical licensing or disciplinary boards. Through mechanisms such as the threat of exposure, imposition of financial sanctions, or withdrawal of accreditation or licensure status, they may be able to deal with outliers (and especially to remove them). They may also be helpful by assessing the quality of the internal quality improvement process and, where appropriate, offering technical assistance. Often, however, external programs will be less well suited to improving the average performance of providers, and most are not in a position to identify exemplary providers or to offer assistance in reaching higher levels of quality care.

Some external programs may have uniform data collection and reporting methods that allow comparisons across settings and institutions; information can be shared with organizations entitled to their own data. External programs can force attention to problems that would not otherwise be addressed, pressure providers to correct problems, and make it harder for incompetent practitioners to move from one facility or organization to another.

For external programs, successful review is feasible only if standards enable accurate assessment of the variations in individual organizations. External review must protect those under review when the reviewers belong to antagonistic or competitive groups. Review of care rendered by physicians in prepaid group practices by those in fee-for-service practice is an example of potential conflict among practitioners who by all other accounts may be considered peers.

Both internal and external quality assurance programs are necessary for a comprehensive approach to quality assurance; neither presents a sufficient response to quality problems. The distinctions may seem somewhat arbitrary because, at one level, everything outside the patient-practitioner pair is external to the interaction. Denoting a hospital or HMO program as internal and the Medicare or a state's program as external, or agreeing on

TABLE 2.1 Desirable Attributes of a Quality Assurance Progra

- Addresses overuse, underuse, and poor technical and interpersonal
- Intrudes minimally into the patient-provider relationship
- Is acceptable to professionals and providers
- Fosters improvement throughout the health care organization and system
- Deals with outlier practice and performance
- Uses both positive and negative incentives for change and improvement in performance.
- Provides practitioners and providers with timely information to improve performance
- Has face validity for the public and for professionals (i.e., is understandable and relevant to patient and clinical decision making)
- Is scientifically rigorous
- Positive impact on patient outcomes can be demonstrated or inferred
- Can address both individual and population-based outcomes
- Documents improvement in quality and progress toward excellence
- Is easily implemented and administered
- Is affordable and is cost-effective
- Includes patients and the public

who can legitimately be considered a peer, is related more to almost incidental traditional professional boundaries of accountability than to intrinsic ones. One challenge in devising a strategy for quality assurance is to combine the strengths of both internal and external approaches yet avoid replication and counterproductive effects, such as the poisoning of the atmosphere for professional involvement in internal programs.

CRITERIA FOR JUDGING AN EFFECTIVE QUALITY ASSURANCE PROGRAM

What are the attributes of a successful quality assurance effort that would be acceptable to those with a stake in the process (i.e., patients, providers, payers, and policymakers)? This section outlines our view of the criteria that a successful quality assurance program, either internal or external, should strive to meet (see Table 2.1). Some of these criteria may appear contradictory (such as minimal intrusion into the patient-provider relationship and ability to deal effectively with outlier providers), but the mark of a good program is an appropriate balance between such elements. We use these attributes later in this chapter to evaluate two conceptual models of quality assurance.

A successful quality assurance program has the following 15 attributes):

1. It is able to address a full range of quality problems—poor technical quality, overuse, and underuse. Reviews of the literature and discussions with providers of care during the study site visits led us to understand that problems of all three kinds occur to varying degrees in different settings of care (e.g., underuse of home health services and overuse of hospital or outpatient surgical procedures) (Chapter 7). Hence, an effective quality assurance program should have a range of methods such that it can prevent, identify, and correct problems of underuse, overuse, and poor technical and interpersonal quality in all patient care settings and under various reimbursement mechanisms. Additionally, an effective quality assurance program should be flexible enough to prompt appropriate responses to new problems as settings, reimbursement mechanisms, and clinical practice change over time.

2. It intrudes minimally into the patient-provider relationship. Because the core of health care is the patient-provider relationship, no quality assurance program should jeopardize the relationship of trust or the ability of the practitioner to use his or her best judgment to guide the care of the patient. Neither should it diminish the autonomy of patients in seeking and obtaining care that conforms to their preferences.

3. It is acceptable to professionals and providers. The essence of quality assurance is improving the care provided by individuals to individuals, through better decision making, enhanced skills, more adequate support systems, and similar elements affecting health care. To accomplish these goals, a successful program must be accepted by the professionals and organizations in which it is embedded or to which it is directed. The program must support, and be seen as supporting, the goal of the well-motivated health professional to provide compassionate and competent care. This implies that judgments about care and recommendations about change in practice are made by peers.

4. It fosters improvement throughout the health care organization and system. A quality assurance program is incomplete without a focus on improving the processes through which patient care is delivered, and these processes involve individuals throughout the health care organization, practice, or institution. On the broader external level, quality assurance should strive to improve the health care delivery system as a whole.

5. It is able to identify and ameliorate outlier practice. A quality assurance program must be able to identify not only problematic patterns of care in the aggregate, but also the individual outlier practitioner, institution, facility, or agency. It must have the tools to intervene in that provider's practice, when necessary, to prevent actual or future harm to patients.

6. It can invoke positive and negative incentives for change and improve-

ment in performance. To support the goal of providing compassionate and competent care, incentives and rewards for high quality are generally preferable to penalties for poor quality, but both should be available to the quality assurance program. In any case, no quality assurance system can rely solely on coercion through sanctions applied at a time and place remote from the site of care.

7. It provides well-motivated people with timely information to improve their practice. Two essential functions of a quality assurance program are the correction of identified problems and the improvement of care generally. If a quality assurance program is to fulfill these functions, it must be able to provide practitioners with timely data at a level of aggregation or disaggregation clinically relevant to their practice. This implies that the data should be based if at all possible on rates, so that comparisons can be made to standards of practice. When problems in individual care are detected, interventions must be sufficiently timely to prevent further harm to that patient and to others who might be at risk.

8. It has face validity to public and professionals. A quality assurance program must be understandable and reasonable to the public and to the health professionals who are subject to assessment; it must reflect their quality objectives and respond to their quality complaints. The program's methods should have clinical relevance to practitioners for the kind of care they provide, and it should include appropriate adjustments for nonpractitioner-related variables. For the public it should illuminate decision making relevant to those aspects of health care under patient or regulatory control.

9. Its individual elements meet requirements for reliability, validity, and generalizability. A successful quality assurance effort should demonstrate scientific rigor of its methods, beyond simple face validity to practitioners or providers. In so doing, it should minimize the need for separate and unique programs among various external organizations.

10. It improves patient outcomes. The focus of compassionate and competent health care is patient well-being and outcomes. Ultimately, therefore, a quality assurance program should affect patient outcomes in ways that can be measured and evaluated over time. When outcomes cannot be measured or evaluated directly and when the process of care is the appropriate aspect of care to be assessed, there should be a demonstrated link between those health care processes and expected patient outcomes such that the impact on patient outcomes of improving the process of care can be inferred.

11. It can address both individual patient and population-based outcomes. The outcomes of care for both individual patients and populations (e.g., collections of patients enrolled in HMOs or the Medicare beneficiary

population as a whole) are important targets of quality assurance. This orientation helps ensure that underuse of services, especially as it is reflected in poor access to care in the first place, receives due attention as part of a quality assurance effort.

12. It documents improvement in quality and progress toward excellence. A quality assurance program must be able to track and evaluate the effect of its efforts. Documenting improvement implies that quality-related information will be analyzed with appropriate statistical tools over time and that such information will be shared among appropriate staff and organizations.

13. It is easily implemented and administered. A successful quality assurance strategy must find a middle ground between (on the one hand) an excessively simplistic system that has little specificity, relevance, or involvement of professionals but is relatively easy to mount and administer and (on the other) an excessively complex, costly, labor-intensive system that may itself detract from the ability of providers to render adequate patient care. Thus, although we do not intend by this criterion to discount the need for considerable investment in a Medicare quality assurance program, we do want to emphasize the need for ease of implementation and administration.

14. It is affordable and cost-effective. Determining whether a quality assurance program is acceptable in cost and is cost-effective is very difficult; in the public sector the history of evaluations of the Professional Standards Review Organizations makes that clear. Nevertheless, the use of public monies to assure quality requires accountability. Part of the challenge of the Medicare quality assurance strategy will be to develop mechanisms to evaluate the costs and cost-effectiveness of that program; this requires articulating criteria for acceptability and effectiveness in this domain and applying those methods and criteria objectively.

15. It includes patients and the public. An effective program must have a mechanism to listen to and respond to complaints and suggestions and a mechanism for change to act as a safety valve. Considering the size and complexity of the Medicare program, this is especially important for the external quality assurance efforts.

QUALITY ASSURANCE CONCEPTUAL MODELS

Designing a strategy for quality assurance for the Medicare program requires us to describe the program we expect to be in place and the steps we believe are necessary to implement that program. This in turn requires a clear conceptual framework and a set of program goals. This section summarizes important conceptual models relating to quality of health care and introduces concepts and terms that we will rely on throughout this report.

The Traditional Structure-Process-Outcome Model

Avedis Donabedian has articulated what continues to serve as the unifying conceptual framework for quality measurement and assurance. His widely accepted model of structure, process, and outcome has guided two decades of research and program development (Donabedian, 1966, 1980, 1982, 1984, 1988a, 1988b, 1988c). We do not depart significantly from this conceptualization.

Structure

Structural measures, the characteristics of the resources in the health care delivery system, apply to individual practitioners, to groups of practitioners, and to organizations and agencies. They are essentially measures of the presumed capacity of the practitioner or provider to deliver quality health care, not of the care itself. Deficiencies in structural measures are not evidence of poor care (and certainly not of poor outcomes); they may, but do not necessarily, point to crucial areas requiring improvement or reform.

For health care professionals, these variables include demographic factors (e.g., age) and professional characteristics (e.g., specialty, licensure and certification, practice setting and style). For facilities and institutions, they include size, location, ownership and governance, and licensure and accreditation status. They can also include many physical attributes (e.g., special units and computer capabilities) and a large set of organizational factors (e.g., staff-to-staff or staff-to-patient ratios; employee morale and turnover).

Quality assurance programs acquire information on structural measures in several ways. The simplest is probably through mechanisms of licensure, certification, or accreditation that are maintained by states, professional associations, or third-party payers. Provider surveys can also provide relevant information.

Some observers question the relationship of structural measures to either process or outcome variables because of inadequate measures and little empirical evidence of direct connections; they tend to downplay the importance of structural characteristics of health care organizations as markers of quality. Nevertheless, over the last decade various elements of the quality assurance field have more explicitly emphasized accountability, governance, and lines of authority, especially for hospitals. Regulatory agencies such as states, voluntary associations such as the Joint Commission, and institutional quality assurance officials are much more likely to repose the ultimate responsibility for quality care in boards of trustees or directors and equivalent organizational executives. Consequently, structural measures that reflect organizational patterns, lines of authority, and communication within health care delivery systems command attention in quality assurance programs.

Process

The process of care embodies what is done to and for the patient. Process measurement is the most common approach to quality assessment and assurance today. The relative merits of process measurement versus outcome measurement have been debated vigorously over the years; the consensus is that both are necessary but that neither is sufficient to successful quality assurance (Table 2.2).

Process measurement can be directed at individual practitioners, teams of practitioners, or entire systems of care. It can include aspects of whether and how patients seek and obtain care. Process measures seek information to identify problems that occur during the delivery of care. Elements of care delivery are evaluated against criteria that reflect professional standards of good quality care and, increasingly, patient-oriented measures of satisfaction.

Data about processes can be obtained in numerous ways. These include patient reports of care rendered, direct observation of care, review of medical records (or abstracts of records) and similar documents, and analysis of insurance claims or other utilization data.

The presumed advantages of process-of-care evaluation are several. It has great appeal to practitioners because it is directly related to what they do. It is easy to explain and to interpret the approach and its findings. Reliable, valid criteria and methods are available. In some cases, review of care against process criteria can be nearly "real time," meaning that corrective actions can be very timely. Data can be analyzed by individual providers or aggregated in various ways that support comparisons of practice patterns across communities or health delivery systems. For certain settings, process measurement may be the preferred strategy (compared to outcome measurement), such as for ambulatory office practice (Palmer, 1988). Finally, process measurement can point directly to specific areas needing performance improvement, which is a fundamental aim of quality assurance.

Process-of-care assessment is not without its limitations. Resource costs can be high, which explains the considerable attractiveness of using administrative or insurance claims data sets. For some settings, such as home health care, the data sources are poor; for others, such as long-term-care facilities (Kane and Kane, 1988), process measures may be less informative than some alternative outcome measures because of the repetitive nature of much that is done in such settings. Process measures may focus on issues

TABLE 2.2 Strengths of Process and Outcome Measurement on Selected Dimensions

Dimensions	Type of Measurement[a]	
	Process	Outcome
Relevance to goal of health care	−	++
Appeal to practitioners and institutions	++	+
Appeal to patients and public	+	++
Can detect problems of overuse	++	−
Can detect problems of underuse	+	+
Can detect poor technical or interpersonal quality	++	−
Real time review and timely intervention possible	++	−
Points directly to specific areas needing performance improvement	++	−
Reflects important trends over time	+	++
Particularly useful for certain settings		
physician office care	++	−
hospital care	++	++
post-hospital care (e.g., home health)	+	+
Minimizes intrusiveness for providers	−	++
Minimizes intrusiveness for patients	++	−
Reliable and valid assessment methods	+	+
Reliable and valid evaluation criteria	+	−
Relevant informaton recorded in administrative (billing or utilization) data	+	− −
Consensus on best practices	++ to − −	NA
Consensus on best outcomes	NA	++
Can account for biological variability	−	+
Can account for patient preferences	− −	+
Can account for patient behavior	− −	−
Can assign accountability for performance when care is from multiple providers over time	−	− −
Costs of measurement	+ to −	+ to − −

[a]Code: ++, strong in this dimension; +, adequate in this dimension; −, fair in this dimension; − −, poor in this dimension. NA means not applicable.

that contribute little to outcomes. Finally, for many clinical areas, practitioners and researchers may be unable to reach consensus on best practices.

Outcomes

Measuring the outcomes of care is the third approach to quality assessment in the classic paradigm. Outcomes are the end results of care—the effect of the care process on the health and well-being of patients and populations. One outcomes list comprises "the five Ds"—death, disease, disability, discomfort, and dissatisfaction (Elinson, 1987). More positively they may be thought of as survival, states of physiologic, physical, and emotional health, and satisfaction (Lohr, 1988).

The philosophical shift in orientation from process measurement to outcomes has been dramatic in the late 1980s.[4] For instance, the Joint Commission has launched an ambitious and far-ranging restructuring of its survey and accreditation procedures—the Agenda for Change—that is expected to rely heavily on outcome measurement (Joint Commission, 1987; Roberts, 1988). Ellwood (1988) has proposed a radical shift to "outcomes management," by which he means collaborative action involving patients, payers, and providers in national information gathering and analysis to facilitate better, more "rational" decision making. He defines outcomes management as a "permanent national medical data base that uses a common set of definitions for measuring quality of life to enable patients, payers, and providers to make informed health choices" (p. 1555), and he puts particular emphasis on understanding the relationships between medical interventions and health outcomes and between health outcomes and money.

This emphasis on outcomes is a critical one. It will not, however, be easy to put into action, and it should never be seen as fully displacing process-of-care assessment. Greenfield (1989), for instance, cautions about the importance of choosing the right kinds of measures.

Outcomes offer a vast range of units of measurement: for example, death; hospital complication rates; functional capacities and performance; emotional health; cognitive functioning; and patient satisfaction, knowledge, and compliance.[5] Such outcomes are measured directly and indirectly. Direct assessments rely on patient examination, physiologic data, patient self-report, and physician or other professional reports or records. Indirect evaluations can be based on utilization records (e.g., encounter forms and insurance claims), vital and health statistics, surveys, and the like; data sources can be the same as those used for process measures in some instances. Almost none of the outcomes mentioned above is amenable to measurement exclusively by insurance claims data, so researchers and policy makers have given substantial attention lately to nonintrusive outcomes, such as mortality or readmissions to hospitals. These proxy measures, typically taken from administrative data, are intended to signal probable levels of quality (usually poor care) (Lohr et al., 1988).

Numerous aspects of outcome measurement should be understood before being considered appropriate for a quality assurance program. The choice of long-run outcomes, intermediate outcomes, or secular patterns of functional change is one important dimension. Some outcomes are more costly to measure than others. Health status is determined in part by factors outside of the clinical intervention, so taking acount of external, environmental and personal variables can be crucial.

The relative goodness of various outcomes and patient preferences (or utilities) for different combinations of quantity and quality of life and health must be taken into account. Articulating and documenting patient preferences are difficult exercises, and they become more so as the circumstances that influence these preferences and their relative importance change over time. Incorporating value judgments, such as patient utilities, in an outcome-oriented quality assurance program presents special challenges in analyzing individual and aggregate data (as would be true for process assessment also).

Some advantages of measuring outcomes mirror those for the process of care. Some outcome measures are comparatively easy to explain and interpret (e.g., death, recovery of function, and reduction in pain) and are of interest to practitioners and their patients. The ready availability of some methods and tools (e.g., functional status instruments and measures of activities of daily living) should not be overlooked, although those that are available are not widely used today in quality assurance programs. Finally, they can be used as screening mechanisms to indicate where more in-depth (process-of-care) measurement is warranted.

Several disadvantages are associated with outcome measurement, however. The focus on aggregate data rather than on individual or case-by-case analysis limits its usefulness in changing practice behavior for the individual practitioner. Review is by definition historical, that is, after care has been delivered; instant intervention in serious situations where immediate action is justified to prevent a potentially bad outcome is not possible. The lack of demonstrated relationships between outcomes and process of care for many aspects of the management of patients is a major barrier to reliance on outcome measurement for quality assurance programs.

Analytic complications arise when patients receive care from multiple sources, when they are lost to follow-up, when noncompliance is an issue, and when patients are unable to represent themselves. For chronic conditions in particular, outcome analysis might best be done on aggregate data over periods that reflect patterns of care; assigning accountability and responsibility for outcomes becomes more complex in the absence of clear points of entry and exit to the health care system. Outcome measurement is limited by the fact that outcomes are not routinely or uniformly recorded, especially when those data are not needed for reimbursement purposes. Finally, outcome measurement can incur high resource costs in time, manpower, and dollars, especially to overcome the problems caused by incomplete documentation of what transpired.

Within the traditional model, more effort has been directed toward quality assessment than quality assurance. Formal methods exist for completing the full cycle, using the information from the assessment to assure quality. No single assurance system, however, parallels the structure, process, and outcome framework.

Continuous Quality Improvement

Within the last five years or so, a model of quality improvement that had its start in the manufacturing field has begun to be applied in the health field. It goes by various names, including "quality improvement process," "total quality management," "organization-wide quality improvement" (called Total Quality Control in Japan), and similar phrases; "continuous improvement" may be the most universally recognized term (Batalden and Buchanan, 1989; Berwick, 1989). The philosophic and technical basis for this model evolved from a set of management and statistical control methods pioneered decades ago by U.S. statisticians and engineers (but implemented chiefly by post-World War II Japanese industrialists) for application in industry, primarily manufacturing (Deming, 1986; Walton, 1986; Garvin, 1986, 1988; Juran et al., 1988). These concepts, as translated for health care delivery, are described below.

Four Core Assumptions

First, people involved in delivering health care work mainly in organizations; therefore, quality improvement uses the energy and lines of accountability of an organization for improvement. To do so, top leadership must be committed to quality improvement. Second, health care workers—administrators, physicians and other professionals, paraprofessionals, and support staff—wish to perform to the best of their capacity. Third, when workers cannot attain their best performance, wasteful, needlessly complex, and undependable systems or organizational methods of work are often to blame. Fourth, the interaction of individuals and the organizations and systems within which they practice can always improve.

Eight Key Constructs

First, the emphasis is on external customers or recipients of care. All that is done is done for the benefit of the patient.

Second, all that precedes the benefit to the patient—for example, facilities, equipment, providers, support staff, and organizational policies—must be involved in a relentless, systematic, and cooperative effort to improve care. The continuous improvement model calls on all involved parties to participate in quality monitoring and to shift the quality curve upward rather than just eliminate the outliers. Continuous improvement, by its very name, assumes that there is no permanent threshold to good performance; in health care, it implies that health professionals and the settings in which they practice should never be content with present performance.

Third, as illustrated in Figure 2.1, activities are cyclic, involving continuous "planning, doing, checking, and acting" (PDCA). One expert has described the PDCA cycle as the "democratization of the scientific method," making it possible for all to participate in the application of these methods to daily work (Paul Batalden, citing George Box, personal communication, 1989). In health care, this implies attention to processes of care that are responsive to patients' needs. It recognizes that the only way to improve outcomes is to work on what produced them.

Fourth, it views the work of individuals and departments within health care organizations as interconnected. One supplies "work products" to others; one also receives from others. As such, people and departments serve as their own internal "suppliers" and "customers," and their interconnected activities are intended to benefit the external customer. Patients may be the key external customers but, for example, subspecialty physicians may be

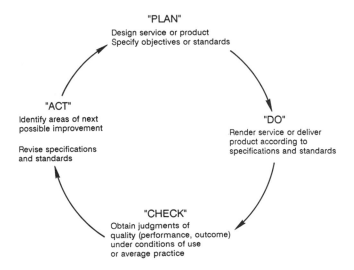

FIGURE 2.1 A Simplified Diagram of the Continuous Improvement Model for Both Internal and External Customers

customers of primary care physicians, and pharmacy staff may be suppliers for nursing staff. In short, "I am a supplier for people who depend on what I do, and I am a customer when I depend on what others in the organization do" (Donald Berwick, personal communication, 1988).

Fifth, it places considerable emphasis on systems or "processes" as the way care gets delivered (Paul Batalden, personal communication, 1989). (See the flow diagram in Figure 2.2.) Suppliers provide inputs that are transformed by a series of actions into outputs. These are received by customers who have needs, expectations, and values by which they judge outcomes, that is, ascribe benefit to that output.[6] Organizations such as hospitals or physician offices are viewed as large networks of interrelated processes with thousands of internal customer-supplier relationships. Constant improvement of every production process by everyone involved is the central focus. In this view, every health worker has two roles: first, doing his or her job and, second, improving the job.

Sixth, improvement occurs by integrating the voices of customers and of processes of care into the cyclical redesign of service and care (Figure 2.1). Both the customer and those serving the customer must contribute to information gathering—the former through surveys, complaint procedures, and similar channels (often external to the organization) and the latter through continual internal monitoring of procedures, resource use, and patient care.

Seventh, active, visible commitment of the highest leadership of the organization is necessary. Because this view holds that the major impediment to improving quality is found in the way people and organizations work together, engagement in quality improvement must permeate an organization, starting at the top.

Eighth, the continuous improvement approach uses a set of practical

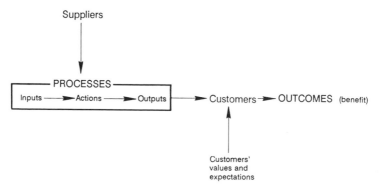

FIGURE 2.2   Flow Diagram of the Process-Outcome Relationship in the Continuous Improvement Model

techniques that facilitate learning and action. These tools (e.g., flow charts, fishbone diagrams, and run charts) have been adapted from the decades of organization-wide efforts at quality control in industry and are intended for use by people at all levels of the organization. All can be used to identify and analyze the various processes of health care delivery and to monitor the effectiveness of quality improvement interventions in organizations.

Applications

Outside the health field, the industries represented by companies that have implemented various quality control programs using this model vary widely: automobile manufacturers, public utilities, communications, and consumer products. In 1987, Congress established the Malcolm Baldrige National Quality Award (P.L. 100-107), which is patterned after the prestigious Deming prize awarded in Japan since 1951.[7] Its aim is to encourage quality accomplishments and excellence in U.S. manufacturing and service companies and small businesses by awarding a prize to companies that pass a rigorous examination of their quality measurement program and demonstrable accomplishments.[8]

As the continuous improvement model is increasingly being diffused in the nonhealth sectors of the U.S. economy, its appeal to the health care community is spreading.[9] For instance, the Joint Commission's Agenda for Change (Joint Commission, 1988; Jurkiewicz, 1988) has adopted a new set of "Principles of Organization and Management Effectiveness" that strongly emphasizes total organizational commitment to the continuous improvement of the quality of patient care.[10] Several hospitals and hospital chains have already implemented various forms of quality improvement activities. For instance, West Paces Ferry, a hospital owned by the Hospital Corporation of America, has embarked on a quality improvement plan (National Demonstration Project, 1989); the hospital has focused specifically on "improving the mean rather than only policing some lower margin of acceptable performance" (Chip Caldwell, personal communication, 1989).[11]

Quality Assurance Concepts from an International Perspective

The commitee sought information on international aspects of quality assurance for the purpose of learning whether concepts and methods in other countries might be helpful to the United States. In preparing this brief discussion we draw on a paper prepared for the study (Reerink, 1989).

After analyzing the efforts of several countries Reerink concludes that the United States is the front runner in the field of quality assurance. In a great majority of countries, the Netherlands being a notable exception, quality assurance is viewed with disdain or mistrust. By comparison, in the

United States quality assurance in health care is studied and implemented with considerable intensity. Some countries have followed the U.S. example and developed (or are in the process of developing) their quality assurance programs on the traditional structure-process-outcome model. In a few countries (e.g., the Netherlands and Malaysia), performance indicators and health accounting are dominant elements of the quality assurance programs. Reerink reports that the most important facets of quality assurance in countries he studied are the dominant role taken by health professions in establishing quality assurance systems and the widely held perception of the necessity of health professional leadership for successful quality assurance programs.

TRADITIONAL AND CONTINUOUS IMPROVEMENT MODELS COMPARED

Several aspects of the continuous improvement model resemble those of contemporary systems of quality assurance or performance monitoring described a decade or more ago for the health care field. These systems include the bi-cycle concepts of Brown and Uhl (1970) and the health accounting approach of Williamson[12] (1978, 1988), both of which have cycles quite analogous to the planning-doing-checking-acting (PDCA) approach. Moreover, both approaches incorporate notions of structure (e.g., organizational factors and high-level accountability), process (e.g., patient care activities), and outcomes (e.g., patient well-being or satisfaction). For instance, both the traditional and the continuous improvement models of quality assurance stress the importance of outcomes (or achievable benefit); Williamson's health accounting approach, for instance, starts with achievable benefit not being achieved and works back to the process of care. The main distinction is that the latter more explicitly involves patient (i.e., customer) values as a critical element of outcomes. Both approaches also acknowledge the importance of information that links processes to outcome. Thus, in many ways the continuous improvement approach is consistent with traditional notions of quality assurance.

The two concepts depart from each other mainly in five ways. The continuous improvement model, first of all, emphasizes continual efforts to improve performance and value even when high performance standards appear to be met. In the latter case, traditional quality assurance activities would cease or shift attention elsewhere. Second, continuous improvement stresses the evaluation of simple and complex systems from the perspectives of the customers. This has the effect, among other things, of directing attention to the way people and departments in organizations work together and, thus, to sources of variation and multidisciplinary quality-of-care issues that traditional quality assurance approaches might not detect or target for change.

Third, it emphasizes understanding the views of patients and other customers about the care process and their outcomes. This tends to draw more attention to patient satisfaction than has been heretofore the case.

Fourth, the continuous improvement model is designed to improve the overall (or average) performance of individuals and the organization more than to remove outliers. That is, poor practitioners or institutions are not the target. Finally, although both approaches would place the accountability for quality high in the organization's leadership, the continuous improvement model explicitly vests ultimate responsibility for quality and quality improvement at the very top of the management structure while still emphasizing the personal responsibility of all members to contribute to quality improvement.

In contrast to traditional quality assurance, however, the utility of the continuous improvement model in dealing with clinical problems encountered in ordinary medical practice is yet to be learned. For instance, its applicability to problems of poor physician decision making in choosing diagnostic or therapeutic modalities is unproven, and its ability to deal with issues of overuse or underuse remains to be shown. Most of the health applications to date have targeted organizational processes and customer or patient satisfaction. Whether health care institutions and facilities can successfully implement the continuous improvement approach with a focus on meaningful medical, nursing, and other professional quality-of-care issues will have to be tested rigorously over the next few years.

Earlier in this chapter we identified 15 attributes of quality assurance programs. How do the two models reviewed in this chapter—the traditional and the continuous improvement models—stand when judged against these criteria?

Both approaches doubtless have the ability to address overuse, underuse, and poor technical and interpersonal quality, to minimize intrusion into the patient-provider relationship, to deal with outlier practice and performance, and to provide practitioners and providers with timely information to improve performance, although they would do so with varying degrees of success. For health care, neither the traditional nor the continuous improvement approach can be proven, at the moment, to be especially rigorous scientifically, to have a consistently positive impact on patient outcomes, to document improvements in quality and progress toward excellence, to be easy to implement or administer, or to be affordable or cost-effective.

The traditional approaches appear valid and are acceptable to professionals and providers, at least for internal programs. They are more suitable for non-organization-based practitioners (such as independent, fee-for-service practitioners) and for population-based outcomes of care. The continuous improvement approach more explicitly includes patients and the public, fosters improvement throughout the health care organization and system, attempts to use the scientific method, and applies both positive and negative incentives for change and improvement in performance.

SUMMARY

This review and comparison of the traditional and continuous improvement models for quality assurance sets forth concepts and terms used throughout the report. The two models are also judged against 15 attributes the committee identified as desirable for a quality assurance program.

The lesson is that no single approach or conceptual framework is likely either to suit our purposes or to meet the criteria we have identified for an effective quality assurance program. The study committee had widely divergent views on the benefits of the continuous improvement model given the limited knowledge about its application to clinical problems and settings of care outside the hospital; the lack of consensus on the committee about a "best" approach to quality assurance and quality improvement is a microcosm of the larger debate in the health care community on concepts and models of quality assurance.

The continuous improvement model has already had a considerable impact on the quality assurance field. The committee's debate underscored the need for flexibility and innovation in the Medicare quality assurance program over the coming decade. Caution was taken to avoid locking the Medicare program into, on the one hand, an older, familiar conceptual model or, on the other, a very appealing yet unproven new system. Rather, we draw on all the elements of these approaches to fashion a program for quality assurance in Medicare (Chapter 12) that we believe will foster improvement in the quality of health care as it was defined in Chapter 1.

NOTES

1. The quality-of-care literature is enormous. The few historical overviews of quality assurance programs include: Egdahl, 1973; Williamson, 1977, 1988; Williams and Brook, 1978; Lohr and Brook, 1984; and Donabedian, 1989.
2. The mechanics of quality assurance may be tailored to specific categories of quality problems or to given settings, such as efforts designed to address problems of underuse of outpatient or inpatient care in a health maintenance organization (HMO) or those intended to improve nursing aide care in a home health agency. Chapters 7, 8, and 9 discuss these points at greater length; examples of methods are found in Volume II, Chapter 6.
3. The term outliers typically refers to clinicians or institutions that render seriously substandard or unorthodox care. A rough rule of thumb might be that it refers to the worst 1 percent or 5 percent of providers on a quality measure, although it can be defined in strictly statistical terms.

4. Outcome measurements are not new. One of the earliest documented efforts to monitor outcomes is that conducted by the surgeon Ernest A. Codman in the early 1900s. Codman's approach, known as the "end result system," included a retrospective review of the outcomes of each of his surgery patients one year following the operation (Brook et al., 1976; Nash and Goldfield, 1989).

5. The literature on the assessment of health status and quality of life is very large. For recent overviews of this field, see Bergner, 1985; Bergner and Rothman, 1987; Katz, 1987; Lohr and Ware, 1987; Lohr, 1989; Greenfield, 1989; Kane and Kane, 1989; Mosteller and Falotico-Taylor, 1989; and Sabatino, 1989. Avery et al., 1976 and Brook et al., 1976 provide landmark overviews of quality assessment using outcome measures.

6. These uses of the terms process and outcomes are not the same as in the familiar triad of structure, process, and outcome, but they are not in conflict. For example, as depicted in Figure 2.2, this use of outcome includes the value set of the customer or recipient of the output of the process. Process includes inputs (which in turn may include structural elements), actions (which may be conditioned by structural factors), and technical outputs.

7. In 1989, Florida Power & Light Co. became the first non-Japanese company to win Japan's Deming award.

8. Several firms participated in the 1988 and 1989 competition rounds. In 1988 awards were given to Westinghouse Electric Corporation's Commercial Nuclear Fuel Division; Motorola, Inc.; and Globe Metallurgical, Inc. The 1989 awards went to Milliken & Company and Xerox Corporation's Business Products and Systems.

9. Several firms participated in an innovative project begun in 1987—the National Demonstration Project on Industrial Quality Control and Health Care Quality—designed to permit high-ranking quality assurance professionals to collaborate on ways to improve the state of health care quality assurance (National Demonstration Project, 1989). The current phase of this project involves a series of courses on quality improvement and studies of clinical and administrative problems tackled through continuous improvement techniques (Donald Berwick, personal communication).

10. The new principles will be elaborated in standards for accreditation of health care providers. They are intended to encourage organizations to weave continuous improvement attitudes and methods throughout the organization, specifically in strategic planning, allocation of resources, role expectations, reward structures, performance evaluations, and the role of the organization in the community. To elaborate these principles, the Joint Commission also appointed a Task Force charged to develop principles for continuous improvement; its work will continue into 1990.

11. One technique the West Paces Ferry program stresses is "benchmarking," which Camp (1989a, 1989b) defines as a process "for uncovering . . . best industry practices . . . ." Camp argues for seeking best practices wherever they might exist (e.g., levels of performance attainable in another setting or industry).

12. The system supported by CBO, the National Organization for Quality Assurance in Hospitals in the Netherlands, incorporates many elements common to Williamson's health accounting approach (Reerink, 1989).

REFERENCES

Avery, A.D., Lelah, T., Solomon, N.E., et al. *Quality of Medical Care Assessment Using Outcome Measures: Eight Disease-Specific Applications.* R-2021/2-HEW. Santa Monica, Calif.: The RAND Corporation, August 1976.

Batalden, P.B. and Buchanan, E.D. Industrial Models of Quality Improvement. Pp. 133-159 in *Providing Quality Care: The Challenge to Clinicians.* Goldfield, N. and Nash, D.B., eds. Philadelphia, Pa.: American College of Physicians, 1989.

Bergner, M. Measurement of Health Status. *Medical Care* 23:696-704, 1985.

Bergner, M. and Rothman, M.L. Health Status Measures: An Overview and Guide for Selection. *Annual Review of Public Health* 8:191-210, 1987.

Berwick, D.M. Sounding Board. Continuous Improvement as an Ideal in Health Care. *New England Journal of Medicine* 320:53-56, 1989.

Brook, R.H., Avery, A.D., Greenfield, S., et al. *Quality of Medical Care Assessment Using Outcome Measures: An Overview of the Method.* R-2021/1-HEW. Santa Monica, Calif.: The RAND Corporation, August 1976.

Brown, C.R., Jr. and Uhl, H.S.M. Mandatory Medical Education: Sense or Nonsense? *Journal of the American Medical Association* 213:1660-1668, 1970.

Camp, R.C. Benchmarking: The Search for Industry Best Practices That Lead to Superior Performance. Part III. Why Benchmark? *Quality Progress* 22:76-82, March 1989a.

Camp, R.C. Benchmarking: The Search for Industry Best Practices That Lead to Superior Performance. Part IV. What to Benchmark. *Quality Progress* 22:62-69, April 1989b.

Deming, W.E. *Out of the Crisis.* Cambridge, Mass.: Massachusetts Institute of Technology Press, 1986.

Donabedian, A. Evaluating the Quality of Medical Care. *Milbank Memorial Fund Quarterly* 44:166-203, July (part 2) 1966.

Donabedian, A. *Explorations in Quality Assessment and Monitoring.* Volumes I-III. Ann Arbor, Mich.: Health Administration Press, 1980, 1982, 1984.

Donabedian, A. Quality Assessment and Assurance: Unity of Purpose, Diversity of Means. *Inquiry* 25:173-192, 1988a.

Donabedian, A. The Quality of Care. How Can it be Assessed? *Journal of the American Medical Association* 260:1743-1748, 1988b.

Donabedian, A. Monitoring: The Eyes and Ears of Healthcare. *Health Progress,* 69:38-43, November 1988c.

Donabedian, A. Reflections on the Effectiveness of Quality Assurance. Paper prepared for the Institute of Medicine Study to Design a Strategy for Quality Review and Assurance in Medicare, 1989.

Egdahl, R.H. Foundations for Medical Care. *New England Journal of Medicine* 288:491-498, 1973.

Elinson, J., quoting himself in Donabedian, A., et al. Advances in Health Assessment Conference Discussion Panel. *Journal of Chronic Diseases* 40(Supplement 1):183S-191S, 1987.

Ellwood, P. Outcomes Management. A Technology of Patient Experience. *New England Journal of Medicine* 318:1549-1556, 1988.

Garvin, D.A. A Note on Quality: The Views of Deming, Juran, and Crosby. *Harvard Business School Note* Publication No. 9-687-011. Cambridge, Mass.: Harvard College, 1986.

Garvin, D.A. *Managing Quality. The Strategic and Competitive Edge.* New York, N.Y.: The Free Press, A Division of Macmillan, 1988.

Greenfield, S. The State of Outcome Research: Are We on Target? *New England Journal of Medicine* 320:1142-1143, 1989.

Joint Commission (Joint Commission on Accreditation of Healthcare Organizations). Agenda for Change. *Update* 1:1,6, 1987.

Joint Commission. Agenda for Change. *Update* 2:1,5, 1988.

Juran, J.M., Gyrna, F.M., Jr., and Bingham, R.S., Jr. *Quality Control Handbook.* Fourth edition. Manchester, Mo.: McGraw-Hill, 1988.

Jurkiewicz, M.J. Spectrum 1988. The Joint Commission and the Agenda for Change. *American College of Surgeons Bulletin* 73:20-25, 1988.

Kane, R.A. and Kane, R.L. Long-Term Care: Variations on a Quality Assurance Theme. *Inquiry* 25:132-146, 1988.

Kane, R.A. and Kane, R.L. Reflections on Quality Control. *Generations* 13:63-68, Winter 1989.

Katz, S., guest ed. The Portugal Conference: Measuring Quality of Life and Functional Status in Clinical and Epidemiological Research. *Journal of Chronic Diseases* 40:459-650, 1987.

Lohr, K.N. Outcome Measurement: Concepts and Questions. *Inquiry* 25:37-50, 1988.

Lohr, K.N., guest ed. Advances in Health Status Assessment: Conference Proceedings. *Medical Care* (Supplement) 27:S1-S294, March 1989.

Lohr, K.N. and Brook, R.H. Quality Assurance in Medicine. *American Behavioral Scientist* 27:583-607, 1984.

Lohr, K.N. and Ware, J.E., Jr., guest eds. Proceedings of the Advances in Health Assessment Conference. *Journal of Chronic Diseases* 40:1S-193S, (Supplement 1) 1987.

Lohr, K.N., Yordy, K.D., and Thier, S.O. Current Issues in Quality of Care. *Health Affairs* 7:5-18, Spring 1988.

Mosteller, F. and Falotico-Taylor, J., eds. *Quality of Life and Technology Assessment.* Monograph of the Council on Health Care Technology. Washington, D.C.: National Academy Press, 1989.

Nash, D.B. and Goldfield, N. Information Needs of Purchasers. Pp. 5-24 in *Providing Quality Care: The Challenge to Clinicians.* Goldfield, N. and Nash, D.B., eds. Philadelphia, Pa.: American College of Physicians, 1989.

National Demonstration Project on Quality Improvement in Health Care. *Quality Improvement in Health Care.* A Newsletter. Boston, Mass.: Harvard Community Health Plan. Premiere Issue, 1989.

O'Leary, D. Quality Assessment: Moving from Theory to Practice. *Journal of the American Medical Society* 260:1760, 1988.

Palmer, R.H. The Challenges and Prospects for Quality Assessment and Assurance in Ambulatory Care. *Inquiry* 25:119-131, 1988.

Reerink, E. Study on International Aspects of Quality Assurance. Paper prepared for the Institute of Medicine Study to Design a Strategy for Quality Review and Assurance in Medicare, 1989.

Roberts, J. S. Quality Assurance in Hospitals: From Process to Outcomes. Pp. 48-62 in *Quality of Care and Technology Assessment.* Lohr, K.N. and Rettig, R.A., eds. Report of a Forum of the Council on Health Care Technology. Washington, D.C.: National Academy Press, 1988.

Sabatino, C. Homecare Quality. *Generations* 13:12-16, Winter 1989.

Walton, M. *The Deming Management Method.* New York, N.Y.: Dodd, Mead & Company, 1986.

Weiss, C.H. *Evaluation Research.* Englewood Cliffs, N.J.: Prentice Hall, 1972.

Williams, K.N. and Brook, R.H. Quality Measurement and Assurance: A Literature Review. *Health & Medical Care Services Review* 3:1, 3-15, May/June 1978.

Williamson, J.W. *Improving Medical Practice and Health Care: A Bibliographic Guide to Information Management in Quality Assurance and Continuing Education.* Cambridge, Mass.: Ballinger, 1977.

Williamson, J.W. *Assessing and Improving Outcomes in Health Care: The Theory and Practice of Health Accounting.* Cambridge, Mass.: Ballinger, 1978.

Williamson, J.W. Future Policy Directions for Quality Assurance: Lessons from the Health Accounting Experience. *Inquiry* 25:67-77, 1988.

3

The Elderly Population

This chapter reviews key descriptors of the elderly population. It documents their continued growth and aging, thus highlighting the demands for health care by this population. It also underscores the complexities of providing that care, given the special challenges faced by the elderly such as multiple chronic illnesses and inadequate means for maintaining many older persons in independent-living situations.

SIZE AND GROWTH OF THE ELDERLY POPULATION

Traditionally, the "elderly" are considered to be those persons age 65 and older. By that definition, in 1987 there were just over 30 million elderly people in the United States, more than 12 percent of the total U.S. population of nearly 252 million (Table 3.1). This group makes up the vast majority, almost 96 percent, of Medicare recipients.[1]

The rate of growth of the elderly segment of the U.S. population has been much more rapid than the rate of growth in the overall population, a phenomenon often referred to as "the graying of America." Data from the National Center for Health Statistics (NCHS) indicate that, from 1960 to 1986, the population age 65 and older increased by 75 percent, from almost 17 million people to over 29 million people, while the population under 65 increased only 30 percent (NCHS, 1989). Among those over age 65 in 1986, about three-fifths were between age 65 and 74; about one-third were 75 to 84, and one-tenth were 85 and older. The rate of growth of the subgroups of the elderly population between 1960 and 1986 was substantially higher for the older age groups (i.e., 75 to 84 and 85 and older) than for the 65 to 74 age group.

Between 1987 and 2030, the total U.S. population is projected to in-

TABLE 3.1 Number and Percentage Distributions of the Population, by Age: United States, Selected Calendar Years 1987-2030

Age	1987	2000	2010	2020	2030
Population in millions[a]					
Under 20 years	73.4	75.9	73.8	74.2	74.4
20-64 years	148.1	165.8	179.6	180.6	175.9
65 years or over	30.2	35.6	40.0	52.8	66.5
65-69 years	9.8	9.6	12.2	17.6	19.0
70-74 years	7.8	8.9	9.1	13.8	17.3
75-79 years	5.8	7.4	7.1	9.2	13.3
80-84 years	3.7	5.1	5.6	5.8	9.0
85 years or over	3.0	4.6	6.0	6.5	7.9
Total	251.8	277.3	93.4	307.7	316.8
Percent distribution of total population					
Under 20 years	29.2	27.4	25.2	24.1	23.5
20-64 years	58.8	59.8	61.2	58.7	55.5
65 years or over	12.0	12.8	13.6	17.2	21.0
65-69 years	3.9	3.5	4.2	5.7	6.0
70-74 years	3.1	3.5	4.2	5.7	6.0
75-79 years	2.3	2.7	2.4	3.0	4.2
80-84 years	1.5	1.8	1.9	1.9	2.8
85 years or over	1.2	1.7	2.0	2.1	2.5
Total	100.0	100.0	100.0	100.0	100.0
Percent distribution of aged population					
65-69 years	32.5	27.0	30.5	33.3	28.6
70-74 years	25.8	25.0	22.7	26.1	26.0
75-79 years	19.2	20.8	17.8	17.4	20.0
80-84 years	12.3	14.3	14.0	11.0	13.5
85 years or over	9.9	12.9	15.0	12.3	11.9
Total	100.0	100.0	100.0	100.0	100.0

[a]Social Security area populations as of July 1.

NOTES: Social Security Administration data were used for this table. Population growth is taken from the intermediate (II-B) assumptions used to prepare the 1989 Annual Report of the Board of Trustees of the Federal Old-Age and Survivors Insurance and Disability Insurance Trust Fund. Columns may not sum to totals and percentages may not sum to 100.0 due to rounding.

SOURCE: Waldo et al., 1989.

crease by 26 percent from 252 million to 317 million, while the population age 65 and older is expected to increase by more than 100 percent from the present 12 percent of the total population to nearly 21 percent of the total population (67 million) (Waldo et al., 1989).

SOCIODEMOGRAPHIC CHARACTERISTICS

Sex Ratios in the Elderly Population

The ratio of males to females varies dramatically with age. For example, in 1986, for every 100 males under age 20, there were 96 females—a ratio of nearly 1:1. In the same year, the male to female ratio for persons over age 65 was almost 1:1.5, and the ratio just for those 85 and older was 1:2.5, highlighting the numerical predominance of women over men in these older age ranges (Special Committee on Aging, 1987-1988).

Race and Ethnicity of the Elderly Population

Table 3.2 summarizes information on the population by age and ethnic group (white, black, and hispanic). In 1986, about 89 percent of the elderly and about 80 percent of the nonelderly were white. The white population has a higher proportion of elderly than do other ethnic groups (13 percent versus 8 and 5 percent for black and hispanic populations, respectively) and a higher proportion of the older old (i.e., those 75 years and older). The proportion of the elderly population who are minority is expected to grow considerably over the next decade (Special Committee on Aging, 1987-1988).

Elderly Support Ratios

The elderly support ratio is defined as the ratio of persons age 65 and older to persons of working age, between 18 and 64 years old. Owing to higher life expectancy and smaller families, the ratio of elderly to working-age persons is increasing dramatically. In 1900, there were about 7 elderly persons for every 100 working-age persons; in 1986 the ratio was about 20 per 100. This ratio is projected to increase to 37 elderly per 100 working-age persons by the year 2030 (Special Committee on Aging, 1987-1988). The elderly support ratio is important in economic terms because the working population can be thought of as supporting the nonworking age groups, although the rise in retirement age might mitigate the economic effects somewhat.

TABLE 3.2 Population by Age and Race: 1986

Age	White Number[a]	Percent[b]		Black Number[a]	Percent[b]		Hispanic Number[a]	Percent[b]	
0-54	158,733	79	(78)	24,926	12	(85)	16,532	8	(89)
55-64	19,641	86	(10)	2,106	9	(7)	1,060	6	(6)
Total									
nonelderly	178,374	80	(87)	27,032	9	(92)	17,592	5	(95)
65-74	15,529	88	(8)	1,491	8	(5)	572	3	(3)
75-84	8,220	89	(4)	691	7	(2)	333[c]	3[c]	(2)[c]
85+	2,549	92	(1)	213	8	(1)			
Total									
elderly	26,298	89	(13)	2,395	8	(8)	905	3	(5)
Total	204,672	81	(100)	29,427	12	(100)	18,497	7	(100)

[a]Numbers are in thousands.

[b]Percentages are of the total in each age group. Percentages shown in parentheses are of the total in each racial and ethnic group. Percentages may not sum to 100 due to rounding.

[c]Data are for persons age 75+.

SOURCE: Special Committee on Aging, 1987-1988. (Data do not match precisely those in Table 3.1 because this table was based in part on unpublished estimates from the U.S. Bureau of the Census.)

Geographic Distribution of the Elderly Population

Almost half of the elderly in the United States live in eight states: Florida, Pennsylvania, New York, Ohio, Illinois, Michigan, California, and Texas. In the first four of these states, the percentage of the state's population that is elderly exceeds the national average of 12.1 percent (Table 3.3), with Florida having the highest concentration of persons over age 65. Other than Florida, many states with a large share of elderly are in areas where the high concentration arises more from out-migration of the young than from shifts in the residence of the elderly population.

Several areas of the country, most notably the Sunbelt, are experiencing an aging of their population because of the in-migration of older persons at retirement. According to data from the Census Bureau, of the 1.7 million Americans age 60 and older who moved out of state between 1975 and 1980, nearly 50 percent moved to Florida, California, Arizona, Texas, or New Jersey. Arizona, Texas, and Florida experienced increases of 215, 191 and 110 percent, respectively, in that same age group between 1960 and 1980 (Special Committee on Aging, 1987-1988).

Recent evidence of a trend called "counter-migration" indicates that a small number of older people who have moved to another state at retirement move back home where family members live. Findings from the Retirement Migration Project show that Florida lost a significant number of elderly migrants to states outside the Sunbelt, namely Michigan, New York, Ohio, and Pennsylvania, which are among the states that have a significant number of migrants to Florida (Special Committee on Aging, 1987-1988).

Living Arrangements for the Elderly

Community Residents

The Commonwealth Fund has recently supported a major Commission to examine issues relating to the elderly population. Special attention has been given to the 8.5 million elderly who live alone (Commonwealth Fund, 1987, 1988). The material cited below (unless otherwise noted) is taken from Commission publications available to date.

The vast majority of elderly (95 percent) live in the community. Of this group, 54 percent live with a spouse, almost 30 percent live alone, and the remaining 16 percent share a home with children, other relatives, or friends. Consistent with widowhood, the percentage of elderly living alone increases with age. For example, of persons age 65 to 74, approximately 24 percent

TABLE 3.3 Percentages of the Elderly Population in Selected States: 1986

State	Persons Age 65+ (thousands)	Persons Age 65+ as Percentage of State Population
Florida	2,071	17.7
Pennsylvania	1,736	14.6
New York	2,283	12.8
Ohio	1,320	12.3
Illinois	1,386	12.0
Michigan	1,039	11.4
California	2,848	10.6
Texas	1,583	9.5

SOURCE: Special Committee on Aging, 1987-1988.

live alone; the figures for those 75 to 84 and for those age 85 and older are 39 and 45 percent, respectively.

Women account for four-fifths of all elderly living alone. The proportion living alone is at least twice as high for women as for men in every age category. Since women have a longer life expectancy than men, widowhood is the reason that three of four women age 65 to 74, and four of five women age 75 and older, live alone. Hispanics are the least likely of the major ethnic groups (white, black, and hispanic) to live alone; 23 percent of elderly hispanics live alone compared to 30 percent of elderly whites and 33 percent of elderly black people.

Elderly persons who live alone are more likely to be poor or near-poor than those who live with others. Among the 8.5 million elderly living alone, 19 percent are poor and 24 percent are near-poor; among all elderly families, 12 percent are poor, 16 percent near-poor. Furthermore, for those who live alone, poverty rates increase with age.

Nursing Home Residents

Only about 5 percent of the elderly live in nursing homes at any given time, although one study estimates that the nursing home population will grow from 1.3 million to about 2 million by the year 2000 (5.7 percent of the elderly population) and to 4.4 million by 2040 (6.6 percent) (Manton and Liu, 1984). This 5-percent figure does not reflect flows into and out of nursing homes; a significant number of people enter nursing homes for recuperative care and leave shortly thereafter (Cohen et al., 1986).

Nearly half of nursing home residents are 85 years of age and older, three-quarters are female, and more than nine-tenths are white (Table 3.4). The proportion of each age group requiring nursing home care increases with age, from about 1 percent of those age 65 to 74 to 22 percent of those age 85 and older (NCHS, 1987a).

The risk of institutionalization after age 65 is widely debated, with recent estimates ranging from 36 percent to 65 percent (Special Committee on Aging, 1987-1988). Cohen et al. (1986), using data from more than 4,400 Medicare beneficiaries, have estimated the upper bound for the lifetime risk of entering a nursing home at age 65 to be approximately 43 percent. The risk of institutionalization increases with age until around age 80 and begins to decline at age 85. At every age, the lifetime risks for females is twice that of males (Cohen et al., 1986).

Health Insurance for the Elderly

Most Americans are automatically entitled, on reaching age 65, to health insurance benefits under the Medicare program. Today almost 96 percent

TABLE 3.4 Number and Percentage of Nursing Home Residents and Rate per 1,000 Population Age 65 and Older, By Age, Sex, and Race: 1985

Age, Sex and Race	Number of Nursing Home Residents	Percent Distribution	Number of Nursing Home Residents per 1,000 Population Age 65+ and Over
Age			
65-74 years	212,100	16.1	12.5
75-84 years	509,000	38.7	57.7
85 years and over	594,700	45.2	219.4
Sex			
Male	334,000	25.4	29.0
Female	981,900	74.6	57.7
Race			
White	1,224,900	93.1	47.6
Black	82,000	6.2	35.0
Other	8,900	0.7	20.1
All nursing home residents	1,315,800	100.0	46.1

SOURCE: NCHS, 1987a.

of the nation's elderly have Medicare coverage. Refer to Chapter 4 for a more thorough description of the Medicare program.

ECONOMICS OF AGING

Elderly Income

People age 65 and older have less income on average than those under age 65, and the disparity increases as the elderly grow older. For example, compared to persons age 65 to 69, the average income is 33 percent lower for persons age 75 to 84 and 36 percent lower for those age 85 and older (Special Committee on Aging, 1987-1988). In 1986, the median income of a family with an elderly head of the household was $19,932, whereas the median income for families with a nonelderly head of the household (age 25 to 64) was approximately $32,368 (Special Committee on Aging, 1987-1988). However, the true disparity between these figures may not be that great when differences in expenditure needs between elderly and nonelderly households are taken into account.

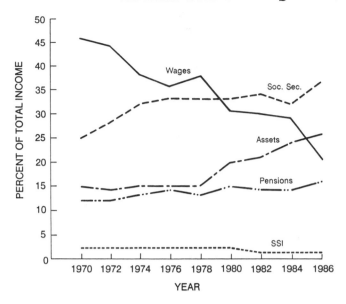

FIGURE 3.1 Composition of Income for Families with Head of Household Age 65+, 1970-1986

Composition of Income

The elderly rely more on Social Security than on any other source for their income, and Social Security is becoming an increasingly important component of income of the elderly while other sources are declining in importance (Figure 3.1). In 1986, 38 percent of income of the elderly came from Social Security; for 31 percent of the aged, Social Security represents at least 80 percent of their income.

Assets account for about 26 percent of the income of the elderly. Other sources of income of the elderly include wages (17 percent of total income), pensions (16 percent), and other sources (2 percent).

Trends in Elderly Income

Elderly incomes differ by sex, by marital status, and by race (Table 3.5). In 1986, the median income of elderly women was nearly 45 percent lower than the median income of elderly men. Although the greatest difference exists between married men and married women (where the household income can be considered to be a combination of the two), widowed males still report a median income nearly 25 percent greater than widowed females. White elderly have higher median incomes than their black and hispanic counterparts. In 1986, incomes for black elderly men and for

TABLE 3.5 Median Income of Persons Age 65 and Older by Demographic Characteristics and Sex: 1986

Demographic Characteristic	Both Sexes	Male	Female
Marital Status			
Married	$9,041	$12,265	$5,253
Single	$8,381	$8,867	$8,122
Widowed	$7,313	$9,258	$6,993
Divorced	$7,406	$7,826	$7,000
Race			
White	$8,544	$12,131	$6,738
Black	$5,030	$6,757	$4,508
Hispanic	$5,510	$7,369	$4,583
All 65+	$8,154	$11,544	$6,425

SOURCE: Special Committee on Aging, 1987-1988.

hispanic elderly men were 56 and 61 percent, respectively, of incomes for white males; the figures for elderly black and hispanic women show a similar pattern.

Although incomes of the elderly are lower than those of the nonelderly, they have been rising steadily. Between 1980 and 1984 income growth of the elderly population was higher than that of other subgroups of the population (Moon, 1988). After adjusting for family size and tax liability, the disposable income of the elderly is comparable to that of the adult population (age 18 to 64).

As a result of this growth in income, poverty rates among the elderly have been declining (Figure 3.2). In recent years, the average level of economic well-being of the elderly has improved substantially, and in general, the elderly appear to be as least as well off as the nonelderly (Hurd, 1989). However, the elderly population is not a homogenous group, and one needs to look beyond overall averages to understand the diversity in economic status of this population (CRS, 1988; Moon, 1988).

Gains have not been shared equally by all elderly. For instance, because of rising wages and increases in Social Security, individuals turning 65 (those just joining the ranks of the elderly) tend to have higher incomes, on average, than those already in the elderly category. Conversely, those who die each year tend to have lower incomes. Therefore, the average income level of the elderly increases as a function of demographic change.

Many elderly people are just above the poverty line. In 1986, the poverty line for a single elderly person was $5,255 and the near-poverty line, or

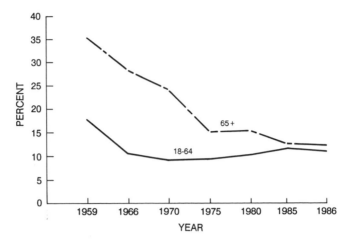

FIGURE 3.2   Percentages of the Adult Non-Elderly and Elderly Populations Below the Poverty Level, Selected Years

125 percent of the poverty threshold, was $6,569; for a couple, the values were $6,630 and $8,288. The data in Table 3.6 can be interpreted as showing that, in 1986, about one in eight elderly persons was at or below the poverty threshold, one in five was below 125 percent of that threshold, and just over one in three was below 150 percent. Although these are still large percentages, they are not as dramatic as the figures two decades earlier, when, for instance, one in four elderly persons was in poverty.

The poverty rate among the elderly would be higher than it is currently if the poverty standards for elderly and nonelderly persons were the same. In

TABLE 3.6   Percentages of the Elderly Below Selected Income Thresholds: Selected Years

	Percent of the Elderly Below		
Year	Poverty Threshold	125% of Poverty	150% of Poverty
1969	25.1	35.2	43.3
1975	15.3	25.4	34.9
1980	15.7	25.7	34.4
1983	14.1	22.5	30.2
1986	12.4	20.5	28.0

SOURCE: Special Committee on Aging, 1987-1988.

TABLE 3.7 Percentages of the Elderly Population with Annual
Incomes Below the Poverty Level by Sex and Age Group: 1986

	Age			
Sex	65-74	75-84	85+	Total 65+
Both Sexes	10.3	15.3	17.6	12.4
Male	7.0	10.7	13.3	8.5
Female	13.0	18.1	19.7	15.2

SOURCE: Special Committee on Aging, 1987-1988.

that case, the proportion of poor elderly would increase from about 13
percent to about 15.2 percent of the total elderly group. At that point, the
poverty rate would be higher for the elderly than for the overall population
(Villers Foundation, 1987).

Poverty rates are higher for elderly women than elderly men, especially
among the younger elderly (Table 3.7). In addition, poverty rates are higher
among minority elderly than white elderly.

USE OF THE HEALTH CARE SYSTEM

Hospital Services

Throughout the 1970s, the hospital discharge rate increased almost 12
percent for all age groups and nearly 23 percent among those persons age
65 and older. Conversely, during the same time period, average length of
stay declined, with the greatest declines among the elderly. The change in
utilization patterns during the 1970s has been attributed partially to implementation of the Medicare program and partially to advances in medical
technology (NCHS, 1987b).

After the implementation of the Medicare prospective payment system
(PPS), the hospital discharge rate for the U.S. population began to decline.
Data from the NCHS National Health Interview Survey suggest that the
drop experienced in the mid-1980s began to subside in 1987 (NCHS, 1988c).
Similarly, the decline in the average length of stay for the U.S. population
since PPS has also begun to level off (Table 3.8).

Physician Services

The number of physician contacts among the elderly population has increased significantly since the beginning of the Medicare program, owing in

part to the increased access to health care resulting from the program. Additionally, from 1983 to 1987 the average number of physician visits for persons age 65 and older increased 17 percent from 7.6 to 8.9 visits per person per year, owing in part to the implementation of PPS and the resulting emphasis on outpatient rather than inpatient care (Table 3.9).

The use of physician services increases with age. For example, in 1987, persons age 45 to 64 averaged 6.4 physician contacts a year, whereas persons age 65 and older averaged 8.9 physician contacts per year (Table 3.9). Within the elderly population, although those 85 and older consume 2 times more hospital care and 23 times more nursing home care than those age 65 to 74, the consumption of physician services is relatively even among the different age groups (Waldo et al., 1989).

Almost 75 percent of physician visits by the elderly are made to a doctor's office. The remaining visits are to hospital emergency rooms, outpatient offices, home and telephone consultations, and other places outside a hospital.

TABLE 3.8 Discharges, Days of Care, and Average Length of Stay in Nonfederal, Short-Stay Hospitals, Selected Age Groups: Selected Years

Age	1980	1982	1984	1986	1987
Discharges per 1,000 population					
65+	384	399	400	367	351
65-74	316	324	320	297	281
75+	489	511	520	470	452
All Ages	159	159	148	133	128
Days of care per 100,000 population					
65+	4,098	4,026	3,575	3,120	3,030
65-74	3,148	3,101	2,711	2,364	2,294
75+	5,577	5,424	4,856	4,228	4,098
All Ages	1,137	1,102	960	833	809
Average length of stay in days					
65+	10.7	10.1	8.9	8.5	8.6
65-74	10.0	9.6	8.5	8.0	8.2
75+	11.4	10.6	9.3	9.0	9.1
All Ages	7.1	7.0	6.5	6.3	6.3

SOURCE: NCHS, 1989.

TABLE 3.9 Physician Visits Per Person
by Age Group: 1983 and 1987

Age Group	Year	
	1983	1987
Under 15	4.6	4.5
15-44	4.4	4.6
45-64	5.8	6.4
65+	7.6	8.9
65-74	7.3	8.4
75+	8.2	9.7
All Ages	5.1	5.4

SOURCE: NCHS, 1989.

The aging of the population will affect the demand for physician care. That demand is expected to increase 22 percent by the year 2000 to 305 million contacts per year, and 125 percent by the year 2030 to 562 million contacts per year, based on 1986 physician contact rates and projections of the noninstitutionalized population (Special Committee on Aging, 1987-1988).

Long Term Care Services

Long term care refers to the array of medical, social, and support services for individuals in nursing homes or in the community who, for an extended period of time, depend on others for physical assistance (GAO, 1988). More than 11 million Americans were estimated to need some form of long term care in 1985. Of this group, approximately 6.5 million were elderly (or 23 percent of the total elderly population), 2 to 3 million were developmentally disabled or mentally retarded, and 1 to 2 million were partially or totally disabled due to chronic mental illness (Scanlon, 1988).

Nursing Home Care

Of the total elderly population needing long term care in 1985, approximately 20 percent resided in nursing homes and other institutions (GAO, 1988). Almost 40 percent lived in the community with their spouses. The other 40 percent were fairly evenly divided between those living with others and those living alone in the community.

The demand for nursing home care is increasing, although the lengths of stay, at least in skilled nursing facilities, are dropping (Gornick and Hall,

1988). This pattern reflects an increase in shorter stays and a decrease in longer stays.

From 1977 to 1987, aggregate nursing home expenditures increased from $13 billion to over $40 billion, an increase of 12.1 percent annually. Almost 90 percent of nursing home expenditures were for people age 65 and older (Waldo et al., 1989). Despite the large amounts of funding for nursing homes, growth in the number of beds has evidently not kept pace with the growth of the elderly population (Scanlon, 1988). This apparent discrepancy may, however, reflect a shift in the locus of care to other long-term-care settings, rather than a shortage of nursing home beds (Gornick and Hall, 1988; NCHS, 1988a).

Home Health Care

Although expenditures for home health benefits represented only about 3.6 percent of total Medicare outlays in 1986, they have been one of the fastest growing components of the program. The number of Medicare-certified home health agencies grew from slightly over 2,200 in 1972 to almost 6,000 in 1986 (Gornick and Hall, 1988). Home health services covered under Medicare include nursing care, physical, speech, and occupational therapy, home health aide services, and some medical supplies and equipment. There is no limit to the number of covered visits for beneficiaries confined to their homes (i.e., those people meeting the strict "homebound" requirements as defined by the Medicare program) and no prior hospitalization or cost-sharing requirements are imposed.

Between 1974 and 1986, Medicare reimbursements for home health care increased from $141 million to $1.8 billion (while total visit charges increased from $137 million to $2.1 billion in the same period), with an average annual growth rate of 24 percent (Ruther and Helbing, 1988). Following PPS implementation, the growth rate of home health expenditures and persons served has declined, as has the number of visits per person (Table 3.10). For example, from 1980 to 1983, the number of persons served increased at an average annual rate of 12.2 percent; however, the average annual rate of growth of persons served after 1983 was only 5.8 percent (Ruther and Helbing, 1988).

The slower rate of growth in the use of Medicare home health services since PPS may be the result of movement toward equilibrium following the growth spurt before PPS. For example, the percent of patients using covered home health services within 60 days of hospital discharge increased 55 percent from 1981 to 1983, but increased only 27 percent between 1983 and 1985 (Gornick and Hall, 1988). Further, the decline in short-stay hospital use among Medicare beneficiaries since PPS is often cited as a reason for the related decline in home health care, although the reduced lengths of

TABLE 3.10 Trends in Use and Costs of Home Health Agency Services
Under Medicare: Selected Years

Year	Number of Persons Served (thousands)	Number of Visits (thousands)	Visits per Person	Charges per Visit (dollars)	Total Visit Charges (dollars)	Total Medicare Reimbursement (thousands)
1974	393	8,070	21	$17	$ 37,406	$ 141,464
1976	589	13,335	23	22	292,697	289,851
1980	957	22,428	23	33	734,718	662,133
1983	1,351	36,844	27	43	1,596,989	1,398,092
1985	1,589	39,742	25	51	2,040,697	1,773,048
1986	1,600	38,359	24	55	2,102,253	1,795,820

SOURCE: Ruther and Helbing, 1988.

hospital stay following PPS should in theory have had the practical consequence of a greater need for home health services. Other factors in this
leveling may be a strict interpretation of the homebound provisions and an
inability of the home care market to expand sufficiently to meet the immediate demand.

A detailed examination of 1986 home health statistics (Table 3.11) shows
that service use increases with age, measured as visits per 1,000 enrollees;
visits per elderly person are about the same at every age (visits per nonelderly person are considerably higher than for elderly). The proportion of
females using home health services is 29 percent higher than that of males.

Community-Based Services

In 1985, 80 percent of the elderly who required assistance with activities
of daily living (ADLs) lived at home. Women outnumbered men 2 to 1 in
this population (GAO, 1988).

Formal community-based services help address the needs of persons with
activity limitations and include a broad range of health and social services
such as home health care, rehabilitation programs, homemaker and chore
services, personal care services, adult day care, and meals on wheels. Some
nursing home patients do not require the level of care provided in an institutional setting and could remain at home assuming that appropriate services
could be provided (Rice and Estes, 1984). Community-based services, therefore, are intended to help the elderly (among others) cope with independent
or community living, so as to improve the quality of individuals' lives and
forestall institutionalization.

TABLE 3.11 Home Health Agency Services Under Medicare: 1986

Age and Sex	Number of Persons Served (thousands)	Visits per 1,000 Enrollees	Visits per Person	Total Visit Charges (dollars)	Charges per Person (dollars)	Charges per Visit (dollars)
Age						
<65	102	982	28.6	$ 158,816	$1,562	$55
65-66	102	578	22.3	126,946	1,242	56
67-68	94	609	22.8	119,603	1,266	56
69-70	109	757	23.0	139,544	1,277	56
71-72	125	939	23.5	162,754	1,299	55
73-74	133	1,124	23.7	173,131	1,301	55
75-79	350	1,493	23.8	456,208	1,302	55
80-84	301	2,023	24.0	394,139	1,311	55
85+	283	2,352	24.3	371,112	1,310	54
Sex						
Male	579	1,011	23.4	745,178	1,286	55
Female	1,021	1,353	24.3	1,357,075	1,329	55
Total	1,600	1,182	24.0	2,102,253	1,308	55

SOURCE: Ruther and Helbing, 1988.

Most of these services are not covered by Medicare, and a significant number of noninstitutionalized individuals who need such services do not receive them. Of the dependent community-dwelling elderly in 1985, almost 74 percent received all of their care from informal care givers; only a small percentage relied exclusively on formal sources of care of the sort previously mentioned (Scanlon, 1988).

The Federal Government's Role in Support of the Elderly

As a result of legislative changes over the last several decades, federal spending has grown for income protection, health insurance, and other services designed to reduce high levels of poverty among the elderly. The focus of this spending has also shifted. According to the Special Committee on Aging (1987-1988), in 1960, less than 15 percent of the federal budget was spent on the elderly; 90 percent was for retirement income and 6 percent for health care. By contrast, in 1986 an estimated 26 percent of the federal budget (nearly $270 billion) went to programs in direct benefit to older Americans. Retirement income accounted for approximately 67 percent, and Medicare and Medicaid benefits accounted for nearly 27 percent of these monies. The federal government also spends money on general benefit programs through the Older Americans Act (social, nutritional, and employment services), the Social Services Block Grants, and research conducted through the National Institutes of Health.

HEALTH STATUS

Self-Assessment of Health Status

Contrary to stereotype, most older persons view their health in a positive manner. In 1987, almost 70 percent of elderly people living in the community described their health as excellent, very good, or good compared with others their own age (Figure 3.3); only about 30 percent reported their health as poor (NCHS, 1989).

Life Expectancy

The trends in life expectancy both at birth and at age 65 continue upward (Table 3.12). The greatest gains in life expectancy at birth occurred at the beginning of the century, owing to reductions in deaths from infectious disease and in infant and childhood mortality. Most of the increase in life expectancy in the later part of the century (since 1970) has come from decreased mortality from chronic conditions among the middle-aged and the elderly populations.

Life expectancy at birth differs by sex; in 1986, life expectancy for males was 71.4 and for females 78.6 (NCHS, forthcoming, Table 20). Since 1900, white females have had the highest life expectancy and black males have had the lowest (NCHS, 1989, Table 13). The probability of surviving

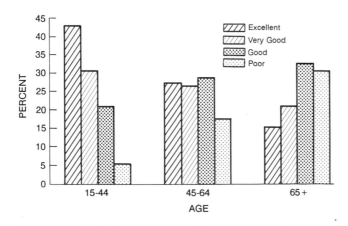

FIGURE 3.3   Self-Assessment of Health by Age Group, 1987

TABLE 3.12 Life Expectancy at Birth and Additional Years of Life Expectancy at Age 65, by Sex: Selected Years

Year	Male	Female
Life Expectancy at Birth		
1900	46.3	48.3
1950	65.6	71.1
1980	70.0	77.4
1985	71.2	78.2
1990	71.6	79.2
2000	72.9	80.5
2050	75.5	83.6
Additional Years of Life Expectancy at Age 65		
1900-1902	11.5	12.2
1950	12.8	15.0
1980	14.1	18.3
1985	14.6	18.6
1990	15.0	19.5
2000	15.7	20.5
2050	17.4	23.1

SOURCES: Special Committee on Aging, 1987-1988; NCHS, 1989.

to age 65 has increased substantially for all race-sex groups since 1900 (NCHS, 1988b).

Life expectancy at age 65 is more pertinent to the elderly population since it estimates additional years of life anticipated after entering the elderly population. Although the differences in life expectancy at age 65 by race are small, the differences by sex are large. According to NCHS (forthcoming, Table 20), life expectancy in 1986 at age 65 for males was 14.8 years and for females, 18.6 years. Males' life expectancy at age 65 ranks tenth among countries with at least one million population, and females share the rank of seventh.

Mortality

Age-specific death rates for the elderly have improved dramatically in the last several decades (Table 3.13), although the amount of improvement varies for individual age-race-sex groups. For example, declines in death rates have been more dramatic for those age 65 to 84 than for those age 85 and older. Additionally, decreases for older females are greater than those for older males.

The top ten causes of death in the United States have changed since 1900, the most striking change being the shift from infectious to noninfectious diseases. Today, heart disease, cancer, and cerebrovascular disease and stroke are the three leading causes of death for the elderly; two of three persons die of one of these conditions. The death rate from stroke has been decreasing over the past 30 years, probably owing to improved control of hypertension and better diagnosis, management, and rehabilitation of stroke

TABLE 3.13 Death Rates for All Causes per 100,000 Population, by Age, Race, and Sex: Selected Years

Age	1960	1970	1980	1986
All races				
55-64	1,735	1,659	1,346	1,255
65-74	3,822	3,583	2,995	2,801
75-84	8,745	8,004	6,693	6,348
85+	19,858	17,539	15,980	15,399
White male				
55-64	2,225	2,203	1,729	1,573
65-74	4,484	4,810	4,036	3,635
75-84	10,300	10,099	8,830	8,342
85+	21,750	20,393	19,097	18,576
White female				
55-64	1,079	1,015	876	853
65-74	2,780	2,471	2,067	2,032
75-84	7,697	6,699	5,402	5,109
85+	19,478	16,730	14,980	14,503
Black male				
55-64	3,316	3,257	2,873	2,546
65-74	5,799	5,803	5,131	4,790
75-84	8,605	9,455	9,232	9,291
85+	14,845	14,415	16,099	15,488
Black female				
55-64	2,511	1,986	1,561	1,470
65-74	4,064	3,861	3,057	2,892
75-84	6,730	6,692	6,212	6,149
85+	13,053	12,132	12,367	12,510

SOURCE: NCHS, 1989.

TABLE 3.14 Death Rates for Three Major Causes of Death per 100,000 Population: Selected Years

Age	1960	1970	1980	1986
Heart disease				
65-74	1,741	1,558	1,219	1,043
75-84	4,089	3,684	2,993	2,638
85+	9,318	8,468	7,777	7,179
All ages[a]	286	254	202	175
Malignant neoplasms				
65-74	714	754	818	847
75-84	1,127	1,168	1,232	1,287
85+	1,450	1,417	1,595	1,612
All ages[a]	126	130	133	133
Cerebrovascular disease				
65-74	469	384	220	164
75-84	1,491	1,254	789	574
85+	3,681	3,235	2,289	1,763
All ages[a]	80	66	41	31

[a]Rates are age-adjusted.

SOURCE: NCHS, 1989.

victims. The death rate from heart disease has also been decreasing over the last several decades, but the death rate from cancer has been increasing.

The greatest number of deaths still occur from heart disease, but deaths from cancer continue to rise relative to that number (Table 3.14). Eliminating deaths from heart disease would add an estimated five years of life expectancy at age 65 (NCHS, 1988c). By contrast, if cancer were eliminated as a cause of death, the average life span would be extended by less than two years.

Although many elderly experience declines in organ functioning and physiologic processes, this is not necessarily an inherent part of the aging process (Manton, 1986; Guralnik and Kaplan, 1989). Since the elderly have experienced improvements in life expectancy and declines in mortality, an important issue to consider is whether these declines in mortality are accompanied by similar declines in morbidity, resulting in an elderly population with improved health status and physical functioning.

Chronic Illness and Impairment

More than four of five older persons have at least one chronic condition, and many have several, although these conditions do not necessarily limit significant daily activities. The most prevalent chronic conditions (expressed in terms of morbidity from these conditions) in the elderly population include arthritis, hypertension, hearing impairments, and heart conditions (Table 3.15).

Older women experience chronic conditions (such as arthritis and osteoporosis) more frequently than men, and older men experience acute conditions (such as heart attacks) more often than women. In general, the health situation of elderly blacks is poorer than that of elderly whites.

Activity Limitations

Most elderly people do not need long-term-care assistance, but many suffer from some form of impairment that limits their ability to perform basic activities of daily living (ADLs) (Rowland et al., 1988). A broad set of ADLs includes eating, toileting, dressing, bathing, transferring, going outside, and walking; a "core set" of five ADLs includes all those except walking and going outside. ADLs categorize levels of functional impairment and thus have many health care planning, research, and policy purposes, such as increasing our understanding of the population at risk of institutionalization (or alternatively, in need of long-term-care services).

Functional impairment can be defined in many ways—ranging from difficulty with at least one ADL in the broad set (e.g., difficulty bathing) to

TABLE 3.15 Prevalence per 1,000 Population of Top Ten Chronic Conditions, by Age Group: 1986

Condition	All Ages	Age 45-64	Age 65+	Age 65-74	Age 75+
Arthritis	131	285	480	443	540
Hypertension	123	251	394	385	409
Sinusitis	145	187	169	169	171
Orthopedic impairment	115	162	173	158	196
Hearing impairment	88	136	296	244	378
Heart disease	78	123	277	250	319
Diabetes	28	64	98	92	109
Tinnitus	27	49	85	83	88
Visual impairment	35	46	95	69	136
Cataracts	21	21	141	84	233

SOURCE: NCHS, 1987c.

difficulty with two or more ADLS in the core set. Some experts also use "instrumental" ADLs (IADLs), which attempt to assess cognitive as well as physical impairment and thus include various home care management activities (e.g., using the telephone, managing finances, and taking medications).

Data from the 1984 National Health Interview Survey Supplement on Aging show that, of the population age 65 and older living in the community, 6 million (23 percent) had difficulty with one or more personal care ADLs inventoried (Table 3.16); this figure is expected to reach 7.3 million by the year 2000. Close to 1.2 million community residents had difficulty with three or more ADLs.

Walking was the most frequently reported limitation, affecting 4.9 million elderly (19 percent of the population surveyed). The severity of ADL limitations is associated with age (Table 3.16). Nevertheless, even at very high levels of impairment, a significant number of community residents with ADL limitations manifest long-term improvements in functioning (Manton, 1988).

Mental Health

Mental health problems of the elderly are significant in frequency and in their influence on the overall well-being of the individual. Between 15 and 25 percent of older persons have serious symptoms of mental disorders (Special Committee on Aging, 1987-1988), and the elderly make up a considerable fraction (well beyond their proportion in the population) of the institutionalized mentally ill. For example, among all state mental hospital patients, 27 percent are age 65 and older (Special Committee on Aging, 1987-1988).

Depression is the psychiatric illness that occurs most commonly in old age; it is more prevalent than all forms of dementia and psychosis (Frengley, 1987). Symptoms of depression have been described in as many as 15 percent of community residents (Special Committee on Aging, 1987-1988). This rate may be misleading, however, because it represents primary depression, or depression that occurs for reasons other than physical causes or drug side effects, rather than secondary depressions due to illness or drug side effects. The elderly are more at risk for secondary depressions than any other age group.

Alzheimer's disease is the leading cause of cognitive impairment in old age. Several studies have shown the prevalence of Alzheimer's disease in the older adult population to range from approximately 6 percent (Special Committee on Aging) to more than 10 percent (Evans et al., 1989). In addition, the prevalence rate is strongly associated with age. For example, one study of the prevalence of Alzheimer's disease in a noninstitutionalized

TABLE 3.16 Age and Sex Distribution of the Elderly Population by
Level of Impairment: 1984

| | | Percent Distribution | | | | |
| | | Age | | | Sex | |
Level of Impairment	Number (millions)	65-74	75-84	85+	Female	Male
One of Seven ADLs[a]	6.0	47	38	15	66	34
One Plus, Core ADLs[b]	3.7	44	38	18	68	32
Two Plus, Core ADLs[b]	2.0	42	37	21	67	33
Three Plus, Core ADLs[b]	1.2	39	39	22	68	32
Total elderly	26.4	62	31	75	9	41

[a]One or more activities of daily living (ADL) limitations based on seven ADLs (walking, getting outside, bathing, transferring, eating, toileting, and dressing).

[b]One, two, or three or more ADL limitations based on the core set (bathing, transferring, eating, toileting, and dressing).

SOURCE: Rowland et al., 1988.

community sample revealed that 3.0 percent of those age 65 to 74 had probable Alzheimer's disease compared with 18.7 percent of those age 75 to 84 (Evans et al., 1989).

Suicide is a more frequent cause of death among the elderly than any other age group (owing to the high suicide rate of older white men). In 1984, the suicide rate for white men age 65 and older was 41.6 deaths per 100,000 population, which was four times the national rate and six times the rate for white women age 65 and older (NCHS, 1988b).

SUMMARY

The United States will experience continued growth of the total population and the elderly population, especially among the oldest age groups. Between the years 2000 and 2040, the "baby boom" generation will turn 65, thus increasing the demands on the Medicare program and the long-term-care system.

The ratio of females to males in the elderly population will continue to rise. In addition, elderly women on average have a higher prevalence of limitations in activities of daily living, visit physicians more frequently, and are more predominant users of hospital and nursing home care than men. These trends have significant implications for demands on the Medicare program and the long-term-care system.

Because of increases in life expectancy and declining fertility rates, the ratio of elderly persons to working-age persons is increasing. This has significant economic implications, insofar as working-age persons support their own children, help support their own parents, provide for their own retirement (and health care), and provide the tax base for that portion of Medicare services covered by payroll taxes and general revenues (rather than those services covered by premiums). The increase in life expectancy also manifests changes in the social circumstances of our population. For instance, there are now four generations of persons, and informal caregivers are themselves older. With more women in the work force, the demand for professional long-term-care services rather than hands-on, informal support is higher. Together these two phenomena may move health care towards a more formalized system of care.

The incidence and prevalence of chronic illness increase with age, and chronic ailments are a major cause of disability requiring medical care. The new elderly population, however, may be healthier than previous cohorts of elderly because they will have experienced a lifetime of different and better medical care. These factors will have complex effects on future mortality rates, utilization of services, and health care expenditures.

Although the average level of economic well-being of the elderly has improved substantially over the past few decades, the incomes of the elderly are still less, on average, than those of the nonelderly. In addition, there are major disparities among subgroups of the elderly population with respect to economic well-being. These factors, too, will affect health, demand for care, and ability to pay for care out-of-pocket.

Health care expenditures for the elderly are expected to increase in the future, although at a slower rate than in the past. With respect to health services utilization, the hospital discharge rate and average length of stay are declining for the elderly population, while the use of physician and outpatient visits and other ambulatory services (such as outpatient surgery) is increasing. These shifts arise from several factors: the advent of PPS and the related incentives to hospitals for changes in behavior; cost containment initiatives fostering a movement from inpatient to outpatient care; expanding coverage for services rendered outside institutions; and the aging of the population.

These changes all increase the potential for overuse of certain services (e.g., procedures done in ambulatory settings) and underuse of other services (e.g., home health care), and they may have unpredictable effects on the technical quality of care.

The availability and adequacy of noninstitutional long-term, or post-acute, care is a specific concern. As the elderly population increases in both size and age, the need for noninstitutional services will be greater. Furthermore, since the beginning of PPS, length-of-stay reductions have been the greatest for patients 85 years of age and older, precisely those who may need outside assistance the most. In addition to the higher discharge acuity, death or institutionalization of a spouse prompts concern about post-acute care because many elderly will then live alone and be likely to face special care needs. Finally, other social and economic trends occurring simultaneously are sure to affect the demand for and supply of long-term-care services. Among these trends are a decrease in family size and an increase of women in the work force, both of which lower the pool of women available to provide informal health care services in the home setting.

In summary, continuing rapid increases in the size and the age of the elderly population are expected over the next several decades. By the year 2000, the elderly population will stand at nearly 35 million, of whom almost 18 million will be ages 65 to 74, 12 million ages 75 to 84, and 5 million ages 85 and older. Taking these factors into account and assuming that current demand for care and utilization patterns remain stable, a myriad of services including alternatives to inpatient care such as outpatient physician care and innovative approaches to long-term and home health care services, will need to increase to meet the needs of the elderly. These changes all have major implications for the quality of and access to needed health care over the coming decade and beyond.

NOTE

1. Patients with end-stage renal disease (ESRD) and disabled patients are the remaining 4 percent of the Medicare enrolled population.

REFERENCES

Cohen, M.A., Tell, E.J., and Wallack, S. The Lifetime Risks and Costs of Nursing Home Use Among the Elderly. *Medical Care* 24:1161-1172, 1986.

The Commonwealth Fund Commission on Elderly People Living Alone. *Old, Alone, and Poor.* Baltimore, Md.: The Commission, 1987.

The Commonwealth Fund Commission on Elderly People Living Alone. *Aging Alone: Profiles and Projections.* Baltimore, Md.: The Commission, 1988.

CRS (Congressional Research Service, U.S. Library of Congress). *Financing and Delivery of Long Term Care Services for the Elderly.* 88-379 EPW. Washington, D.C.: U.S. Government Printing Office, May 25, 1988.

Evans, D.A., Funkenstein, H.H., Albert, M.S., et al. Prevalence of Alzheimer's Disease in a Community of Older Persons: Higher Than Previously Reported. *Journal of the American Medical Association* 262:2551-2556, 1989.

Frengley, J.D. Depression. *Generations* 7(1):29-33, 1987.

GAO (General Accounting Office). *Long-Term Care for the Elderly: Issues of Need, Access, and Cost.* GAO/HRD-89-4. Washington, D.C.: General Accounting Office, November 28, 1988.

Gornick, M. and Hall, M.J. Trends in Medicare Use of Post-Hospital Care. *Health Care Financing Review* (Annual Supplement):27-38, 1988.

Guralnik, J.M. and Kaplan, G.A. Predictors of Healthy Aging: Prospective Evidence from the Alameda County Study. *American Journal of Public Health* 79:703-708, 1989.

Hurd, M. The Economic Status of the Elderly. *Science* 244:659-664, 1989.

Manton, K.G. Past and Future Life Expectancy Increases at Later Ages: Their Implications for the Linkage of Chronic Morbidity, Disability, and Mortality. *Journal of Gerontology* 41(5):672-681, 1986.

Manton, K.G. A Longitudinal Study of Functional Change and Mortality in the United States. *Journal of Gerontology* 43(5):163-61, 1988.

Manton, K. and Liu, K. The Future Growth of the Long-Term Care Population: Projections Based on the 1977 National Nursing Home Survey and the 1982 Long-Term Care Survey. Paper prepared for the Third National Leadership Conference on Long-Term Care Issues, Washington, D.C., 1984.

Moon, M. *Emerging Wealth and Continuing Hardship: The Ecomonic Consequences of Aging Differently.* Washington, D.C.: American Association of Retired Persons, 1988.

NCHS (National Center for Health Statistics). Use of Nursing Homes by the Elderly: Preliminary Data From the 1985 National Nursing Home Survey. *Advancedata.* No. 135. DHHS Publ. No. (PHS) 87-1250. Public Health Service. Hyattsville, Md.: National Center for Health Statistics, May 14, 1987a.

NCHS. Recent Declines in Hospitalization: United States, 1982-1986. Data From the Nation Hospital Interview Survey and the National Hospital Discharge Survey. *Advancedata.* No. 140. DHHS Publ. No. (PHS) 87-1250. Public Health Service. Hyattsville, Md.: National Center for Health Statistics, September 24, 1987b.

NCHS. Dawson, D.A., and Adams, P.F. *Current Estimates From the National Health Interview Survey, United States, 1986.* Vital and Health Statistics. Series 10, No. 164. DHHS Publ. No. (PHS) 87-1592. Public Health Service. Washington, D.C.: U.S. Government Printing Office, October 1987c.

NCHS. Nursing and Related Care Homes as Reported From the 1986 Inventory of Long-Term Care Places. *Advancedata.* No. 147. DHHS Publ. No. (PHS) 88-1250. Public Health Service. Hyattsville, Md.: National Center For Health Statistics, January 22, 1988a.

NCHS. *Health, United States, 1987.* DHHS Publ. No. (PHS) 88-1232. Public Health Service. Washington, D.C.: U.S. Government Printing Office, March 1988b.

NCHS. 1987 Summary: National Hospital Discharge Survey. *Advancedata.* No. 159 (Rev.). DHHS Publ. No. (PHS) 88-1250. Public Health Service. Hyattsville, Md.: National Center for Health Statistics, September 28, 1988c.

NCHS. *Health, United States, 1988.* DHHS Publ. No. (PHS) 89-1232. Public Health Service. Washington, D.C.: U.S. Government Printing Office, March 1989.

NCHS. *Health, United States, 1989.* Public Health Service. Washington, D.C.: U.S. Government Printing Office, forthcoming.

Rice, D.P. and Estes, C.L.   Health of the Elderly: Policy Issues and Challenges. *Health Affairs* 3(4):25-49, Winter 1984.

Rowland, D., Lyons, B., Neuman, P., et al.   Defining the Functionally Impaired Elderly Population.   Center for Hospital Finance.   Baltimore, Md.: The Department of Health Policy and Management, School of Hygiene and Public Health, The Johns Hopkins University.   Report prepared under a grant from the American Association of Retired Persons, 1988.

Ruther, M. and Helbing, C.   Use and Cost of Home Health Agency Services Under Medicare. *Health Care Financing Review* 10(1):105-108, 1988.

Scanlon, W.J.   A Perspective on Long-Term Care for the Elderly. *Health Care Financing Review* (Annual Supplement):7-15, 1988.

Special Committee on Aging, U.S. Congress, Senate. *Aging America: Trends and Projections.* Washington, D.C.: U.S. Department of Health and Human Services, 1987-1988 Edition.

The Villers Foundation. *On The Other Side of Easy Street.* Washington, D.C., 1987.

Waldo, D.R., Sonnefeld, S.T., McKusick, D.R., et al.   Health Expenditures by Age Group, 1977 and 1987. *Health Care Financing Review* 10(4):111-120, 1989.

4

The Medicare Program

In an effort to increase access to health care while reducing the financial burden of care for the aged, Congress enacted the Medicare program, Title XVIII of the Social Security Act, into law on July 30, 1965. Key aspects of this new program included free choice of provider by the beneficiary and no interference by the government with the routine practice of medicine. Although the initial Medicare program was intended solely to benefit elderly persons, the Social Security Amendments of 1972 (P.L. 92-603) expanded benefit coverage to include disabled persons receiving social security benefits and persons with end-stage renal disease (ESRD). The Medicare program is one of our more successful public programs providing broad health care coverage to a very vulnerable population; indeed, many elderly would have greater cost, access, and possibly even quality problems in the absence of such a program (Blumenthal et al., 1988). Table 4.1 summarizes major legislation related to the development of the Medicare program and the genesis of corresponding cost and utilization efforts.[1]

Before the enactment of Title XVIII, experts predicted that demand for and use of health care services would increase under a publicly funded program of health insurance (Klarman, 1966). The actual increases, however, were far greater than anticipated and resulted from many factors: (1) a rise in wage and price levels within the health care industry; (2) incentives within the payment system for use of hospitals and physicians; (3) increases in the supply of certain services (especially ancillary services); (4) changes in the organization of care (such as growth of intensive care units and long-term-care institutions); (5) development of new and costly technologies; (6) growth of third-party reimbursement systems that removed the patient from the direct cost of care; and (7) rising expectations in the nation with regard to health care services.

The federal sector responded to the increasing costs of health care by attempting to develop programs to curb expenditures in all arenas of the health care system, with special attention on the Medicare program. The primary goals of such programs were to control duplication of services and the provision of unnecessary services and to reform payment methodologies. These included health planning efforts, the Certificate of Need program, and price freezes for physicians and hospitals as part of the Economic Stabilization Program in 1971 (Luft, 1985). The Social Security Amendments of 1972 mandated several other cost containment measures including the Professional Standards Review Organizations (PSROs), whose charges were to assure that Medicare services were provided in an efficient and cost-effective manner and to eliminate unnecessary hospital utilization. The PSRO program was not successful, however, in curbing spiraling use and costs (Lohr, 1985). In 1982, legislation was adopted that replaced the PSROs with Utilization and Quality Control Peer Review Organizations (PROs), whose emphasis was to include monitoring the quality, as well as utilization, of Medicare services. A series of steps up to 1983 led to the implementation of Medicare's Prospective Payment System (PPS), which radically restructured hospital payments by introducing prospective payment on the basis of diagnosis-related groups (DRGs).

STRUCTURE, ELIGIBILITY, AND BENEFIT COVERAGE OF THE MEDICARE PROGRAM

The Medicare program was designed as a national, federally administered program with uniform eligibility and benefits. The program has two distinct parts: Part A, Hospital Insurance (HI) and Part B, Supplementary Medical Insurance (SMI).

Hospital Insurance

Medicare Part A (HI) provides benefits for inpatient hospital services, care rendered in a skilled nursing facility (SNF), and home health visits, subject to deductible and coinsurance limits. Persons age 65 and older who are eligible for Social Security cash benefits or payments from the Railroad Retirement System are automatically entitled to HI benefits, as are disabled persons eligible for Social Security or Railroad Retirement benefits for 24 months and ESRD patients. In addition, elderly people who are otherwise ineligible for HI benefits may enroll voluntarily by paying a monthly premium equal to the full actuarial cost of coverage (estimated to be $165 per month in 1990). The voluntary HI enrollee must also obtain SMI coverage.

TABLE 4.1 Major Legislation Relating to the Medicare Program

Year	Title and Description
1935	**SOCIAL SECURITY ACT** Extended the federal government's role in underwriting health care for the elderly by providing monthly cash payments from federal funds for medical expenses.
1965	**SOCIAL SECURITY AMENDMENTS** Title XVIII, Medicare, established compulsory Hospital Insurance (Part A) and optional Supplementary Medical Insurance (Part B) for persons age 65 and older. Benefits for Part A are financed by a payroll tax through the Social Security System, and Part B benefits are financed through a monthly premium.
1972	**SOCIAL SECURITY AMENDMENTS** (P.L. 92-603) Extended Medicare benefits to the disabled and end-stage renal disease patients. Voluntary enrollment in Part A through a premium payment was made available to people age 65 and older otherwise not eligible for Part A. Established the Professional Standards Review Organization (PSRO) program to control health care costs and improve quality of care through utilization and quality monitoring.
1981	**OMNIBUS BUDGET RECONCILIATION ACT** (OBRA) (P.L. 97-35) Eliminated the carryover from the previous year of incurred expenses for meeting the Part B deductible and raised the deductible from $60 to $75 per year. Raised the Part A deductible and coinsurance rate.
1982	**TAX EQUITY AND FISCAL RESPONSIBILITY ACT** (TEFRA) (P.L. 97-248) Established a cost-per-case basis for reimbursement and placed a limit on the annual rate of increase in hospital revenues. Extended Medicare coverage to all federal employees who previously had not been eligible. Replaced the PSRO program with the Utilization and Quality Control Peer Review Organization (PRO) program for utilization and quality monitoring.
1983	**SOCIAL SECURITY AMENDMENTS** (P.L. 98-21) Established the Prospective Payment System (PPS) for reimbursement of hospital services. The hospital is paid a single price per discharge based on prices set prospectively for diagnosis-related groups (DRGs).

1984 **DEFICIT REDUCTION ACT**
(P.L. 98-369)
Established PROs as the quality and utilization monitors for the Medicare reimbursement system (PPS and DRGs) established by the Social Security Amendments of 1983. Placed a freeze on Medicare payment levels for physician services. Introduced the concept of "participating physicians" to constrain the rate of growth of Part B expenditures.

1985 **COMPREHENSIVE OMNIBUS BUDGET RECONCILIATION ACT**
(COBRA) (P.L. 99-272)
Mandated 100 percent review of certain surgical procedures as a result of several studies on medical practice variation.

1986 **OMNIBUS BUDGET RECONCILIATION ACT**
(OBRA) (P.L. 99-509)
Extended PRO review beyond the inpatient setting to include review of ambulatory care, skilled nursing facilities, home health agencies, and health maintenance organizations and competitive medical plans.

1987 **OMNIBUS BUDGET RECONCILIATION ACT**
(OBRA) (P.L. 100-203)
Extended PRO contract cycles from two to three years, and allowed a one-time contract extension (for up to two years) for existing contracts to achieve more efficient renewals.

Supplementary Medical Insurance (SMI)

Enrollment in Medicare Part B (SMI) is voluntary and covers physician services, including visits in the home, office, and hospital. It also covers outpatient services rendered in hospitals and in rural health, community health, and renal dialysis centers, as well as physical and occupational therapy services. Beneficiaries pay a monthly premium for SMI coverage ($27.90 in 1989). During each calendar year, enrollees must exceed the deductible before being reimbursed for additional services. After the deductible is met, Medicare pays 80 percent of the allowable charges for covered services; the beneficiary is responsible for the remainder.

Two terms characterize physician payment relationships: assignment and participation. Assignment means that a physician agrees to accept as payment-in-full the amount Medicare reimburses for the service (i.e., 80 percent of the allowable charge) plus the coinsurance for which the beneficiary is liable (20 percent). In this case, the physician receives payment for services directly from Medicare. If the physician does not accept assignment, in addition to the standard 20-percent coinsurance of the allowable charge, the beneficiary is also responsible for the difference between the physician's charge and the allowable charge. In this case, Medicare reimburses the beneficiary for covered services, who then makes payment directly to the physician. Physicians are either participating or nonparticipating in the Medicare program. Participating physicians voluntarily sign an agreement to accept assignment for all services provided to Medicare beneficiaries; nonparticipating physicians can accept assignment on a claim-by-claim basis.

Size of the Medicare-Enrolled Population

Today about 96 percent of the nation's population over 65 years of age have Medicare coverage (CRS, 1988). In 1977, the enrolled population of approximately 23 million represented 10.4 percent of the U.S. population; in 1989, the enrolled population of slightly more than 29 million represented more than 12 percent of the population (Table 4.2). Approximately 99 percent of those people with HI coverage have also enrolled for SMI coverage. In addition to aged enrollees, the Medicare program covered approximately 144,000 ESRD patients and 3 million disabled persons in 1989 (Committee on Ways and Means, 1989).

Alternatives to Fee-for-Service Health Care Under the Medicare Program

There are several structural and financial alternatives to the traditional fee-for-service system for providing health care to the elderly population under the Medicare program. These alternatives, mainly prepaid health plans, take many forms. They are expected to grow in number and popularity although their effects on quality of care are as yet unknown, mainly because of the small size of their market share relative to fee-for-service.

Health Maintenance Organizations and Competitive Medical Plans (HMOs and CMPs)

Before the Social Security Amendments of 1972 (P.L. 92-603), prepaid health plans had little incentive to enroll Medicare patients because they were reimbursed for these members on the basis of the cost of services rendered. In 1972, Congress authorized risk contracts for HMOs in which the costs per beneficiary in prepaid plans were compared to the estimated costs per beneficiary in fee-for-service settings, known as the Average Adjusted Per Capita Charge or AAPCC (Langwell and Hadley, 1986). If the actual costs to the HMO per Medicare member were lower than the AAPCC,

TABLE 4.2 Medicare Eligible Enrollees and Beneficiaries, Age 65 and Older (in thousands)

Year	Eligible Enrollees	Beneficiaries[b]	Average Benefit per Enrollee
		Part A	
1977	22,941	5,370	$575
1980	24,571	6,940	853
1986	27,831	6,370	1,558
1989[a]	29,423	6,740	1,727
1990[a]	29,966	6,950	1,866
		Part B	
1977	22,737	13,256	$220
1980	24,422	16,119	347
1986	27,607	21,119	799
1989[a]	29,204	23,604	1,184
1990[a]	29,758	24,208	1,389

[a]Estimated
[b]Beneficiaries receiving reimbursed services.

SOURCE: Committee on Ways and Means, 1989, citing data from HCFA, Division of Budget.

the HMO could share in the savings up to 10 percent of the AAPCC. If actual costs were greater than the AAPCC, however, the HMO absorbed all the excess costs, with no maximums. Given this one-sided encouragement, the incentives to enroll Medicare beneficiaries in prepaid health plans were low.

The Tax Equity and Fiscal Responsibility Act (TEFRA) of 1982 (P.L. 97-248) changed the incentives to enroll Medicare beneficiaries in prepaid health plans by authorizing prospective reimbursement under risk contracts with HMOs and other organizations at a rate of 95 percent of the AAPCC. This allowed HMOs with costs below 95 percent of the AAPCC to use these savings to reduce copayments or enhance benefits.

TEFRA regulations issued in 1985 also expanded the option of risk contracts beyond the traditional HMO setting to include CMPs. CMPs are federally certified organizations that do not meet the strict requirements applied to federally qualified HMOs but are still capable of providing services to Medicare beneficiaries on a prepaid basis. In 1985, Medicare beneficiary enrollment in HMOs and CMPs reached 1.1 million, or almost 4 percent of all Medicare enrollees (Gornick et al., 1985). As of March 1989, one million Medicare beneficiaries were enrolled in 133 risk-contract HMOs (HCFA, 1989).

Medicare Insured Groups

Another means of financing health care for the elderly is the Medicare Insured Group (MIG). MIG demonstration projects were authorized in OBRA 1987 (P.L. 100-203) and allow risk contracting directly with sponsors, such as employers and unions, for health care coverage to elderly beneficiaries, usually retired employees. The MIG receives payment directly from the government based to a certain extent on the utilization experience of the group. The MIG can then contract with other health care providers including HMOs and CMPs to provide care for its enrollees. OBRA 1987 authorized up to $600 million each year for a maximum of three MIG projects (ProPAC, 1988). Two MIG projects are currently in the developmental phase, one with the American Life Insurance Corporation and another with Southern California Edison.

ADMINISTRATION AND FINANCING OF
THE MEDICARE PROGRAM

Administration

Responsibility for the Medicare program has been delegated from the Secretary of the Department of Health and Human Services (DHHS) to the Administrator of the Health Care Financing Administration (HCFA). Operational activities of the program, including determination of reasonable costs for covered benefits, claims review, monitoring, and payment are performed by fiscal intermediaries (FIs) for Part A services and carriers for Part B services. National, state, public, or private agencies serve as FIs between hospitals and the federal government. Insurance organizations, contracted by the Secretary of DHHS, serve as carriers. Administrative costs of the FIs and carriers are estimated to be approximately 2.5 percent of Medicare outlays (Committee on Ways and Means, 1989).

The Medicare Statistical System (MSS) (see Appendix B), which is part of the Medicare/Medicaid Decision Support System, provides data for analyzing and evaluating the program's effectiveness (HCFA, 1988). It also enables HCFA to conduct a wide variety of research based on the use and reimbursement of Medicare services.

TABLE 4.3 Sources of Revenue for the Hospital Insurance and Supplemental Medical Insurance Trust Funds: Selected Years

Source of Revenue[a]	Fiscal Year				
	1975	1980	1985	1989	1990[b]
Hospital Insurance (HI)					
Payroll tax	11,291	23,244	46,490	64,733	68,776
Transfers from railroad retirement	132	244	371	337	319
Reimbursement for uninsured persons	481	697	766	515	411
Premiums from voluntary enrollees	6	17	38	55	58
Payments for military wage credits	48	141	86	94	95
Interest income	609	1,072	3,182	6,404	7,742
Subtotal HI	12,567	25,415	50,933	72,138	77,401
Supplementary Medical Insurance (SMI)					
Premiums	1,887	2,928	5,524	10,341	11,095
General revenues	2,330	6,932	17,898	31,137	34,242
Interest	105	415	1,155	735	908
SMI catastrophic premiums				1,165	
Subtotal SMI	4,322	10,275	24,577	43,378	46,245
Grand total	16,889	35,690	75,510	115,516	123,646

[a]In millions of dollars
[b]Estimated

NOTE: Columns may not sum to subtotals or total due to rounding.
SOURCE: Committee on Ways and Means, 1989.

Financing

As previously mentioned, Medicare Part A (HI) is financed mainly through a payroll tax on earnings covered under the Social Security Act (Table 4.3). In 1989, the tax rate was 1.45 percent of earnings up to $48,000 per employee (Committee on Ways and Means, 1989). Other sources of revenue include transfers from the Railroad Retirement account, general revenues for uninsured persons and military wage credits, premiums from voluntary enrollees, and interest on investments. These monies are deposited into the HI Trust Fund from which reimbursement for benefits and administrative expenses is made.

Medicare Part B (SMI) funds come mainly from premiums paid by or on behalf of SMI enrollees as well as funds provided by the federal government (Table 4.3). These premiums are based on projected program costs for the coming year and at present are intended to cover 25 percent of the expected outpatient outlays. Other sources of Part B revenues include general revenues and interest on investments. These monies are deposited into the SMI Trust Fund.

Beneficiaries have always been required to share in the costs of the program through deductibles and coinsurance. The Part A inpatient deductible, equal to the average cost of one day of inpatient care, has increased from $40 at the start of the Medicare program in 1966 to $560 in 1988;[2] it is projected to rise to $684 by 1993 (Committee on Ways and Means, 1989). The Part B deductible and premium have also increased since the beginning of the program. For instance, monthly premiums for Medicare Part B increased from $3.00 in 1966 to $24.80 in 1988, or about 725 percent.

Approximately 65 percent of Medicare enrollees have private insurance (usually referred to as Medigap insurance) to cover Medicare deductible and copayment costs, and another 15 percent of the aged are dually eligible for Medicare and Medicaid coverage (CRS, 1988). For those enrollees with Medigap coverage, out-of-pocket costs (namely, copayments and deductibles) are lower, but total insurance premium costs are higher compared to those without Medigap coverage.

EXPENDITURES OF THE MEDICARE PROGRAM

National Health Care Expenditures

In 1965, health care spending by the total U.S. population amounted to almost $42 billion, or 5.9 percent of Gross National Product (GNP) (Table 4.4). By contrast, in 1987 national spending for health care amounted to more than $500 billion or 11.1 percent of GNP (Letsch et al., 1988). Health care spending will total an estimated $647 billion in 1990 and $1.5 trillion in the year 2000, more than 12 percent and 15 percent of GNP, respectively (HCFA, 1987a). Spending for health care continues to escalate despite recent cost-containment efforts. For example, health care spending increased 8.1 percent from 1985 to 1986, and 8.4 percent from 1986 to 1987 (ProPAC, 1988).

Of the $500 billion spent on health care in 1987, almost 89 percent, or $443 billion, was for personal health care (Table 4.4). These are total

TABLE 4.4 National Health Expenditures: Selected Years

Category of Expenditure[a]	1965	1970	1980	1985	1987
Health services and supplies	$38.4	$69.6	$236.2	$403.4	$483.2
Personal health care	35.9	65.4	219.7	368.3	442.6
Hospital care	14.0	28.0	101.6	166.7	194.7
Physician services	8.5	14.3	46.8	81.4	102.7
Drugs and medical supplies	5.2	8.0	18.8	28.5	34.0
Nursing home care	2.1	4.7	20.4	34.7	40.6
Other[b]	6.1	10.3	32.1	57.1	70.5
Program administration and cost of health insurance	1.7	2.8	9.2	22.6	25.9
Government public health activities	0.8	1.4	7.3	12.5	14.7
Research and construction of medical facilities	3.5	5.4	11.9	15.6	17.1
Total	41.9	75.0	248.1	419.0	500.3

[a]In billions of dollars
[b]Includes: dental services, other professional services, eyeglasses and appliances, and other health services.

NOTE: Columns may not sum to subtotals or total due to rounding.
SOURCES: HCFA, 1987a; Letsch et al., 1988.

health care expenditures minus the costs of research, government public-health activities, and administration; components include hospital care, physician services, nursing home care, dental services, drugs and medical supplies, and other personal health care services. Although persons age 65 and older make up 12 percent of the total population, they account for more than 36 percent (or $162 billion) of all personal health care expenditures.

Medicare Expenditures

Total Medicare expenditures reached almost $88 billion in 1988 (Table 4.5)—up from almost $3.4 billion in 1967. They are estimated to be nearly $114 billion in 1990. Medicare is one of the fastest-growing components of the federal budget, rising from 3.9 percent in 1975 to 7.6 percent of the total budget in 1989 (CRS, 1989). By themselves, Medicare expenditures represented 1.8 percent of GNP in 1989.

From 1978 to 1983, total Medicare spending has increased 128 percent from over $25 billion to almost $57 billion (Table 4.5). Between 1983 (when PPS was enacted) and 1988, however, the percentage increase of

TABLE 4.5 Medicare Benefit Payments and Percent Change, 1978-1988

Year	Part A		Part B		Total Dollars
	Dollars[a]	Percent Increase[b]	Dollars[a]	Percent Increase[b]	
1967	2,597	—	799	—	3,396
1978	17,862	17.5	7,356	16.0	25,218
1979	20,343	13.9	8,814	19.8	29,157
1980	24,288	19.4	10,737	21.8	35,025
1981	29,260	20.5	13,228	23.2	42,488
1982	34,864	19.2	15,560	17.6	50,424
1983	38,624	10.8	18,311	17.7	56,935
1984	42,108	9.0	20,372	11.3	62,480
1985	48,654	15.5	22,730	11.6	71,384
1986	49,685	2.1	26,217	15.3	75,902
1987	50,803	2.3	30,837	17.6	81,640
1988	52,730	3.8	34,947	13.3	87,677
CBO[c] estimates					
1989	58,777	11.5	39,753	13.8	98,530
1990	66,266	12.7	47,671	19.9	113,980

[a]In millions
[b]Percent increase over prior year
[c]Congressional Budget Office

SOURCE: Committee on Ways and Means, 1989

total Medicare expenditures was only about 54 percent, from $57 billion to almost $88 billion.

An examination of the 10 year period from 1978 to 1988 shows fairly constant percentage increases for Parts A and B in the earlier part of the decade (Table 4.5). However, during the later part of that 10 year period, trends in expenditures for Parts A and B have been quite different. Especially since 1985, the rate of growth for Part B expenditures has been far greater than that for Part A (Guterman et al., 1988; ProPAC, 1988; Committee on Ways and Means, 1989), and the annual percentage increases in Part B outlays have continued nearly unabated. By contrast, the rate of growth for Part A expenditures slowed significantly between 1983 and 1987, although recent trends indicate that Part A costs are again beginning to rise.

PPS may have helped to reduce the relative growth in the health care sector (ProPAC, 1988). From 1980 to 1983, the average inflation-adjusted growth rate was 1.0 percent for GNP compared with 5.9 percent for health care expenditures. From 1984 to 1987, however, the growth rate for GNP was 2.9 percent while the growth rate for health care expenditures was 5.2 percent. Thus, although the growth rate of the general economy has accelerated in the 1984-1987 period, the growth rate of the health care sector has decelerated slightly.

During the 1980s, growth in enrollment in both programs (Parts A and B) of Medicare has been fairly steady, averaging about 2 percent per year. The percentage of Part A enrollees using services has decreased slightly, perhaps as a result of a substitution of outpatient services for inpatient hospitalization. The percentage of enrollees receiving reimbursable services under Part B has increased substantially. The latter proportion is sensitive to the proportion of outpatient expenditures exceeding the deductible.

Part A payments now make up about 60 percent of Medicare expenditures (Table 4.5). Of these, inpatient hospital services constitute the largest spending category and will continue to do so, but their proportion of total Part A spending is changing. For instance, in 1975, inpatient hospital services constituted about 70 percent of Part A benefit payments, whereas in 1986 their proportion of the total had decreased to 61 percent (Guterman et al., 1988). Home health expenditures, once the fastest-growing component of Medicare spending, are showing slower rates of increase.

For Part B (the other 40 percent of all Medicare spending), physician services constitute the largest spending category. During the last 20 years, the rate of growth of reimbursement for physician services has been almost equal to the rate of growth in reimbursement for inpatient hospital services (Gornick et al., 1985), and although these expenditures have declined as a proportion of total spending over time, they have increased in the last few years as payments for outpatient hospital services have increased. This is believed to be partially attributable to the implementation of PPS and the resulting substitution of outpatient care for inpatient hospitalization.

The Prospective Payment System (PPS) is cited as a major factor in moderating the growth of inpatient expenditures for the Medicare program, but other trends have affected the use of services by Medicare and non-Medicare patients. For instance, the average length of stay in hospitals began declining in the late 1970s before the implementation of PPS. However, the decrease in average length of stay accelerated slightly after PPS for all patients, not just the elderly. The greater availability of home health care, improvements in technology, and stricter utilization review by third parties may have contributed to the decrease in the length of stay.

A drop in hospital admissions has been a second major change affecting Medicare expenditures. In the early 1980s, admissions for patients under age 65 were dropping, but admissions for patients over age 65 were still rising; the decline in admissions for the elderly did not occur until after the implementation of PPS. During the first three years of PPS, admissions per Medicare enrollee fell by 15.9 percent (Guterman et al., 1988). This decline was not an anticipated result of PPS; instead, admissions had been expected to increase either generally or in certain types because of the limits on reimbursement from each individual admission. The substitution of outpatient care was a response to changes in medical technology, higher payments for certain outpatient services than for inpatient services, and programs to deny authorization for hospitalization for certain procedures.

Finally, an examination of the sources and uses of total health care dollars reveals a contrast between those of the total population and the elderly population. For instance, in 1987, for the total population, private sources paid for 48 percent of hospital care, 69 percent of physician services, and 51 percent of nursing home care; public sources paid for the remainder in each category. As seen in Figure 4.1 by contrast, public sources paid for the majority of hospital and physician services for the elderly population. For example, public sources (both Medicare and Medicaid) paid for approximately 85 percent of hospital care, 64 percent of physician services, and 40 percent of nursing home care (Waldo et al., 1989).

THE PROSPECTIVE PAYMENT SYSTEM (PPS)

The PPS, established by the Social Security Amendments of 1983 (P.L. 98-21), was probably the most revolutionary change in the method of financing health care since the beginning of the Medicare program. It changed the economic incentives that motivate hospital behavior, moving from a cost-based retrospective reimbursement system for the hospital to a diagnosis-based prospective reimbursement system.

The PPS went into effect for most acute hospitals beginning October 1, 1983, and involved a three-year transition period to phase in a national payment rate for hospital care based on DRGs. Payment rates are determined by classifying the patient at discharge into one of nearly 500 DRGs. A weight is assigned to each DRG, based on data that reflect the relative resource consumption of the DRG. Actual payment for each DRG is determined by multiplying a standardized payment rate by the DRG weight with adjustments for urban and rural cost differentials, area wage rates, and institutions with certain characteristics such as sole community hospitals, teaching hospitals, and disproportionate share hospitals. This pricing system applies to all inpatient acute care, with adjustments for extremely long lengths of stay and extremely high costs per case. Institutions currently exempt from the PPS system include psychiatric, children's, long-term-care, and rehabilitation hospitals.

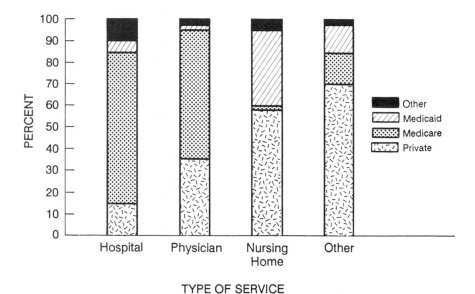

TYPE OF SERVICE

FIGURE 4.1 Personal Health Care Expenditures For People Age 65+, by Source of Funds and Type of Service, 1987

PPS was developed in an effort to contain rising health care costs while maintaining access to quality care and providing incentives for efficiency, flexibility, innovation, planning, and control (ProPAC, 1989). Before PPS, there was general concern about the effects this new payment system might have on the medical-care delivery system and on the quality of care. These concerns included the possibility of shorter lengths of stay, which was viewed at the time as having negative consequences for the elderly population, increases in admissions of certain types (those cases expected to be at or below the DRG cost), readmissions for medically unrelated problems that could have been handled in the first admission, and fewer support staff per patient (Lohr et al., 1985). To date, no concrete evidence has been amassed to document that quality of care for Medicare patients has declined as a result of PPS (HCFA, 1987; Guterman et al., 1988; ProPAC, 1988).

Medicare-Related Commissions

Concerned about the need to monitor and update the PPS system, Congress established the Prospective Payment Assessment Commission (ProPAC) in 1983. The 17 members of ProPAC are appointed by the director of the congressional Office of Technology Assessment (OTA) for a 3-year term. The Commission has two major responsibilities; first, it recommends annual changes in the hospital payment rates to the Secretary of DHHS and second, it recommends changes in the DRG classifications. It has discharged this responsibility through regular Commission meetings, which are generally open to the public, and detailed annual reports and technical documents. The statute limits the number of staff to 26, and the annual budget for the ProPAC activities approaches $4 million.

Physician payment under Medicare has come under close scrutiny in recent years. Concern is being heard among physicians, beneficiaries, and government officials about the tremendous growth of physician expenditures over the last several years, the increasing fiscal burden on beneficiaries and taxpayers, and diminished access to quality care for Medicare enrollees who, under the constraints of limited financial resources, avoid seeking services that may not be reimbursed.

As a result, Congress established the Physician Payment Review Commission (PPRC) in 1986 (P.L. 99-272) to advise on reforms to the physician payment system under the Medicare program (PPRC, 1988, 1989). The PPRC is modeled on ProPAC and members include physicians, other health professionals, experts from other disciplines, and representatives of consumers and the elderly. This Commission has four major roles (PPRC, 1988). First, it provides advice to the Secretary of DHHS. Second, it seeks the views of physicians, beneficiaries, and others concerning its recommendations. The conduct of analyses on which to base policy decisions is the third role of the Commission. Finally, it undertakes the work necessary to implement the recommended policy changes.

PPRC has initiated several research projects to develop a Medicare fee schedule for physician payment based on the relative value of resources used by the physicians to produce the services rendered to the patient (see Hsiao et al., 1988). It has also called for practice guidelines to help physicians understand better when services, especially procedures, are appropriate and when they are not.

QUALITY ASSURANCE IN MEDICARE

The Utilization and Quality Control
Peer Review Organization Program (PRO)

In addition to managing Medicare outlays, HCFA is charged with ensuring the quality of care rendered to Medicare beneficiaries. Thus, the PRO program, implemented as part of TEFRA 1982 (P.L. 97-248) and administered by HCFA, is intended to ensure quality of care within the Medicare program while reducing unnecessary and inappropriate utilization of services covered by Medicare. (Refer to Chapter 6 and Volume II, Chapter 8 for a broader description of the PRO program.)

Conditions of Participation

The oldest form of quality assurance for Medicare is based on "structural" properties of organizations wishing to be eligible for reimbursement for services rendered to Medicare enrollees. Specifically, such organizations must meet certain "Medicare Conditions of Participation." Hospitals can meet these conditions by being accredited mainly by the Joint Commission on Accreditation of Healthcare Organizations (and hence be accorded "deemed status") or by being certified by state agencies. (Refer to Chapter 5 and Volume II, Chapter 7 for a broader discussion of the Medicare Conditions of Participation.)

Utilization Management

Another outgrowth of cost-containment pressure is the development of utilization management. This refers to a set of tools designed to monitor both the appropriateness of a given treatment and the treatment site to control unnecessary use of health care services by prior review and authorization for services (especially procedures and hospital admission). Integrating utilization management with other strategies for balancing cost, quality, and access may improve the effectiveness and efficiency of the health care system as a whole (Gray and Field, 1989). The private sector has been more aggressive about implementing utilization management into health care plans for the nonelderly than the government has been with respect to Medicare and the elderly, although this is changing as government decision makers look to the private sector for ideas and models to help shape Medicare policy (PPRC, 1988).

SUMMARY

Central to any discussion of national health policy in general, or the Medicare program in particular, are the issues of cost, access, and quality. Of major concern to the public and to policymakers are the rising costs of health care and the rising expenditures of the Medicare program, at a rate well beyond that for general goods and services.

High-quality health care costs money. What has not been determined, however, is whether allocating additional amounts of money to the health care system necessarily guarantees better quality of care or improved health. Similarly, it is not known whether providing fewer, or different, resources in the health care system necessarily means poorer quality and worse health outcomes.

These issues have special significance for Medicare in light of the revolution that has occurred in the organization and financing of health services in the last decade. Major shifts have occurred in the settings in which care is delivered. Payment modes have changed for hospital services and are expected to change for physician services. New, capitated alternatives to fee-for-service care are emerging. We do not know, and may never know, the full impact of these and other changes on the quality of health care.

The basic purpose of this study has been to develop a quality assurance program, and a strategy for implementing that program, that will permit rapid identification of any threats to the quality of care for the elderly, and, indeed, will be able continuously to improve the quality of that care.

NOTES

1. Appendix A briefly describes the Medicare Catastrophic Coverage Act of 1988 (MCCA) (P.L. 100-360), which was enacted in July of that year and represented the most significant expansion of Medicare benefits since the inception of the program in 1965. The MCCA was repealed in November 1989 as a result of pressure from the elderly concerning the financing of the new benefits.
2. By comparison, the Consumer Price Index, a general measure of inflation, has increased from a base of 100 in 1967 to 340.4 in 1987. Similarly, the Medical Care Price Index rose from 100 in 1967 to 462.2 in 1987 (NCHS, 1989).

REFERENCES

Blumenthal, D., Schlesinger, M., and Drumheller, P.B. *Renewing the Promise: Medicare and Its Reform*. New York: Oxford University Press, 1988.

Christensen, S. and Kasten, M. Covering Catastrophic Expenses Under Medicare. *Health Affairs* 7:79-93, Winter 1988.

Committee on Ways and Means, U.S. Congress, House of Representatives. *Background Material on Programs Within the Jurisdiction of the Committee on Ways and Means*. Washington, D.C.: U.S. Government Printing Office, March 1989.

CRS (Congressional Research Service, U.S. Library of Congress). Catastrophic Health Insurance: Medicare. CRS IB-87-106. Washington, D.C.: U.S. Government Printing Office, June 1988.

CRS. Medicare: Its Use, Funding, and Economic Dimensions. 89-143 EPW. Washington, D.C.: U.S. Government Printing Office, March 1989.

Division of National Cost Estimates, Office of the Actuary, Health Care Financing Administration. National Health Expenditures, 1986-2000. *Health Care Financing Review* 8:1-36, Summer 1987.

GAO (General Accounting Office). *Medicare Catastrophic Act. Options for Changing Financing and Benefits*. GAO/HRD-89-156. Washington, D.C.: General Accounting Office, September 1989.

Gornick, M., Greenberg, J.N., Eggers, P.W., et al. Twenty Years of Medicare and Medicaid: Covered Populations, Use of Benefits, and Program Expenditures. *Health Care Financing Review* (Annual Supplement):13-58, 1985.

Gray, B.H. and Field, M.J., eds. *Controlling Costs and Changing Patient Care? The Role of Utilization Management.* Washington, D.C.: National Academy Press, 1989.

Guterman, S., Eggers, P.W., Riley, G., et al. The First Three Years of Medicare Prospective Payment: An Overview. *Health Care Financing Review* 9:76-77, Spring 1988.

HCFA (Health Care Financing Administration). Office of Research and Demonstrations. *Impact of the Medicare Hospital Prospective Payment System, 1985 Annual Report to Congress.* HCFA-03251. Washington, D.C.: U.S. Government Printing Office, August 1987.

HCFA. Bureau of Data Management and Strategy. *Medicare Statistical Files Manual.* HCFA Publication No. 03272. Baltimore, Md.: U.S. Department of Health and Human Services, Health Care Financing Administration, July 1988.

HCFA. Enrollment in TEFRA Risk HMOs/CMPs. Unpublished monthly compilations, March 1989.

Hsiao, W.C., Braun, P., Yntema, D., et al. Estimating Physicians' Work for a Resource-Based Relative Value Scale. *New England Journal of Medicine* 319:835-841, 1988.

Klarman, H. Policies and Local Planning for Health Services. *Milbank Memorial Fund Quarterly* 54:1-28, Winter 1966.

Langwell, K.M. and Hadley, J.P. Capitation and the Medicare Program: History, Issues, and Evidence. *Health Care Financing Review* (Annual Supplement):9-20, 1986.

Letsch, S.W., Levit, K.R., and Waldo, D.R. National Health Expenditures: 1987. *Health Care Financing Review* 10:109-122, Winter 1988.

Lohr, K.N. *Peer Review Organizations: Quality Assurance in Medicare.* P-7125. Santa Monica, Calif.: The RAND Corporation, July 1985.

Lohr, K.N., Brook, R.H., Goldberg, G.A., et al. *Impact of Medicare Prospective Payment on the Quality of Medical Care. A Research Agenda.* R-3242-HCFA. Santa Monica, Calif.: The RAND Corporation, March 1985.

Luft, H.S. Competition and Regulation. *Medical Care* 23:383-400, 1985.

NCHS (National Center For Health Statistics). *Health United States, 1988.* DHHS Pub No. (PHS) 89-1232. Public Health Service. Washington, D.C.: U.S. Government Printing Office, March 1989.

PPRC (Physician Payment Review Commission). *Annual Report to Congress.* Washington, D.C.: Physician Payment Review Commission, 1988.

PPRC. *Annual Report to Congress.* Washington, D.C.: Physician Payment Review Commission, 1989.

ProPAC (Prospective Payment Assessment Commission). *Medicare Prospective Payment System and the American Health Care System: Report to Congress.* Washington, D.C.: Prospective Payment Assessment Commission, June 1988.

ProPAC. *Report and Recommendations to the Secretary, U.S. Department of Health and Human Services.* Washington, D.C.: Prospective Payment Assessment Commission, March 1, 1989.

APPENDIX A
THE MEDICARE CATASTROPHIC COVERAGE ACT OF 1988

Despite concerns with escalating Medicare costs and utilization extending over nearly two decades, Congress enacted The Medicare Catastrophic Coverage Act of 1988 (MCCA) (P.L. 100-360) in July of that year. This Act substantially increased protection for beneficiaries who incur large health care expenses by limiting the amount of out-of-pocket costs for covered services. It was the largest benefit expansion in the history of the program. It also significantly affected Medicaid coverage for low-income elderly, disabled persons, pregnant women, and children.

However, 16 months after its passage, Congress repealed all the Medicare provisions of the Act. It did so in response to considerable dissent among the elderly and lobbying efforts on their behalf concerning the increased premiums (an income-related surtax) they faced to finance these expanded benefits. The Medicaid benefits are the only provisions remaining from the original legislation.

Benefits of the Medicare Catastrophic Coverage Act

The MCCA changed the benefit and copayment levels for both parts of the program (Part A, hospital insurance, and Part B, supplementary medical insurance) (refer to Table A.1) and added a third distinct component known as catastrophic drug insurance (CDI). Provisions of the law became effective on January 1, 1989 when Part A benefits began, and implementation was to extend through 1993 when the prescription drug benefits and Medicaid benefits were to be completely phased-in.

Financing

As described in Chapter 4, Part A (Hospital Insurance) of the Medicare program is funded primarily as social insurance through a payroll tax levied equally on employers and employees (that is, people pay into the system while they are working and become eligible for benefits when they retire or become disabled). Part B (Supplementary Medical Insurance) is funded partially through premiums paid by the beneficiaries (25 percent) with the remainder (75 percent) being funded by the federal government.

The MCCA included three new premiums (Committee on Ways and Means, 1989; GAO, 1989). The first was to be paid by all beneficiaries and was referred to as the catastrophic coverage premium. This premium was $4.00 per month in 1989 and was expected to increase to $7.18 per month in 1993. The second, referred to as the prescription drug premium, was to be required of all beneficiaries upon complete phase-in of the program in 1993.

TABLE A.1 Comparison of Medicare Benefit Structure Before and After Implementation of the Medicare Catastrophic Coverage Act of 1988

Before Catastrophic Coverage	After Catastrophic Coverage
HOSPITAL INSURANCE (PART A)	
Coverage	
Hospital inpatient care	Same, with changes noted below
Short-term skilled nursing care	
Intermittent home health care	
Hospice care for terminally ill	
Limits	
Hospital stays limited to 90 days per benefit period with lifetime reserve of 60 days	No limit on covered inpatient days
Skilled nursing facility stays limited to 100 days per benefit period. Three-day prior hospitalization required	Skilled nursing facility limits changed to 150 days per year, no prior hospitalization required
Consecutive days of home health care limited to 21	Consecutive days of home health care limited to 38
Hospice limit of 210 days	Hospice benefits extended beyond 210 days with physician certification of terminal illness
Deductibles	
Inpatient deductible for first stay in each benefit period	Deductible for first stay each year
Blood deductible up to three units each benefit period	Blood deductible up to three units each year
Coinsurance	
Hospital coinsurance required for days 61 to 90 (25% of deductible) and lifetime reserve days (50% of deductible)	No hospital coinsurance
SNF coinsurance for days 21 to 100 (12.5%)	SNF coinsurance for days 1 to 8 each year (20% of daily cost)
SUPPLEMENTARY MEDICAL INSURANCE (PART B)	
Coverage	
Physician's services	Supplementary Medical Insurance (SMI) program expanded to cover screening mammography and respite care
Hospital outpatient department	
Ambulatory surgicenters	
Laboratory services	

Table A.1 continues

TABLE A.1 Continued

Before Catastrophic Coverage	After Catastrophic Coverage
Intermittent home health care	New Part B drug program introduced to cover prescription drugs, insulin, and drugs for transplant patients
Limits	
Preventive services generally not covered	Respite care limited to 80 hours per year and available only to those who exceed SMI copayment cap or drug deductible in the previous 12 months
Reimbursement limit of $1,100 per year for outpatient psychiatric services	
Deductibles	
Annual SMI deductible of $75	Same, plus separate drug deductible set to affect 16.8% of enrollees
Coinsurance	
Coinsurance of 20% of reasonable charges above deductible amount (50% for outpatient psychiatry)	Same, subject to SMI copayment cap
Copayment Cap	
No copayment cap	SMI copayment cap set to affect 7% of enrollees No drug copayment cap

SOURCE: Christensen and Kasten, 1988.

The premium was to be $1.94 per month in 1991, increasing to $3.02 per month in 1993. The third new premium was related to beneficiary income and was referred to as the supplemental Medicare premium. The amount of this premium depended on federal tax liability; those beneficiaries with less than $150 of tax liability in a year would pay no supplemental premium. An estimated 40 percent of the beneficiaries would be required to pay the premium in 1989. The maximum supplemental premium in 1989 was $800 and was slated to increase to $1,050 in 1993.

Repeal of Catastrophic Coverage

One title of The Deficit Reduction Act of 1989, The Medicare Catastrophic Coverage Reform Amendments of 1989, repealed all of the benefits provided by the MCCA except the provisions related to the Medicaid program. The repealed benefits include: (1) unlimited hospital coverage after payment of the annual deductible; (2) the out-of-pocket cap on expenses under Part B; (3) coverage of outpatient prescription drugs; (4) expanded coverage of home health, hospice, and skilled nursing care as well as the respite benefit; and (5) coverage for screening mammography.

APPENDIX B
THE MEDICARE DECISION SUPPORT SYSTEM

HCFA develops its "basic records groups" of the Medicare/Medicaid Decision Support System (M/MDSS) from several different sources including the Social Security Administration, insurance claims, and records of providers eligible for Medicare reimbursement. The Medicare Statistical System (MSS), which is part of the M/MDSS, has as its main objective the provision of data necessary to measure and evaluate the effectiveness of the Medicare program and to improve the decision-making process. Extensive, systematic, and continuous information about the amount and kind of hospital and medical care services used by beneficiaries and the related costs of such services are derived from the benefit payment operation.

The M/MDSS has five basic record groups. First, the Health Insurance Master File (HIM) contains demographic information (such as name, sex, date of birth and death, geographic location) on the entire Medicare enrolled population—approximately 29 million elderly and 3 million disabled. This file also includes the dates of enrollment in HMOs and state buy-in programs.

Second, the Provider of Service Record (POS) contains information on all institutional Medicare providers such as hospitals, skilled nursing facilities (SNFs), home health agencies, independent laboratories, ambulatory surgery centers, and other Medicare providers. Each is assigned a unique provider number. Approximately 6,700 hospitals, 6,100 SNFs, 5,200 home health agencies, 3,900 independent laboratories, and 1,600 other types of facilities are included in this file.

Third, the Utilization Record contains Medicare Part A (Hospital Insurance) and B (Supplementary Medical Insurance) billing information including days of care, diagnoses, procedures, physician visits, charges, and payments. Approximately 11 million inpatient hospital, 800,000 SNF, 42 million outpatient, 5 million home health agency, and 360 million physician and supplier payment records are processed annually.

Fourth, Provider Cost Report Records contain data from institutional providers about costs, accounting information, and general provider characteristics. Fifth, Special Program Data are collected on specific programs within Medicare (e.g., end-stage renal disease).

Within the basic records groups are four major record files. First, the

Medicare Provider Analysis and Review (MEDPAR) file includes information on 100 percent of Part A inpatient discharges (1986 to present). This file contains person-level data with unique identifiers (to allow linkage with other files), demographic data, clinical data, and information on days of care, charges, and provider of service. The diagnoses and procedures in this file are coded with ICD-9-CM codes (International Classification of Diseases, Ninth Revision, Clinical Modification). The MEDPAR file contains approximately 10 million records per year and is updated quarterly.

Second, the Medicare Automated Data Retrieval System (MADRS) contains 100 percent of Part A and B files, linked together. This file also contains person-level data with unique identifiers, demographic data, information on all institutional services, Part B payment records (summary level only), and limited medical information. MADRS is triggered by the inpatient admission, contains 250 million records, and is updated monthly.

Third, the Health Insurance Master Accretion (HIMA) contains 100 percent information on all Medicare enrollees (approximately 32 million). This file contains person-level data with unique identifiers, demographic data, name and address of the beneficiary, and dates of entitlement. HIMA is updated daily.

Finally, the Part B Medicare Annual Data (BMAD) file contains a 5-percent sample of beneficiaries and includes over 21 million records. The data are on a person level with unique identifiers. They include physician and supplier Part B claims for services and expense information (dates, place, and type of services rendered). The procedures in this file are coded with the HCFA Common Procedure Coding System (HCPCS), which is based on the CPT-4 (Current Procedure Terminology) system. BMAD is updated annually.

5

Hospital Conditions of Participation in Medicare

Since the passage of Medicare legislation in 1965, Section 1861 of the Social Security Act has stated that hospitals participating in the Medicare program must meet certain requirements specified in the act and that the Secretary of the Department of Health and Human Services (DHHS) may impose additional requirements found necessary to ensure the health and safety of Medicare beneficiaries receiving services in hospitals. On this basis, the Conditions of Participation, a set of regulations setting minimum health and safety standards for hospitals participating in Medicare, were promulgated in 1966 and substantially revised in 1986. This chapter, in response to the congressional request, discusses the adequacy of the federal Conditions of Participation for hospitals in assuring quality of care. Limitations of the accreditation and certification methods are reviewed and recommendations are set forth for strengthening the Conditions of Participation program.

Since 1965, under authority of Section 1865 of the Social Security Act, hospitals accredited by the Joint Commission on the Accreditation of Healthcare Organizations (Joint Commission) or the American Osteopathic Association (AOA) have been automatically "deemed" to meet all the health and safety requirements for participation except the utilization review requirement, the psychiatric hospital special conditions, and the special requirements for hospital providers of long term care. As a result of this deemed status provision, most hospitals participating in Medicare do so by meeting the standards of a private body governed by representatives of the health providers themselves (i.e., the Joint Commission or the AOA). Both the federal conditions and the Joint Commission standards also require hospitals to be licensed by their states. (A more detailed discussion of the Conditions of Participation and deemed status is provided in Volume II,

Chapter 7, from which much of the information in this chapter was taken. Options covering the Conditions of Participation program, and their respective implications, considered by the committee in developing its conclusions on the certification and accreditation of hospitals are delineated in the Volume II chapter.)

The Joint Commission is a private nonprofit organization governed by a board with 21 representatives of hospital and medical associations and 3 public representatives. The American Medical Association (AMA) and the American Hospital Association (AHA) each appoint 7 members.

About 5,400 hospitals are accredited by the Joint Commission, about two-thirds of which are in metropolitan areas. Of the 5,388 currently accredited, 36 percent are facilities of fewer than 100 beds, 55 percent 100 to 499 beds, and 9 percent 500 or more beds (Joint Commission, personal communication, 1989). Another 1,600 hospitals are certified by state inspectors to meet the federal Conditions of Participation. Most certified hospitals are small and located in nonmetropolitan areas; they usually do not wish to pay the expense of accreditation and often do not feel the need for the stamp of approval that accreditation implies because they are the only hospitals in their areas.

Although one is governmental and the other private, both the Health Care Financing Administration (HCFA) (as the administrative branch within DHHS responsible for the Medicare program) and the Joint Commission are regulatory in their approach. Each attempts to assure quality of care by influencing individual and institutional behavior. As in any regulatory system, quality assurance in health delivery organizations has three components (IOM, 1986). First, standards have to be set that relate to quality of care. Second, the extent of compliance of hospitals with the standards must be monitored. Third, procedures for enforcing compliance are necessary.

STANDARDS AND CONDITIONS

Historical Background

The current federal standards for hospitals participating in Medicare are presented in the Code of Federal Regulations as 24 "Conditions of Participation," containing 75 specific standards (Table 5.1). Another regulation automatically permits hospitals that meet the Medicare Conditions of Participation to participate in Medicaid. The Health Standards and Quality Bureau (HSQB) of HCFA is responsible for administering and enforcing the Conditions of Participation. In addition to overseeing the Medicare accredited and certified hospitals, HSQB enforces separate sets of Conditions of Participation for over 25,000 other Medicare providers. The actual compliance of hospitals with the Conditions of Participation is monitored for the federal government by each state through periodic on-site surveys by personnel of the state agency that licenses hospitals and other health facilities (or, in a few cases, by an equivalent agency).

Responsibility for revising the Conditions of Participation lies with HCFA's Bureau of Policy Development, a unit separate from the HSQB. The conditions were first drafted in 1966, by the Bureau of Health Insurance of the Social Security Administration's Medicare Bureau with technical assistance from the Public Health Service, to ensure that hospitals have a minimum capacity to deliver quality care. The conditions were criticized from the beginning for only looking at the capacity of a hospital to provide adequate quality of care rather than monitoring the hospital's actual performance or effect on patient well-being. After several unsuccessful efforts to update the conditions and associated standards in the late 1970s and early 1980s, a new set of regulations was promulgated in 1986, which includes a new quality assurance condition that mandates an extensive program for evaluating patient care services.

In 1966, at the time the Conditions of Participation were first drafted, Donabedian (1966) identified three aspects of patient care that could be measured in assessing the quality of care: structure, process, and outcome. Theoretically, structure, process, and outcome are related, and, ideally, a good structure for patient care (e.g., safe and sanitary building, necessary equipment, qualified personnel, and properly organized staff) increases the likelihood of a good process of patient care (e.g., the right diagnosis and best treatment available), and a good process increases the likelihood of a good outcome (e.g., the highest health status possible) (Donabedian, 1988).[1]

Generally, the conditions in effect from 1966 until 1986 emphasized structural (rather than process or outcome) measures of organizational and clinical capacity, such as staff qualifications, written policies and procedures, and committee structure. These were usually specified at the standard level. The process aspects of quality-of-care standards were usually suggested as explanatory factors that could be used to evaluate compliance with the standard.[2]

The revised conditions were put into final form in 1986 (51 CFR 22010); they were based in part on conditions proposed in 1983 (48 CFR 299) and 1980 and reflected input from the public through an extensive rulemaking process. In line with the Reagan administration's emphasis on deregulation, the resulting regulations carried further the process of eliminating prescriptive requirements specifying credentials or committees, departments, and other organizational arrangements; to increase administrative flexibility, the 1986 revisions reflected more general statements of desired performance or outcome. In contrast, some activities were elevated to the condition level to give them more emphasis in the certification process; these included infec-

TABLE 5.1   Current Medicare Conditions of Participation and Standards for Hospitals

Conditions of Participation	Standards
1. Provision of emergency services by nonparticipating hospitals	
2. Compliance with Federal, State, and local laws	(a) Federal laws (b) State licensure (c) Personnel licensure
3. Governing body	(a) Medical staff (b) Chief executive officer (c) Care of patients (d) Institutional plan and budget (e) Contracted services (f) Emergency services
4. Quality assurance	(a) Clinical plan (b) Medically related patient care services (c) Implementation
5. Medical staff	(a) Composition of the medical staff (b) Medical staff organization and accountability (c) Medical staff bylaws (d) Autopsies
6. Nursing services	(a) Organization (b) Staffing and delivery of care (c) Preparation and administration of drugs
7. Medical record services	(a) Organization and staffing (b) Form and retention of record (c) Content of record
8. Pharmaceutical services	(a) Pharmacy management and administration (b) Delivery of services
9. Radiologic services	(a) Radiologic services (b) Safety for patients and personnel (c) Personnel (d) Records
10. Laboratory services	(a) Adequacy of laboratory services (b) Laboratory management

Conditions of Participation	Standards
	(c) Personnel
	(d) Blood and blood products
	(e) Proficiency testing
	(f) Quality control
11. Food and dietetic services	(a) Organization
	(b) Diets
12. Utilization review	(a) Applicability
	(b) Composition of utilization review committee
	(c) Scope and frequency of review
	(d) Determination regarding admissions or continued stays
	(e) Extended stay review
	(f) Review of professional services
13. Physical environment	(a) Buildings
	(b) Life safety from fire
	(c) Facilities
14. Infection control	(a) Organization and policies
	(b) Responsibilities of chief medical staff, and director of nursing services
15. Surgical services	(a) Organization and staffing
	(b) Delivery of services
16. Anesthesia services	(a) Organization and staffing
	(b) Delivery of services
17. Nuclear medicine services	(a) Organization and staffing
	(b) Delivery of service
	(c) Facilities
	(d) Records
18. Outpatient services	(a) Organization
	(b) Personnel
19. Emergency services	(a) Organization and direction
	(b) Personnel
20. Rehabilitation services	(a) Organization and staffing
	(b) Delivery of services
21. Special provisions applying to psychiatric hospitals	

Table 5.1 continues

TABLE 5.1 Continued

Conditions of Participation	Standards
22. Special medical record requirements for psychiatric hospitals	(a) Development of assessment and diagnostic data (b) Psychiatric evaluation (c) Treatment plan (d) Recording progress (e) Discharge planning and discharge summary
23. Special staff requirements for psychiatric hospitals	(a) Personnel (b) Director of inpatient psychiatric services; medical staff (c) Availability of medical personnel (d) Nursing services (e) Psychological services (f) Social services (g) Therapeutic activities
24. Special requirements for hospital providers of long-term care services ("swing-beds")	(a) Eligibility (b) Skilled nursing facility services

SOURCE: 42 CFR Part 482, effective September 15, 1986

tion control and surgical and anesthesia services. In addition, quality assurance was made a separate condition.

The new Conditions of Participation took effect September 15, 1986. They were accompanied by interpretive guidelines and detailed survey procedures developed by HCFA to increase consistency of interpretation and application by the state agency surveyors (HCFA, 1986).

Joint Commission standards are contained in its *Accreditation Manual for Hospitals,* parts of which are revised each year through an elaborate process of professional consensus. With the advent of the Conditions of Participation in 1966, which were based on Joint Commission standards of the time, the Joint Commission decided to develop "optimum" standards. An explicit quality-of-care standard first adopted in 1979 has undergone continuous evolution.

Shift from Capacity Standards to Performance Standards

In recent years, HCFA and the Joint Commission have tried to revise their standards in ways that would impel hospitals to examine and to improve the quality of their organizational and clinical performance. For example, both organizations have adopted quality assurance standards that call for hospitals to set up structures and processes for monitoring patient care, identifying and resolving problems, and evaluating the impact of quality assurance activities (GAO, 1988). By and large, these capacity-oriented standards are based on professional consensus, although some are based on research. Under these standards, the medical staff is required to develop or adopt indicators of quality of care, gather information on the indicators, select criteria for deciding when an indicator is signaling a possible problem, and act on those signals. The Joint Commission calls these quality assurance activities "outcome-oriented," although the main emphasis of the new standards is to make hospitals adopt processes for monitoring indicators of the quality of their performance.

In early 1988, the Joint Commission again eased implementation of the quality assurance standards. It no longer gave contingencies if hospitals were using only "generic" rather than department-specific indicators in monitoring and evaluating the quality and appropriateness of care in the various departments and services. The Joint Commission takes the position that health care organizations do not have available a full set of validated indicators for each area of clinical practice because such do not exist in the clinical literature (Joint Commission, 1988a).

The problems that many hospitals experienced in complying with the Joint Commission standards for outcome-oriented monitoring and evaluating quality of care have been part of the impetus for the Joint Commission's current and ongoing effort, called the Agenda for Change, to develop indicators of organizational and clinical performance for the hospitals to use (Joint Commission, 1988b, 1988c, 1988d).

Development of the Quality Assurance Condition of Participation

The quality assurance condition implemented in late 1986 is similar in approach although less elaborate than the Joint Commission's quality assurance standards. The task force of HCFA officials that developed the revised conditions in 1981 and 1982 intentionally sought consistency with the Joint Commission standards (HCFA Task Force, 1982).

The new quality assurance condition as finally promulgated calls for a formal, ongoing, hospital-wide program that evaluates all patient care services. Explicit references to nosocomial infections, medicine therapy, and tissue removal were dropped. The interpretive guidelines state that criteria generated by the medical and professional/technical staffs should guide the information gathered by the hospital to monitor and evaluate the provision of patient care and that information gathered should reflect hospital practice patterns, staff performance, and patient outcomes (Table 5.2).[3]

TABLE 5.2 Medicare's Quality Assurance Condition of Participation

---

Condition of Participation: Quality Assurance (QA)
The governing body must ensure that there is an effective, hospital-wide QA program to evaluate the provision of patient care.

> *Interpretive guidelines:* The condition requires that each hospital develop its own QA program to meet its needs. The methods used by each hospital for self-assessment (QA) are flexible. There are a wide variety of techniques used by hospitals to gather information to be monitored. These may include document-based review (e.g., review of medical records, computer profile data, continuous monitors, patient care indicators or screens, incident reports, etc.); direct observation of clinical performance and of operating systems and interviews with patients, and/or staff. The information gathered by the hospital should be based on criteria and/or measures generated by the medical and professional/technical staffs and reflect hospital practice patterns, staff performance, and patient outcomes.

(a) *Standard:* Clinical Plan.
The organized hospital-wide QA program must be ongoing and have a written plan of implementation.

> *Interpretive guidelines:* Ongoing means that there is a continuous and periodic collection and assessment of data concerning the important aspects of patient care. Assessment of such data enable areas of potential problems to be identified and indicates additional data which should be collected and assessed in order to identify whether a problem exists. The QA program must provide the hospital with findings regarding quality of care.
>
> The QA plan should include at least the following: program objectives; organization involved; hospital-wide in scope; all patient care disciplines involved; description of how the program will be administered and coordinated; methodology for monitoring and evaluating the quality of care; ongoing; setting of priorities for resolution of programs; monitoring to determine effectiveness of action; oversight responsibility—reports to governing body; documentation of the review of its own QA plan.

(1) All organized services related to patient care including services furnished by a contractor must be evaluated.

> *Interpretive guidelines:* "All organized services" means all services provided to patients by staff accountable to the hospital through employment or contract. All patient care services furnished under contract must be evaluated as through they were provided by hospital staff.
>
> This means that all patient services must be evaluated as part of the QA program, that is: dietetic services; medical records; medical staff care—appropri-

ateness and quality of diagnosis and treatment; laboratory service; nursing service; pharmaceutical service; radiology service; hospital-wide functions—infection control, utilization review (for hospitals under PRO review this requirement does not apply), discharge planning programs.

If the hospital offers these optional services, they must also be evaluated: anesthesia services; emergency services; nuclear medicine services; outpatient services; psychiatric services; rehabilitation services; respiratory services; surgical services.

Each department or service should address: patient care problems; cause of problems; documented corrective actions; monitoring or follow-up to determine effectiveness of actions taken.

(2) Nosocomial infections and medication therapy must be evaluated.

(3) All medical and surgical services performed in the hospital must be evaluated as they relate to appropriateness of diagnosis and treatment.

Interpretive guidelines: All services provided in the hospital must be periodically evaluated to determine whether an acceptable level of quality is provided. The services provided by each practitioner with hospital privileges must be periodically evaluated to determine whether they are of an acceptable level of quality and appropriateness,

(b) *Standard:* Medically-related patient care services.
The hospital must have an ongoing plan, consistent with available community and hospital resources, to provide or make available social work, psychological, and educational services to meet the medically-related needs of its patients. The hospital also must have an effective, ongoing discharge planning program that facilitates the provision of followup care.

Interpretive guidelines: To be considered effective, the discharge planning program must result in each patient's record being annotated with a note regarding the nature of post-hospital care arrangements.

(1) Discharge planning must be initiated in a timely manner.

(2) Patients, along with necessary medical information, must be transferred or referred to appropriate facilities, agencies, or outpatient services, as needed, for follow-up or ancillary care.

(c) *Standard:* Implementation
The hospital must take and document appropriate remedial action to address deficiencies found through the QA program. The hospital must document the outcome of the remedial action.

SOURCE: HCFA, 1986.

The term outcome does not appear in the language of the conditions or standards, however, because the majority of the task force did not think that outcome measures could be used in the survey process. The task force report pointed out that although outcome measures were desirable, in part because they promised maximum flexibility to hospitals, they were difficult to assess without undertaking longitudinal studies beyond the given episode of care, which would be too cumbersome for hospitals and surveyors and would be difficult to use in enforcement.

The 1986 revisions of the Conditions of Participation, including the new quality assurance condition, were largely based on work done in the late 1970s and very early 1980s. They resemble the evolution of the Joint Commission standards in the same time period, when the Joint Commission adopted a quality assurance standard and began to revise the other standards to make them more flexible and less prescriptive. However, the Joint Commission's standards have undergone substantial evolution since the early 1980s; the latter's quality assurance standard in particular has undergone a great deal of elaboration in the process of trying to help hospitals understand how to comply with its intent (Roberts, 1988).

INSPECTION AND ENFORCEMENT

Inspection Processes

The HSQB Office of Survey and Certification administers the inspection and enforcement process for hospitals that are not accredited by the Joint Commission. The process relies on inspectors from state health facility licensure agencies to determine and certify compliance with the Conditions of Participation through periodic on-site visits. In the past, certified hospitals have been surveyed about every 24 months, although HCFA is now requiring the states to shorten the cycle to about 18 months.

The federal regulations governing the survey process and HCFA's state operations manual are very general regarding survey agency staffing levels and qualifications. As a result, the size and composition of survey teams vary considerably. The person-days spent in on-site inspections and other survey activities also vary. State inspectors undergo a week of training at HCFA and are provided with survey forms on which they mark "met" or "not met" for each condition, for second-level "standards" associated with each condition, and for third-level "elements" associated with each standard. HCFA also provides "interpretive guidelines" for assessing compliance. HCFA does not, however, furnish criteria for deciding which and how many elements have to be out of compliance for a standard to be marked not met or which combinations of unmet standards call for a deter-

mination that a hospital is out of compliance with a condition. T|
probably leads to significant variations from inspector to inspect
been found in studies of nursing home regulation (IOM, 1986; GAO, 1986).

Accredited hospitals are surveyed every three years. The Joint Commission has standardized the size and composition of its survey teams, depending on the type of hospital (e.g., general acute versus psychiatric, substance abuse, or rehabilitation). It has developed several sets of formal criteria and decision rules for rating compliance with each standard and associated "required characteristics" on a scale from 1 to 5 and for deciding whether the resulting scores justify accreditation. Use of these criteria and decision rules no doubt increases consistency and reliability, but their validity is not known (OTA, 1988).

Enforcement

Typically, 10 to 15 (0.6 to 0.8 percent) of the 1,800 hospitals surveyed each year by the Joint Commission either lose their accreditation or close voluntarily. The trend over the past few years shows an increase in this percentage. Hospitals that lose accreditation can and many do apply for certification from HCFA in order to stay in the Medicare program; however, the number of hospitals that lose accreditation and subsequently are certified is not currently available from HCFA's survey and certification data system. There are also cases in which hospitals are decertified by HCFA but retain Joint Commission accreditation. Generally, 1 to 2 percent of the approximately 800 hospitals inspected for HCFA each year by the state survey agencies are decertified involuntarily [9 in fiscal year (FY) 1987, 20 in FY 1986, and 8 in FY 1985] and most are recertified within a short time. Past comparisons of state surveyor and Joint Commission surveyor findings in the same facilities, however, have found low levels of agreement on specific deficiencies (DHHS, 1988).

Most enforcement occurs during the administrative process, in which hospitals are notified of deficiencies (by HCFA) or contingencies (by the Joint Commission) and are given deadlines for correcting them. In response, the hospitals develop plans of correction that are approved by the state inspection agency or the Joint Commission; follow-up visits are made or written documentation is submitted to show compliance, and, in 98 or 99 percent of the cases, certification or accreditation continues. The Joint Commission reports that 4 to 6 percent (about 80) of the hospitals surveyed each year have problems that put them into a tentative nonaccreditation category; most of them make corrections in time to avoid losing accreditation. Similarly, most of the certified hospitals put in the 23-day, "fast-track" termination category—for problems that pose a serious threat to the health and safety of patients—avoid decertification by making immediate changes.

TABLE 5.3 Numbers of Hospitals with Specified Accreditation Status by the Joint Commission: Four Recent Years

Accreditation Status	Year			
	1986	1987	1988	1989
Total accredited with no contingencies	18	22	11	
Total accredited with contingencies (and no tentative nonaccreditation)	1579	1795	1644	534
Total closed before decision rendered	4	2	8	
Hospitals receiving tentative nonaccreditation				
Open		1	55	38
Accredited with contingency	67	43	37	
Consultative and education decision	2	1	2	
Nonaccreditation decision	2	2	2	
Nonaccreditation decision under appeal		2	3	1
Hospitals closed during tentative nonaccreditation process	1	2		
Total	72	51	99	39
Total surveyed	1673	1870	1762	573

NOTE: Includes full accreditation survey data only and as of 8/14/89.
SOURCE: Joint Commission on Accreditation of Healthcare Organizations, personal communication 1989.

A breakout by year (1986-1989) of the accreditation status granted by the Joint Commission to hospitals is shown in Table 5.3.

The Joint Commission has recently developed formal decision rules for determining whether the levels and pattern of compliance with specific standards and required characteristics are adequate and merit accreditation. The rules are also used to make contingency decisions, including if and when on-site follow-up visits or written progress reports are necessary.

In HCFA's state certification process, a hospital cannot be certified if it fails to meet any Condition of Participation, but decisions on compliance with conditions and standards are left to the judgment of the surveyors, as are decisions concerning the adequacy of plans of correction. If inspectors decide to initiate decertification procedures, hospitals may and usually do remedy the deficiencies in time to avoid actual decertification. Facilities also have extensive legal due process protections that serve as a deterrent to enforcement attempts, as do the difficulties encountered by the surveyors in documenting quality problems (Vladeck, 1988).

Strictly speaking, it is impossible to know, in the absence of research, if this practice of citing numerous deficiencies and contingencies accompanied by little formal enforcement by the Joint Commission or HCFA means that the system is working or that enforcement measures are very weak. Various features of the inspection and enforcement processes used by HCFA and the Joint Commission permit and perhaps encourage under-enforcement.[4] The surveyors and their supervisors are health professionals who generally prefer to be consultants to troubled facilities rather than enforcers. The administrative process allows numerous chances for facilities, even those with serious patient-care problems, to come into compliance before they lose certification or accreditation. The Joint Commission is a private organization governed by the health professions it is regulating. HCFA and the state inspection agencies, on the other hand, are public agencies subject to due process rules and vulnerable to political pressures. The inspection agencies have only one sanction, that is, expulsion, which is too drastic to use credibly in situations short of extreme negligence or clearly wrongful death.

FEDERAL GOVERNMENT'S ROLES AND RESPONSIBILITIES

Federal Oversight

Federal responsibility for applying health and safety regulations in hospitals participating in Medicare is delegated, on the one hand, to the Joint Commission, and, on the other hand, to the state survey agencies. Since 1972, HCFA has been required to have the state agencies conduct validation surveys of a random sample of accredited hospitals each year to ensure that the Joint Commission's surveying of accredited hospitals is equivalent to state agency surveying of unaccredited hospitals. As of late 1989 HCFA was considering a revision of its sampling methodology to improve the effectiveness of its validation efforts (HCFA, personal communication, 1989). HCFA is also authorized to have state inspectors investigate allegations of substantial deficiencies in accredited hospitals. HCFA concludes in its annual reports that the two systems are equivalent, because the percentage of Joint Commission-accredited hospitals found out of compliance with one or more Conditions of Participation (including about 400 a year inspected on the basis of complaints) has been roughly equal to the percentage of unaccredited hospitals found out of compliance (DHHS, 1988).

HCFA also has about 100 federal inspectors based in the DHHS regional offices to conduct validation surveys in state-inspected facilities, but they are primarily devoted to nursing homes and facilities for the mentally retarded. They do not perform enough surveys of hospitals to make any statistical inferences about a state inspection agency's performance.

Federal Resources

HSQB's Office of Survey and Certification enforces separate Conditions of Participation for over 25,000 Medicare provider organizations in addition to the 1,600 certified and 5,400 accredited hospitals. These include 10,000 skilled nursing homes, 5,700 home health agencies, and 4,775 laboratories. Because hospitals are not perceived to have significant problems, compared with nursing homes and home health agencies, and because there is no deemed status for other types of health providers, this HSQB office devotes most of its resources to these other types of facilities. Also, the funding of Medicare certification activities was cut drastically in the early 1980s and the number of federal validation surveyors fell to 60; at the same time, concern about nursing homes and intermediate care facilities for the mentally retarded became acute and regulation was extended to home health agencies. Funds and staff have been increased recently.

Administrative Coordination

Although the Office of Survey and Certification and the Office of Medical Review, which administers the Utilization and Quality Control Peer Review Organization (PRO) program, are both in HSQB and deal with the same Medicare hospitals, they do not interact in terms of information sharing or coordinated action. At the state level, numerous obstacles exist (e.g., legal and administrative) to deter information sharing about a facility or practitioner between a Medicare PRO and the state survey agency.

CONCLUSIONS

The study committee concluded that the Medicare Conditions of Participation and procedures for enforcing them should become a more significant component of and be more consistent with the overall federal quality assurance effort. This position was taken after weighing other options and their respective implications, many of which are stated in Volume II, Chapter 7.

The federal-state and Joint Commission efforts to develop and apply quality assurance standards are hampered in several ways. First, because outcome measures such as functional level are affected by many factors beyond what happens in hospitals, adverse or even improved outcomes are frequently only indicators of possible quality problems or opportunities; as indicators, they can only trigger further investigation to determine if some aspect of hospital care was involved (Roberts, 1988).[5] Medicare and the Joint Commission staff responsible for setting the standards have tried, therefore, to mandate quality assurance processes in which hospitals use indicators of quality—outcome-oriented if possible, but usually process and even structural in nature—to examine quality of care. However, few clinical indicators have been adequately validated through research. Even fewer indicators of the quality of organizational performance exist (Kaluzny and Barnsley, 1988; Donabedian, 1989). Nevertheless, to the extent knowledge exists about how to improve quality or make quality assurance more effective, it should be reflected in the Medicare and the Joint Commission standards and survey processes.

The second barrier to quality assurance through certification and accreditation is the limited surveillance capacity inherent in any system of periodic inspections. A two-day visit every year or two limits the ability of even the best surveyors to see if the process of care conforms to standards of best practice in an adequate sample of cases, let alone see what the outcomes were. This distance problem is another reason why those who set the standards have tried externally to impose quality assurance standards that make the hospital itself conduct such surveillance continuously after the inspectors leave (Vladeck, 1988). The Office of Survey and Certification focuses on the facility and not the individual physician. The quality-of-care screens used by the PROs provide limited information on the actual role of a hospital (rather than a physician) in producing adverse indicators. Sharing of information between the two would facilitate focused review by each; this enhanced information flow could alleviate some of the problems occurring from periodic and thus limited surveillance.

A third impediment to the use of regulatory, or self-regulatory, standards to assure quality is the ambivalent attitude of Medicare officials, the state agencies that actually survey the facilities, and the Joint Commission leaders toward the use of sanctions. The reason for the Joint Commission is professional self-improvement. Federal and state officials are primarily motivated by the desire to make Medicare benefits widely available, and they are also subject to political pressure to keep facilities open, if at all possible. The only formal sanction is loss of formal certification or accreditation, a drastic step that officials are reluctant to take except in extreme cases; some states use less extreme enforcement measures that vary in impact. The due process protections of the legal system also discourage enforcement attempts, as do the difficulties of documenting quality problems more subtle than gross negligence or death. Thus, for a variety of reasons, officials are very reluctant to take formal enforcement actions, especially to the extent of terminating a facility, preferring to work with substandard or marginal facilities over time and bring them into compliance. This approach works well if the hospitals involved have the will and capacity to improve if shown how to do it, but it is ill-equipped to deal with places that cannot or will not improve.

Fourth, whereas the federal government has delegated much of the standard-setting and enforcement to private accreditation bodies on the one hand, it has given away much discretion to the states on the other. The states have always varied greatly in their interpretation of federal standards, and little has been done to increase consistency. HCFA requirements for state survey programs are very loose. It was recognized from the beginning that who does the surveying is critical, "since this greatly influences what the emphasis will be, regardless of what the standard setters think the emphasis should be" (Cashman and Myers, 1967, p. 1112), but little has been done to standardize state survey capacity or process. The development of interpretive guidelines and survey procedures for the new Conditions of Participation was a step in the right direction.

A number of steps should be taken by HCFA to strengthen the Conditions of Participation process, working with both the Joint Commission on deemed status and the state survey and certification agencies for those hospitals not accredited. This initiative should include updating the conditions and their related standards and elements within the next two years and continually thereafter (no more infrequently than every three years). The Department should continue to support the concept of deemed status for hospitals. In addition, the Department should encourage the Joint Commission in its efforts to develop a state-of-the-art quality assurance program and in its program to disclose information to the Department or its agency about conditionally accredited and nonaccredited hospitals in a timely fashion. A reasonable amount of contact with Joint Commission activities will be necessary on behalf of the Department to ensure that the Joint Commission's accreditation program remains consistent with the intentions of the Medicare Program to Assure Quality (MPAQ) as recommended by the IOM study committee in Chapter 12. The Secretary should improve the coordination of federal quality assurance efforts by developing criteria and procedures for referring cases involving serious quality problems from the PROs (or their restructured entities described in Chapter 12 under the proposed MPAQ) to the Office of Survey and Certification (and vice versa).

In addition, the committee identified the following steps to be taken by HCFA to strengthen the state survey and certification system: (1) specify the size and composition of state survey teams; (2) use survey procedures and instruments that focus more on patient care and outcomes and less on medical records; (3) develop explicit (national) decision rules for determining compliance and taking enforcement actions; (4) adopt intermediate sanctions (e.g., fines, suspensions from Medicare admissions, and focused restrictions) that better reflect the problem being addressed; and (5) use more federal inspectors to evaluate state agency performance (through validation surveys) and to inspect state hospital facilities.

SUMMARY

The contents of this chapter and Volume II, Chapter 7 respond to the legislative charge to the IOM to conduct a study on the adequacy of the standards used in hospitals, for purposes of meeting Medicare Conditions of Participation in assuring the quality of services furnished in hospitals.

About 7,000 hospitals provide services to Medicare patients. The Secretary of DHHS has the regulatory authority to promulgate and enforce standards called Conditions of Participation to assure the adequate health and safety of Medicare patients in those hospitals, although the 5,400 hospitals accredited by the private Joint Commission and the 100 hospitals accredited by AOA are deemed to meet the appropriate federal conditions without further inspection by a public agency (except for a small number of accredited hospitals that are subject to validation or complaint surveys each year). In effect, then, Joint Commission standards are the Medicare standards for most Medicare beneficiaries using hospital services. At the same time, the users of 1,600 hospitals rely on the standards in the Medicare Conditions of Participation. These are mostly small, primarily rural hospitals where Medicare's beneficiaries do not have the alternative of going to an accredited hospital. Both sets of standards, therefore, affect a large number of people and should be as effective as possible in achieving the goal of assuring adequate care.

The Medicare program and the Joint Commission hospital standards have evolved from mostly structural standards (aimed at assuring that a hospital has the minimum capacity to provide quality care) to mostly process standards (aimed at making hospitals assess in a systematic and on-going way the actual quality of care provided on their premises). Certain structural standards, such as those for fire safety, that continue to be mandated and enforced through the certification and accreditation standards may not be closely related to patient care but are important factors in patient safety.

The certification and accreditation programs are inherently limited in their capacity to assure quality of care. They are hampered by the lack of knowledge about the relationships between structure and process features of a hospital and patient outcomes. They are limited because periodic inspections cannot reveal much about how well the process of care conforms to the standards of best practice, or what the outcomes of care are. They rely on the subjective judgment of their inspectors and the enforcement attitudes of the inspection agencies.

The committee concludes that the Medicare Conditions of Participation and procedures for enforcing them should become a more significant component of and be more consistent with the overall federal quality assurance effort; thus, the committee articulates a major recommendation in this regard in Chapter 12. A number of steps are identified to strengthen the Conditions of Participation process that call for HCFA to work with both the Joint Commission on deemed status and the state survey and certification agencies for those hospitals not accredited.

NOTES

1. Chapter 2 provides a detailed discussion on quality assessment measures (structure, process, and outcome).
2. For example, no quality-of-care or quality assurance condition or standard existed in the 1966-1986 period. Instead, the medical staff condition had a meetings standard calling for regular meetings of the medical staff "to review, analyze, and evaluate the clinical work of its members," using an "adequate" evaluation method. The explanatory factors that surveyors were supposed to use to determine compliance with the standard included attendance records at staff or departmental meetings and minutes that showed reviews of clinical practice (e.g., selected deaths, unimproved cases, and infections) at least monthly.
3. Chapter 10 discusses attributes of quality-of-care criteria and standards.
4. The *Wall Street Journal* conducted a study of the Joint Commission's accreditation process and concluded that "the Joint Commission is accountable to neither government nor patients . . . yet it commands a quasi-regulatory status." The *Journal* further stated that the federal efforts to monitor the Joint Commission are "disorganized, weak, and ineffective" (Bogdanich, 1988, pp. A-1, A-12).
5. Chapter 9 and Volume II, Chapter 6 examine strengths and weaknesses of selected quality assessment and assurance methods.

REFERENCES

Bogdanich, W. Prized by Hospitals, Accreditation Hides Perils Patients Face. *Wall Street Journal,* pp. A-1, A-12. October 12, 1988.

Cashman, J.W. and Myers, B.A. Medicare: Standards of Service in a New Program—Licensure, Certification, Accreditation. *American Journal of Public Health* 57:1107-1117, 1967.

DHHS (Department of Health and Human Services). Report on Medicare Validation Surveys of Hospitals Accredited by the Joint Commission on Accreditation of Hospitals (JCAH): Fiscal Year 1985. In *Report of the Secretary of DHHS on Medicare.* Washington, D.C.: U.S. Government Printing Office, 1988.

Donabedian, A. Evaluating the Quality of Medical Care. *Milbank Memorial Fund Quarterly* 44:166-203, 1966.

Donabedian, A. The Quality of Care: How Can it be Assessed? *Journal of the American Medical Association* 260:1743-1748, 1988.

Donabedian, A. Reflections on the Effectiveness of Quality Assurance. Paper prepared for the Institute of Medicine Study to Design a Strategy for Quality Review and Assurance in Medicare, 1989.

GAO (General Accounting Office). *Medicare: Improving Quality of Care Assessment and Assurance.* PEMD-88-10, Washington, D.C.: General Accounting Office, May 1988.

HCFA (Health Care Financing Administration). Appendix A, Interpretive Guidelines—Hospitals. Pp. A1-A165 in *State Operations Manual: Provider Certification.* Transmittal No. 190. Washington, D.C.: Department of Health and Human Services, 1986.

HCFA Task Force. HCFA Task Force Recommendations. Unpublished document in files of the Health Standards and Quality Bureau, Health Care Financing Administration, Baltimore, Md., 1982.

IOM (Institute of Medicine). *Improving the Quality of Care in Nursing Homes.* Washington, D.C.: National Academy Press, 1986.

Joint Commission (Joint Commission on Accreditation of Healthcare Organizations). Rules Change on Monitoring and Evaluation Contingencies. *Joint Commission Perspectives* 8:5-6, 1988a.

Joint Commission. *Medical Staff Monitoring and Evaluation: Departmental Review.* Chicago, Ill.: Joint Commission on Accreditation of Healthcare Organizations, 1988b.

Joint Commission. Proposed Clinical Indicators for Pilot Testing. Chicago, Ill.: Joint Commission on Accreditation of Healthcare Organizations, 1988c.

Joint Commission. Field Review Evaluation Form: Proposed Principles of Organizational and Management Effectiveness. Chicago, Ill.: Joint Commission on Accreditation of Healthcare Organizations, 1988d.

Kaluzny, A.D. and Barnsley, J.M. Organizational Indicators of Quality. *Health Matrix* 6:3-7, Summer 1988.

OTA (Office of Technology Assessment). *The Quality of Medical Care: Information for Consumers.* OTA-H-386. Washington, D.C.: U.S. Government Printing Office, 1988.

Roberts, J.S. Quality Assurance in Hospitals: From Process to Outcomes. Pp. 48-62 in *Quality of Care and Technology Assessment.* Lohr, K.N. and Rettig, R.A., eds. Report of a Forum of the Council on Health Care Technology. Washington, D.C.: National Academy Press, 1988.

Vladeck, B.C. Quality Assurance Through External Controls. *Inquiry* 25:100-107, 1988.

6

Federal Quality Assurance
Programs for Medicare

After creating the Medicare program in 1965, Congress mandated efforts for organized quality assurance for Medicare beneficiaries. Successive federal activities have included Experimental Medical Care Review Organizations (EMCROs), Professional Standards Review Organizations (PSROs), and Utilization and Quality Control Peer Review Organizations (PROs). Antedating these efforts were "foundations for medical care," a physician-based movement begun in California in the 1950s. These community-centered organizations of participating physicians monitored the use and quality of both hospital and ambulatory care services before payment by fiscal intermediaries (FIs) (Egdahl, 1973; Harrington, 1973; Lohr et al., 1981).

These activities (and the growth of the Joint Commission on Accreditation of Hospitals) were the most visible examples of a grassroots professional interest in the quality of medical care delivery that emerged following the Second World War. In contemplating the structure and purposes of a quality assurance system for Medicare that will carry into the 21st century, one should realize that organized quality assurance arose initially as a professional effort and that it has a modern-day history half a century old.

The nation's health care providers have devised many ways to assure the quality of health care.[1] The Medicare program has used two main approaches. One is Medicare Conditions of Participation and the closely linked accreditation activities of the Joint Commission on Accreditation of Healthcare Organizations. The second is the program's successive Medicare quality review programs, which are discussed in this chapter. The sources of information include literature reviews, extensive site visits around the country, documents and staff briefings from the Health Care Financing Administration (HCFA), interviews with representatives of relevant organizations and institutions, and personal experience of members of the IOM committee.

The federal programs were fashioned to address incentives of the prevailing financing mechanisms for health care. For instance, when cost-based reimbursement was the predominant mode of hospital payment, utilization review to detect overuse of care had a key place in peer review efforts such as the PSRO program. Prospective payment prompts more attention to underuse and quality of care, as seen in recent activities of the PRO program. Nevertheless, utilization review and quality assurance are closely linked activities; both have been and will continue to be important in any program intended to assure the quality of care for the elderly. In designing the strategy for a new quality assurance program for Medicare (Chapter 12), we hope to create a program with the flexibility and appropriate tools that can respond to whatever incentives emerge from changing Medicare financing and reimbursement schemes. To lay the groundwork for such a program, we here examine past and existing quality assurance efforts for Medicare.

EXPERIMENTAL MEDICAL CARE REVIEW ORGANIZATIONS

Experimental Medical Care Review Organizations (EMCROs) were voluntary associations of physicians who reviewed inpatient and ambulatory services paid for by Medicare and Medicaid. The program, in existence between 1970 and 1975, was administered and funded by the National Center for Health Services Research and Development. Far more a research and development effort than an operational one, the EMCRO mission was to encourage physicians to work together and to upgrade methods for assessing and assuring quality of care. EMCROs were concerned with both inpatient and ambulatory care.

Although no comprehensive evaluation of the EMCRO program was ever done, analyses of data and activities of the New Mexico EMCRO documented important impacts of the program on the appropriate use of injectable drugs and on the quality of ambulatory care in the state's Medicaid program (Lohr et al., 1980). Those results were obtained through a dual approach that emphasized education (development and promulgation of injection guidelines) and economic sanctions (denial of payments for inappropriate services). EMCROs were essentially a prototype for PSROs, established about midway through the EMCRO program.

PROFESSIONAL STANDARDS REVIEW ORGANIZATIONS

Purpose and Structure

Professional Standards Review Organizations (PSROs) were established by the Social Security Amendments of 1972 (P.L. 92-603) to assure that physicians and institutions met their Medicare obligations; such obligations required that services provided or proposed to be provided to Medicare beneficiaries were medically necessary, of a quality that met local professionally recognized standards, and were provided in the most economical manner consistent with quality of care (Goran et al., 1975; Blum et al., 1977). Congress intended PSROs to lower public expenditures for medical care, to counter fee-for-service incentives toward overuse of services, and to help to ensure the quality of care.

PSROs were voluntary, not-for-profit, local physician organizations; each PSRO area covered approximately 35 hospitals and 2,000 to 3,000 physicians, on average, although the range was quite broad. The original PSRO areas numbered 203 (195 in 1977 and thereafter). By mid-1981, of these 195 designated areas, 182 had funded PSROs; of those, 47 were "fully designated," 132 were "conditional," and 3 were in the planning stage. Consequently, length of continuous operation, skills, and experience varied considerably across PSROs, and the history of the fully operational program was relatively short. The program was administered by HCFA's Health Standards and Quality Bureau (HSQB) in the Department of Health, Education and Welfare [later Health and Human Services (DHHS)]. HSQB used a complicated system of annual grants to PSRO entities consisting partly of congressionally appropriated general revenues and partly of Medicare Trust Fund monies.

Aspects of the PSRO Program of Importance to the PRO Program

Briefly, PSROs carried out the following activities: hospital utilization review, development of hospital discharge data (the PSRO Hospital Discharge Data Set), profile analysis, Medical Care Evaluation (MCE) studies and Quality Review Studies, and review of care rendered in other settings (ancillary services, nursing home care, and ambulatory care). Some PSROs contracted to do utilization review for private firms and municipal governments. A few PSROs collaborated in research studies (Chassin and McCue, 1986) and studies of variations in hospital use.

Utilization Review

Hospital utilization review was viewed as distinct from quality assurance and was given highest priority by PSROs. It usually took the form of preadmission certification for elective hospital admissions, certification of nonelective admissions (within three days of admission), and continued stay recertification; both concurrent and retrospective review was done. One lesson of the PSRO program was that 100 percent utilization review was excessive, and PSROs came to "focus out" about 50 percent of the admissions they might have reviewed at the start of the program. No consensus was ever reached, however, either on the appropriate criteria for such focusing out or on the sample sizes needed to achieve cost-effective utilization review. Issues of concurrent versus retrospective review and of focusing out providers or particular types of services are as pertinent for the PRO program as they were a decade ago.

Profile Analysis

Profiling is a form of retrospective review of patient care data to identify patterns of care over a defined period of time. Profiles can be constructed by groups of patients (e.g., diagnostic group), by provider (e.g., hospital or nursing home), or by practitioner (e.g., physician) to determine rates of use of services such as admissions or specific procedures and lengths of stay over time. They can be used to identify "outliers" that fall outside established standards of appropriate care, such as excessively long hospital stays; such providers or practitioners can then be targeted for closer scrutiny or corrective interventions. This targeting was the principal application of profiling in the PSRO program, and profile analysis continues to be a major tool for review.[2]

Quality of Care

Quality-related activities of the PSRO program included MCE studies, which were audits based on medical records of locally identified quality problems, typically related to specific diagnoses, technologies, or procedures. MCEs were done either by individual (delegated) hospitals or by PSROs for nondelegated hospitals or for groups of hospitals. The numbers of MCEs done by (or for) any one hospital were determined partly in conjunction with Joint Commission requirements. Toward the end of the PSRO program, MCEs evolved into Quality Review Studies, which were expected to rely on data beyond the medical record, identify a broader set of topics for study, and document more fully the impact of the review activity on quality of care.

Many innovative PSROs did area-wide MCEs that permitted hospitals to compare their audit outcomes with those of their peers; this was considered a valuable quality assurance mechanism. The difficulty, however, of demonstrating in quantitative terms the impact of MCEs (as contrasted with simply enumerating the number of MCEs conducted) contributed to the inability of the PSRO program to document a meaningful effect on quality of care. Studies of the MCE variety still dominate the quality assurance efforts in hospitals, owing in part to the familiarity of hospital staffs with this activity, but they are not part of the PRO scope of work.

Other Efforts

Often lost in the historical account of the PSRO program is that some PSROs embarked on a considerably broader review agenda than simply hospital utilization review and MCEs. Perhaps as many as one-third of PSROs became involved in hospital-related ancillary services review (e.g., radiology, medications, and laboratory tests), although budget constraints for this were severe. The ancillary services experience relates directly to the procedure-oriented review the PROs do now, but in some respects the PSRO experience represents a broader set of health care services.

Still other PSROs reviewed care in long-term-care facilities; although budget cuts curtailed these efforts, at the peak about 55 PSRO projects were underway in such facilities. Ten PSRO demonstration projects that reviewed nursing home care (which included pre-admission, admission, and continued stay review, quality assurance activities, MCEs, and data systems development) were given special attention in the late 1970s (Kane et al., 1979).

Finally, a few PSROs were involved in various ambulatory care review projects (e.g., physician office care as distinguished from ambulatory surgical procedures done in hospitals or free-standing clinics). Evaluations of these activities were inconclusive about dollar savings to the Medicare program (the key evaluative criterion), and PSROs made little progress in this arena, for several reasons. In the first place, ambulatory care is harder to review than inpatient care; it is more dispersed, involves more providers and sites, reflects many more patient-provider encounters, and has less well-developed methods. Second, the Medicare insurance claims forms of the day would not have provided adequate information for this endeavor. Third, physicians a decade ago were reluctant to facilitate review of their private office practice records. Fourth, the costs of outpatient care were less significant before the Medicare prospective payment system and the considerable shift of hospital care to the nonhospital setting, and ambulatory care offered less opportunity for meaningful savings than hospital care; given that cost control was the principal operational task of PSROs, they had less incentive to attempt ambulatory review. Finally, the program budgets for ambulatory review were quite low.

Delegation

One controversial aspect of the PSRO program was its ability—more accurately, its mandate and related budgetary incentives—to "delegate" certain quality assurance and utilization review functions to individual hospitals judged to be capable of carrying them out. Delegated hospital review was funded through negotiated budgets between the PSRO and the individual hospital. PSROs monitored the performance of delegated hospitals but usually did no ongoing data collection or abstracting in those facilities. By contrast, they did all such tasks directly in nondelegated institutions.

This form of delegation was not judged particularly successful at the time (HCFA, 1980). PSROs lacked administrative and financial control of delegated hospital review. For instance, removing delegated status was administratively very difficult. Further, delegated review costs were simply passed on to the Medicare Trust Fund, whereas nondelegated review was a PSRO line item in the federal budget; thus, the pressure to delegate was very great. Finally, delegated hospitals determined their own procedures, identified their own MCE topics, and in other ways operated quite independently of one another; this complicated the job of evaluating the impact of the program as a whole.

In an environment in which the majority of physicians and hospitals tolerated rather than enthusiastically supported the PSRO program, the performance of delegated hospitals was often a perfunctory exercise in "paper compliance." Another issue was the mismatch between the expectation that the PSRO program act as a regulatory control mechanism for an activity— namely, health care delivery—from which they were twice removed; that is, they neither delivered health care directly nor, for delegated hospitals, directly reviewed the performance of caregivers.

This mirrored the great divergence in expectations for the PSRO program generally—namely, the congressional expectations that they were getting a cost-control program, the PSRO belief that they were doing quality assurance, and HCFA's view that the program did both. The end result was that, as PSROs were phased out and PROs phased in, HCFA regulations eliminated delegation as a program option.

Costs

According to the 1979 HCFA evaluation (HCFA, 1980), the mean dollar cost of hospital-based review per discharge in 1978 (i.e., fiscal year (FY) 1979, when program costs were $147.2 million) was $13.68 for the review activity itself and $7.10 for management and support tasks. The median total review cost for FY 1979 was $12.91, a figure the HCFA evaluation noted was "considerably greater than the target of $8.70" (HCFA, 1980, p. 92).

Mean costs per discharge differed markedly by type of review: $8.81 for concurrent review, $1.28 for MCE review, and $3.61 for areawide review; the highest and lowest cost ranges around these averages were fairly wide.[3] Costs differed by who did the review. Delegated review (e.g., when delegated hospitals did concurrent hospital admission and continued-stay review themselves) was less expensive on a per-discharge basis than was nondelegated review; for instance, the median concurrent review cost for the larger PSROs (those responsible for 50,000 or more discharges) was $6.93 for delegated hospitals and $10.56 for nondelegated hospitals. In short, costs of review were extremely variable (as they remain in the PRO program).

Total PSRO funding rose from $4.3 million in 1973 to $173.7 million in 1981 (CBO, 1981). Funding was unstable over the period; for instance, it increased almost 43 percent between FY 1977 and FY 1978 but just under 2 percent between FY 1978 and FY 1979 and not quite 4 percent between FY 1979 and FY 1980.

Medicare expenditures during the PSRO program ranged from about $9.5 billion in FY 1973 to $42.5 billion in FY 1981. Hospital insurance (Part A) outlays alone were $6.8 and $29.3 billions, respectively (Committee on Ways and Means, 1989). Taking total outlays as the denominator, PSRO program costs by the end of the program amounted to only about one-half of 1 percent (about 0.45 percent) of outlays; the figures reach about 0.7 percent if only Part A expenditures are used as the base. As will be seen, PRO funding has been equally tight, if not more so.

Additional Aspects of the PSRO Program

The National Council

The PSRO legislation provided for a National Professional Standards Review Council, appointed by the executive branch. It consisted of 11 physicians not in the federal government who could represent or were recommended by practicing physicians, consumer groups, and other health care interests. The Council was charged with reporting at least annually to the Secretary of the Department of Health, Education and Welfare and to the Congress on its activities; the report was supposed to review the effectiveness and comparative performance of PSRO operations, develop recommendations concerning ways that the program might be designed more effectively, and provide comparative data indicating the results of review activities. At the time, the Council was regarded with some suspicion because its rather ambiguous charge was seen as a threat to the local autonomy of physicians and as an opening wedge in the establishment of national or model standards of care (Blumstein, 1976), all issues of vastly greater sensitivity 15 years ago than now.

In retrospect, the Council was not demonstrably successful in shaping the long-term policies of the program toward quality of care and away from cost containment. The economic and political forces pushing for control of utilization and costs were too strong. The Council also made little progress toward developing standards of care; again, the climate for such efforts was not receptive.

The Council's value was as a regular public forum for discussion of issues pertinent to the PSRO program. The public meetings were extremely well attended, fostered both formal and informal interaction among the Council, public attendees, and staff, and permitted timely information to be published in the lay press concerning program direction. The Council provided, albeit imperfectly, for some accountability of the program, and it gave some opportunity for early review and consideration of program plans and advice to HCFA by a well-disposed, but external, group of experts.

Sanctions and Regulatory Orientation

PSROs were perceived as essentially regulatory mechanisms for controlling medical practice. HCFA (1980), for instance, characterized PSROs as "formalized externally authorized and mandated local physician organizations expected to function as a regulatory system exercising control via performance evaluations tied to financial and professional sanctions" (p. 141).

The PSRO program was hampered by its relatively limited ability to act on this presumed regulatory power and to bring or recommend sanctions against providers. Aggressive PSROs initiated sanctions generally the way PROs do now, except that sanctions were pursued internally at HCFA, not by the Office of Inspector General (OIG), and with similar results (e.g., very high costs and reversals at the level of administrative law judges). Furthermore, hospitals and other providers were assumed to have a favorable "waiver of liability" status. PSROs could only recommend to the relevant FI that the waiver be revoked, but the decision to do so resided with the FI.[4] In principle, the PROs have a considerably stronger hand in sanctioning physicians and hospitals than did the PSROs, in part because sanctions are now pursued through the OIG and in part because the waiver of liability issue has been muted. In practice (as will be seen), their regulatory power has not been demonstrably enhanced.

To gain the acceptance of the provider community in the early years, some congressional supporters and some executive branch directors of the program emphasized the quality-of-care (rather than the cost-control) thrust of the program (Blumstein, 1976). In quality assurance terms, this translated into an "educational" rather than a "regulatory" program. The ambiguity inherent in an "educational-regulatory" stance was never successfully resolved.

More importantly, a considerable ambiguity arose in the conflicting emphases on containing costs while maintaining quality. The framers of the PSRO legislation and program intended primarily that it lower the inappropriate or unnecessary use of services, as the alarming increase in the cost of medical care at that time was assumed to arise largely from overuse of services. Evaluations at the time were focused mainly on PSRO impacts on costs; for instance, from the General Accounting Office (GAO) in 1979 came *Problems with Evaluating the Cost Effectiveness of Professional Standards Review Organizations,* which was focused exclusively on savings in costs and patient hospital days, and from the Congressional Budget Office (CBO) in 1981 came *The Impact of PSROs on Health-Care Costs.* Evaluations of PSRO impacts on quality of care were never accorded similar status or conducted with equivalent sophistication. A major lesson of the PSRO program was that the conflict between using such agents simultaneously to contain costs and to maintain quality will almost surely shortchange the latter unless strong programmatic steps are taken to protect and emphasize it.

Impact of the PSRO Program

The net impact of PSROs on utilization, expenditures, or quality remains uncertain. Several evaluations of the PSRO program conducted in the late 1970s yielded contradictory findings (e.g., CBO, 1979, 1981; GAO, 1979; HCFA, 1980). Overall, the PSRO program probably saved as many resources as it consumed, but in an era of rapidly escalating health (and Medicare) expenditures, this was not perceived as an adequate level of performance (Lohr, 1985). PSROs did appear to have a slight positive impact on quality of care as measured by documented changes in medical practices rather than by dollar savings (HCFA, 1980; AAPSRO, 1981). Again, however, in an environment concerned chiefly with rising expenditures, these effects were not persuasive as regards the success of the PSRO program.

Among the conclusions that might be drawn about the PSRO experience were the following. Monitoring and evaluating a program that operates through almost 200 individual organizations is difficult. Budget constraints, although a fact of life, will compromise the effectiveness of such a program. Delegating review authority, when not accompanied by the power to remove delegation promptly for poor performance, can undermine the effectiveness of a program. Finally, it is exceedingly difficult to combine cost and quality functions in one organization, especially when expectations and evaluations of the program concentrate on cost issues.

Movement to a New Program

Disappointment at the limited effectiveness of the PSRO program prompted calls for its abolition or restructuring, and it was phased out in the early 1980s as the PRO program was slowly put into place. Despite rhetorical emphasis on assuring quality of care, the principal focus of the new PRO program initially remained on use of services and costs. In other words, philosophically not much changed.

Structurally, much about the program was revamped. The ability PROs to act against overuse of services and to curtail expenditures v strengthened (relative to the PSRO program), and administrative and financing arrangements were changed so that the program could, at least in theory, be better managed at the federal level. Nevertheless, many of the difficulties facing the PSRO program remained, not the least of them being the mismatch between the call for attention to quality of care and the funding for activities designed to control utilization and expenditures. In this vein, it is well to remember that the full name of the PROs is the Utilization and Quality Control Peer Review Organizations.

UTILIZATION AND QUALITY CONTROL PEER REVIEW ORGANIZATIONS (PROs)

The PRO program was a congressional response to considerable discouragement over the performance and impact of the PSRO program as well as an effort to design a system to fit the diagnosis-related group (DRG) prospective payment system (PPS) for hospital care that began in October 1983. Like PSROs, PROs are supposed to ensure that services rendered through Medicare are necessary, appropriate, and of high quality.

PRO activities, however, extend widely into many aspects of the administration of Medicare program. They are by no means confined to issues relating to use, costs, or quality of care, and certainly not just to ensuring the technical quality of care rendered to beneficiaries. PROs serve different purposes for different parties, not all of whom have the same interests or concerns. Given the hostility and disappointment registered about a PSRO program that was vastly less burdened with administrative and outreach responsibilities, this increase in the responsibilities and visibility of the program created to replace PSROs is somewhat ironic.

PROs carry out their complex assignments on a total annual budget that now approximates $300 million per year—a sum that seems large in the abstract but in fact accounts for about 0.3 percent of Medicare Part A and Part B expenditures. Thus, understanding the role and potential impact of PROs on assuring quality of care for Medicare calls for appreciating the many and complex tasks they have been assigned, the specificity of the contract requirements that govern those tasks, and the limited resources they can bring to bear on the required activities. The remainder of this chapter discusses these topics.

PRO Legislation and Regulations

Several pieces of legislation governed the development of the PRO program. The key act was the Tax Equity and Fiscal Responsibility Act (TEFRA) of 1982 [more specifically, the Peer Review Improvement Act, Title I, Subtitle C of TEFRA (P.L. 97-248)], which amended Part B of Title XI of the Social Security Act. Other important legislation included the Social Security Amendments of 1983 (P.L. 98-21), the Deficit Reduction Act (DEFRA) of 1984 (P.L. 98-369), the Consolidated Omnibus Budget Reconciliation Act (COBRA) of 1985 (P.L. 99-272), the Omnibus Budget Reconciliation Acts (OBRA) of 1986 and 1987 (P.L. 99-509 and P.L. 100-203), and the Medicare and Medicaid Patient Program Protection Act of 1987 (P.L. 93-100).

Apart from legislation, numerous regulations and other directives govern the administration and operation of the PROs. The Administrative Procedure Act (APA) requires that regulations be promulgated through notice and comment rulemaking procedures. HCFA follows the APA procedures in some instances. As an adjunct to the cumbersome and often lengthy public rulemaking mechanism, the agency also relies extensively on PRO *Manual* transmittals, contracts and contract modifications, and other, less formal instructions.

PRO Organizational Characteristics

PSRO regions were consolidated into 54 areas (all the states, the District of Columbia, Puerto Rico, the Virgin Islands, and a combined area of American Samoa, Guam, and the Commonwealth of the Northern Marianas). Beginning roughly in 1986, eight PROs covered two areas, and one PRO covered three areas.[5]

Congress tried to retain some semblance of "local" peer review. To qualify as a PRO, the statewide organizations must demonstrate sponsorship by being composed of at least 10 percent of the physicians practicing in the area (known as a physician-sponsored organization), or it must have available for PRO review at least one physician in every generally recognized specialty in the area (known as a physician-access organization); the former have priority. Third-party payers can obtain PRO contracts only if no other eligible organization is available. A PRO may not be a health care facility or other entity subject to review, it must have at least one consumer representative on its governing board, and it must operate with objectivity and without apparent or real conflict of interest.

PRO Contracts

PROs are financed through competitively awarded contracts. The very complex set of review and intervention tasks are specified in great detail in the "Scope of Work" (SOW) in the Request for Proposal for these contracts, and PRO performance is evaluated on the basis of how well they meet these specifications. Compared to a grant mechanism (as in the PSRO program), contracting makes the program more manageable centrally but renders the local entities less able to respond flexibly and sensitively to local problems and needs.

PRO contracts were initially established for two years, but OBRA 1987 extended contract periods to three years to permit somewhat more stability in anticipated financing and planning. PRO contracts can be renewed triennially or cancelled and put up for competitive bidding, or they can be terminated by either the PRO or the Secretary of DHHS at any time. The Secretary, in accordance with a complex set of procedures, has the absolute right either to terminate or to choose not to renew a PRO contract. The Secretary's decisions in this regard are not subject to judicial review and thus cannot be overturned in court.

Third PRO Scope of Work (1988-1990)

The first SOW was used during the first contract cycle (1984 to 1986), the second during the 1986-1988 contract cycle, and the third covers the present period. All PROs were expected to be on the third SOW as of April 1, 1989.[6]

Many PRO activities have remained fairly constant over the three SOWs, although the first SOW emphasized controlling inappropriate utilization and the second and third SOWs gave more attention to assuring quality. To achieve consistency with minimum disruption to ongoing review activities, much of the second SOW remains in the third but with variations in the size of samples. The following section and Table 6.1 describe PRO activities for only the third SOW; Table 6.2 briefly compares key activities for the three SOWs. The focus is on inpatient hospital review, but the activities do not differ appreciably for nonhospital practitioners or settings.

Required Review Activities for Hospital Inpatient Care

The following PRO review activities are required for all inpatient hospital cases reviewed retrospectively: (1) generic quality screening; (2) discharge review; (3) admission review; (4) review of invasive procedures; (5) DRG validation; (6) coverage review; and (7) determination of the application of the waiver of liability provision. These are described in more detail below.

Cases are identified for review through a random sampling process that constitutes 3 percent of all Medicare admissions and, in addition, through selection of cases for many specific reasons that reflect concern about use of services, costs to the Medicare program, or quality. Altogether, the pool of cases under review constitutes almost 25 percent of all Medicare admissions (Table 6.3).

TABLE 6.1 Elements of Required Peer Review Organization (PRO) Activities for the Third Scope of Work

I. Prospective Payment System (PPS) Hospital Cases[a]
   A. Random (the 3-percent sample)
   B. Transfers
      1. PPS to PPS hospitals
      2. PPS to exempt psychiatric units
      3. PPS to exempt swing beds
   C. Readmissions in less than 31 days from discharge from a PPS hospital with review of intervening care
      1. PPS hospital readmission
         a. Identifying all readmissions
         b. Review a random 25-percent hospital-specific sample
      2. Intervening care
         a. Identify all cases in the 25-percent sample with care rendered by skilled nursing facilities, home health agencies, or hospital outpatient departments
         b. Review a 20-percent sample of each hospitals' intervening care universe for quality of care (not medical necessity or overuse of services), with HCFA's generic quality screens
   D. Focused DRGs (100 percent review of DRGs 385-391, 472, 474, 475; 50 percent review of DRG 468; 25 percent review of DRG 462)[b]
   E. Day and cost outliers (25 percent random samples)
   F. Medicare code editor (12 principal diagnoses)[c]
   G. Hospital adjustments (any adjustments to higher weighted DRGs)
   H. Noncovered admissions (with covered level of care later in stay)
   I. FI and HCFA regional office referrals
II. Specialty Hospitals
   A. Exempt units of PPS hospitals
   B. Exempt hospitals
III. Ambulatory Surgery [Hospital Outpatient Areas and Ambulatory Surgical Centers (ASCs)]
IV. Intensified Review
V. Pre-admission and Pre-procedure reviews
   A. Ten procedures[d]
   B. Assistants at cataract surgery
VI. Review of Freestanding Cardiac Catheterization Facilities
VII. Objectives (e.g., based on Generic Quality Screens)
VIII. Development and Use of Explicit Written Criteria
IX. Reconsideration and Review of DRG Changes and Preparing Appeals Folders
X. Data
   A. Reports submitted to HCFA on completed reviews
   B. Profiling
      1. Hospital statistics (by 14 variables)
      2. Physician statistics (by 4 variables)
      3. Other provider statistics (HHA, SNFs, ASCs)
      4. Internal quality control (monitoring of review decisions)
XI. Beneficiary Communications
   A. *Important Message to Medicare Beneficiaries* (from hospitals)
   B. Hospital notices of noncoverage

C. Community outreach
   1. Hotline
   2. Written inquiries responses
   3. Education programs, seminars, and workshops
   4. Informational materials
   5. Coordination with beneficiary groups
XII. Responsiveness to Inquiries and Complaints
XIII. Interaction with Physicians and Providers
   A. Peer review
   B. Opportunity for consultation
   C. Education
   D. Criteria development and dissemination
   E. Communications
   F. Confidentiality and disclosure guidelines
   G. External relationships with concerned organizations
   H. Management responsibilities
XIV. Sanctions
XV. Confidentiality and Disclosure of Information
XVI. Fraud and Abuse Review (of Cases referred by OIG or HCFA)
XVII. Anti-Dumping Review (of Cases referred by HCFA)
XVIII. Private Review
XIX. Civilian Health and Medical Programs of the Uniformed Services (CHAMPUS)
XX. Other Requirements
   A. Cooperation with HCFA
   B. Cooperation with the SuperPRO
   C. Private review
   D. Internal quality control

---

[a]The required review activities include: generic quality screens, discharge review, admission review, invasive procedure review, DRG validation, coverage review, and waiver of liability.

[b]The DRG catagories are as follows: 385, neonates, died or transferred; 386, extreme immaturity, neonates; 387, prematurity with major problems; 388, prematurity without major problems; 389, full-term neonate with major problems; 390, neonate with other significant problems; 391, normal newborn; 462, rehabilitation; 468, unrelated operating room procedures; 472, extensive burns; 474, tracheostomy; and 475, mechanical ventilation through endotracheal intubation.

[c]Diabetes mellitus, without mention of complication, non-insulin dependent and insulin dependent; obesity; impacted cerumen; benign hypertension; left bundle branch hemiblock; other bundle branch hemiblock; positive SRL/VRL HL3; elevated blood pressure reading without diagnosis of hypertension; other and unspecified complications of medical care, not elsewhere specified; and cardiac pacemaker (fitting and adjustment).

[d]Carotid endarterectomy and cataract procedures are required. Eight of the following 11 can also be selected: cholecystectomy, major joint replacement, coronary artery bypass graft, percutaneous transluminal coronary angioplasty, laminectomy, complex peripheral revascularization, hysterectomy, bunionectomy, inguinal hernia repair, prostatectomy, and pacemaker insertion.

SOURCE: Attachment 33, HCFA, 1988.

TABLE 6.2 Comparison of the Three Scopes of Work (SOWs) with Respect to Selected Utilization and Quality Control Peer Review Organization (PRO) Activities (Ordered by Tasks Pertaining to the Third SOW)[a]

I. Prospective Payment System Hospitals Cases
Random Samples
> First SOW: 5 percent admission sample. DRG sample ranging from 3 to 100 percent based on hospital discharge size.
> Second SOW: 3 percent sample (includes 1- and 2-day stays)
> Third SOW: Same as second SOW

Transfers
> First SOW: From PPS to another hospital, exempt unit, or swing bed.
> Second SOW: Same as first SOW, but lower level of review
> Third SOW: PPS to PPS, 50 percent sample; PPS to psychiatric, 10 percent; and PPS to swing bed, 25 percent

Readmissions
> First SOW: All related readmissions within 7 days of discharge
> Second SOW: All related readmissions within 15 days of discharge
> Third SOW: 25 percent of readmissions within 31 days of discharge

Intervening Care
> First SOW: Not in scope of work
> Second SOW: Not in scope of work
> Third SOW: 20 percent of all cases receiving home health agency, hospital outpatient, inpatient, or skilled nursing facility (SNF) care between sampled hospital admissions less than 31 days apart.

Focused DRGs
> First SOW: Review of DRG numbers 462 and 468
> Second SOW: Review of DRG numbers 462, 468, and 088
> Third SOW: Review of DRG numbers 462, 468, 385-391, 472, 474-475[b]

Day and Cost Outliers
> First SOW: Originally 100 percent; reduced to 50 percent during contract period
> Second SOW: 50 percent of day and cost outliers
> Third SOW: 25 percent of day and cost outliers

Medicare Code Editor
> First SOW: 100 percent of nine diagnoses with code editor rejects
> Second SOW: Same as first SOW
> Third SOW: 100 percent of 12 diagnoses with code editor rejects[c]

Hospital Adjustments
> First SOW: 100 percent of all cases adjusted to a higher weighted DRG
> Second SOW: Same as first SOW
> Third SOW: Same as second SOW

FI and HCFA Regional Office Referrals
> First SOW: 100 percent review of cases referred by FI or HCFA regional office for determination of medical necessity
> Second SOW: Same as first SOW
> Third SOW: Same as second SOW

II. Specialty Hospital Review
> First SOW: Proposed by each PRO
> Second SOW: 15 percent of all discharges
> Third SOW: 15 percent random sample for PPS-exempt hospitals and units

III.   Ambulatory Surgery
     First SOW: Not in scope of work
     Second SOW: Not in scope of work
     Third SOW: 5 percent random sample of all cases

IV.   Intensified Review
     First SOW: Trigger: 2.5 percent or 3 cases reviewed (whichever is greater). Review increased to 100 percent or subsets.
     Second SOW: Trigger: 5 percent or 6 cases reviewed (whichever is greater). Review increased to 100 percent or subsets (two consecutive quarters)
     Third SOW: Same as second SOW

V.   Preadmission Review
     First SOW: 5 procedures proposed by each PRO
     Second SOW: Pacemaker plus 4 procedures proposed by the PRO
     Third SOW: 100 percent of 10 procedures (cataract extraction, cartoid endarterectomy plus 8 of 11 others specified by HCFA)[d]

VI.   Assistants at Cataract Surgery
     First SOW: Not in scope of work
     Second SOW: 100 percent review of cases for medical necessity of assistant at surgery
     Third SOW: Same as second SOW

VII.   Objectives
     First SOW: Three admission objectives and five quality objectives. All proposed and validated by the PRO. Very limited areas for focusing objectives
     Second SOW: Five objectives based on PRO data from first 90 days of generic quality screen review. HCFA-identified mortality rate outliers.
     Third SOW: Objectives based on data from generic screens. May be statewide, or focused by physician, DRG, provider, etc.

XI.   Hospital Notices of Noncoverage
     First SOW: 100 percent where patient or physician disagrees; 100 percent where patient is liable; 10 percent random sample
     Second SOW: Same as first SOW
     Third SOW: 100 percent where patient or physician disagrees; 100 percent where patient is liable

     Community Outreach
     First SOW: Not in scope of work
     Second SOW: Each PRO to propose its own program
     Third SOW: Minimum requirements to be met

---

[a]Roman numerals refer to parts in Table 6.1.
[b]For definitions, see Table 6.1.
[c]For definitions, see Table 6.1.
[d]For listing, see Table 6.1.

SOURCE: Adapted from unpublished HCFA documents.

TABLE 6.3 Numbers and Percentages of Cases Reviewed by Peer Review Organizations (PROs) Through May 1989 and Expected for Third Scope of Work

Category of Cases for Review	Number	Percent
Combined retrospective review and pre-admission and prepayment review through February 1989		
Cases selected for review	6,507,133	24
Cases reviewed	7,213,265	26[a]
Total bills and cases	27,397,688	
Estimated number of cases to be reviewed for the third SOW		
Hospital reviews	7,600,066	72
Health maintenance organization reviews	877,739	8
Ambulatory surgery reviews	2,063,985	20
Total	10,541,793	

[a]Technical notes to the data summary indicate that the fact that more cases are shown as reviewed than as selected for review is an artifact of counting practices; for instance, transfer and readmission categories involve reviewing two or more cases, and Medicare Code Editor cases are reported under both pre-admission, pre-payment, and retrospective review.

SOURCE: HCFA, 1989d.

Generic quality screening. Hospital generic quality screens are widely used to detect what are regarded as the most common causes or manifestations of potential quality problems (Table 6.4). Introduced in the second SOW in the fall of 1986 (without pilot-testing), they were carried over into the third SOW. Most changes in generic screens occur in the interpretive guidelines that are issued with the screens, not in the screens themselves. HCFA issued interpretive guidelines in May 1987 and in 1988 met with each PRO to review and critique the screens for modification in the third SOW.

The six required generic quality screens covered the following: (1) adequacy of discharge planning; (2) medical stability of patient at discharge; (3) unexpected deaths; (4) nosocomial infections; (5) unscheduled return to surgery; and (6) trauma suffered in hospital. In addition, PROs can use an optional screen for medication or treatment changes (including discontinuation) within 24 hours of discharge without adequate observation. The third

TABLE 6.4 Generic Quality Screens—Hospital Inpatient

1. Adequacy of Discharge Planning[a]
   No documentation of discharge planning or appropriate followup care with consideration of physical, emotional and mental status needs at time of discharge.
2. Medical Stability of the Patient at Discharge
   a. Blood pressure within 24 hours of discharge (systolic less than 85 or greater than 180; diastolic less than 50 or greater than 100)
   b. Temperature within 24 hours of discharge greater than 101 degrees Fahrenheit (38.3 Centigrade) oral; greater than 102 degrees Fahrenheit (38.9 Centigrade) rectal
   c. Pulse less than 50 (or 45 if the patient is on a beta blocker), or greater than 120 within 24 hours of discharge
   d. Abnormal diagnostic findings which are not addressed and resolved or where the record does not explain why they are not resolved
   e. Intravenous fluids or drugs after 12 midnight on day of discharge
   f. Purulent or bloody drainage of wound or open area within 24 hours prior to discharge
3. Deaths
   a. During or following any surgery performed during the current admission
   b. Following return to intensive care unit, coronary care or other special care unit within 24 hours of being transferred out
   c. Other unexpected death
4. Nosocomial Infection[a] (Hospital-acquired infection)
5. Unscheduled Return to Surgery
   Within same admission for same condition as previous surgery or to correct operative problem
6. Trauma Suffered in the Hospital
   a. Unplanned surgery which includes, but is not limited to, removal or repair of a normal organ or body part (i.e., surgery not addressed specifically in the operative consent)
   b. Fall[a]
   c. Serious complications of anesthesia
   d. Any transfusion error or serious transfusion reaction
   e. Hospital-acquired decubitus ulcer and/or deterioration of an existing decubitus[a]
   f. Medication error or adverse drug reaction (1) with serious potential for harm or (2) resulting in measures to correct
   g. Care or lack of care resulting in serious or potentially serious complications

"Optional Screen"

Medication or treatment changes (including discontinuation) within 24 hours of discharge without adequate observation

[a]PRO reviewer is to record the failure of the screen, but need not refer potential severity Level I quality problems to physician reviewer until a pattern emerges.

SOURCE: HCFA, 1988.

SOW also adds an adequacy-of-care screen to the set of "trauma" screens; it is defined as inappropriate or untimely assessment, intervention, and/or management resulting in serious or potentially serious complications. Generic screens are applied to all hospital charts under review by the PRO for any reason.

Figures 6.1A and 6.1B illustrate the generic screening process. Generic screens are first applied by nurse reviewers, who can determine that a case passes the screens. If a case fails any screen and has a potential quality problem, then it must be referred to a physician advisor for further evaluation; only the physician advisor can "confirm" a quality problem. (A physician advisor is a physician practicing in the state who is hired to do peer review.) Initially, nurse reviewers were required to refer all screen failures to physician advisors; this produced considerable numbers of false-positive cases and appreciable frustration and anger for reviewers and the medical community. HCFA later permitted PRO nurse reviewers to override this rule for screens relating to adequacy of discharge planning, nosocomial infections, falls, and decubitus ulcers as part of the trauma screen; all remaining cases failing a screen and involving a potential quality problem must still be referred to a physician advisor.

Discharge review is intended to flag problems with premature discharge when the patient was not medically stable at discharge or when discharge was not consistent with the patient's continued need for acute inpatient care.

Retrospective *admission review* identifies whether inpatient hospital care was medically necessary and appropriate, by reviewing reasons for admission against pre-established criteria devised or adopted by individual PROs.

Invasive procedure review retrospectively examines the medical necessity of invasive procedures that affect the assignment of a case to one DRG rather than another (which means nearly all such procedures done in the hospital setting). The review is applied to cases already selected for review, not to any other cases. If the procedure is not medically necessary or is not a covered service, and if the procedure was the sole reason for admission, then payment for the entire admission and the procedure is denied. If the procedure is not medically necessary or is not covered, but the admission is medically necessary and other reasonable and necessary services were provided, then the physician's payment for the procedure is denied, and the DRG is changed.

DRG validation assures that cases are accurately classified for Medicare payment under PPS. It also ensures that the responsible physicians have certified that their narrative descriptions of the principal and secondary diagnoses and the major procedures are accurate and complete to the best of their knowledge (a statement known as physician attestation). A Registered Record Administrator or an Accredited Record Technician generally has the

FIGURE 6.1A Overview of the Quality Review Process for Inpatient Hospital, Home Health Agency and Outpatient Surgery Generic Screens[a]

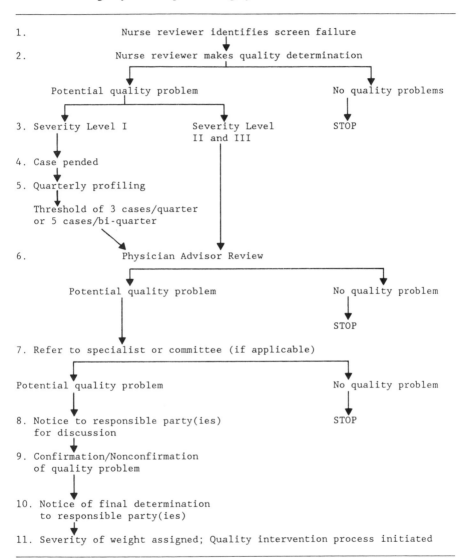

[a]Includes inpatient hospital screens 1, 4, 6b, and 6e and certain home health agency and outpatient surgery screens.

SOURCE: HCFA, 1988.

FIGURE 6.1B   Overview of the Quality Review Process for Other Generic
Screens[b]

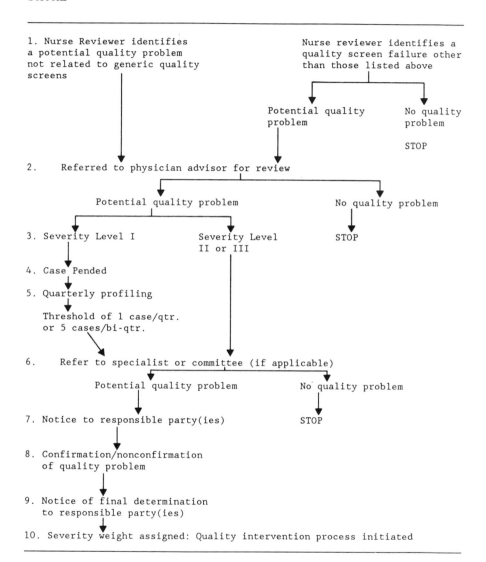

[b]Includes inpatient hospital, home health agency, and outpatient surgery generic
screens not covered by the process in Figure 6.1A.

SOURCE: HCFA, 1988.

responsibility for the validation process at the PRO. The results of DRG validation can be to leave the DRG unchanged or to upgrade or downgrade it, thereby affecting the hospital payment.

Coverage review determines whether items or services normally excluded from Medicare coverage are medically necessary; it is done only in instances when coverage can be extended for specific items and circumstances if certain conditions are met. Under the *waiver of liability* (also referred to as limitation of liability), the PRO must determine whether the beneficiary or provider should be held liable for care not covered under Medicare because either the beneficiary or provider knew, or could reasonably have been expected to know, that such care was not covered.

Pre-admission and Pre-procedure Review

PROs are required to review 10 procedures, generally on a pre-admission or pre-procedure basis, for necessity and for appropriateness of setting (e.g., inpatient or ambulatory). They must review all proposed carotid endarterectomies and cataract procedures and an additional 8 procedures selected from a list of 11 supplied by HCFA.[7] Each PRO establishes its own prior-authorization criteria, sometimes in consultation with local or state physician specialty groups, and some criteria are shared among PROs. Not surprisingly, PROs differ in the types of clinical factors or levels of patient functioning that they require to be present (or absent) before they will approve the procedure (see Table 6.5 for an example).

Rural Providers

Rural physicians and hospitals have vigorously asserted that they are not reviewed by local peers and that their style of practice and the constraints under which they function are not well appreciated or taken into account. To help overcome these criticisms and to bring the peer review effort more fully into areas that were rarely visited, the third SOW mandates that at least 20 percent of all rural hospitals be reviewed on-site. Moreover, during the sanctioning process rural physicians (those in officially designated rural health manpower shortage areas or in counties of fewer than 70,000 residents) are given special protections that put exclusions from the Medicare program on hold until full hearings have been conducted, unless a judge determines that the provider or practitioner poses a serious risk to individuals in those areas if permitted to continue to furnish such services.

Nonhospital Review

Various acts direct PROs to undertake review in several nonhospital settings apart from physician offices. By and large, nonhospital review

TABLE 6.5 Examples of Peer Review Organization (PRO) Criteria for Prior Authorization of Cataract Procedures as Part of Pre-Procedure Review

Delmarva PRO[a]
  Indications for a cataract procedures require:
  1. Visual acuity of 20/50 or worse in the affected eye for distance or visual acuity of 20/40 or worse in the affected eye for near vision;
  2. Three other criteria are also stated:
     a. visual acuity is interfering with the patient's lifestyle,
     b. cataracts are causing another ocular disease, and
     c. cataract is preventing treatment for another disease.
New York PRO
  Indications for the procedure require the patient to meet one specific criterion and one of several additional criteria:
  1. Specific criteria:
     Cataract removal will improve the patient's visual performance for daily activities, employment, or recreation.
  2. Among the remaining additional criteria are: vision in the operative eye is less than 20/60; the non-operative eye is phakic and visual acuity is less than 20/40.

[a]Another set of specifications is given as indications for admission for the procedure.

activities have not been very comprehensive. The main effort to date has been review of a small sample of cases receiving "intervening care"—mainly, care delivered by home health agencies (HHAs) and skilled nursing facilities (SNFs) between two related hospital admissions up to 31 days apart. This effort was not preceded by demonstration or pilot projects or pretesting. Initiatives in the other settings, especially ambulatory physician office care, are getting underway mainly as pilot projects.

For the third SOW, generic quality screens have been developed to review care rendered in the following settings: HHAs, SNFs, hospital outpatient departments (HOPDs), and ambulatory surgery centers (ASCs). The new screens are similar to inpatient generic screens, but they are supposed to be more relevant to the particular setting (Volume II, Chapter 6, Table 8.4). For example, the SNF screens deal with polypharmacy (multiple medication) issues and the mental stability of the resident. Screens for reviewing psychiatric care were issued to PROs in November 1989, and those for rehabilitative services are scheduled for completion in FY 1990.

PRO Responses to Quality or Utilization Problems

PROs can pursue several interventions when they have confirmed a quality or utilization problem. They can notify practitioners or providers of problems, put practitioners and providers on "intensified" review, require a wide variety of corrective actions, or institute sanction procedures. Although these interventions have been available since the start of the PRO program, they are now required to be part of a written quality intervention plan.

Quality Intervention Plan

The quality intervention plan (QIP) is "a prescribed blueprint which requires PROs to implement specific interventions in response to confirmed quality problems" (*Federal Register*, 1989a, p. 1966). The QIP is intended to promote greater consistency among PROs by a more systematic follow-up of identified problem practitioners or providers. (The terms practitioners and providers are used by the PRO program to refer, respectively, to physicians or other individual clinical caregivers and to facilities and institutions such as hospitals.) Minimum QIP requirements set by HCFA include a timeframe for completion of the review process, determination of the source of the problem, assignment of quality problem "severity levels" and weights, profiling, and quality interventions that are related to severity levels.

Timeframe. HCFA has determined a maximum time frame for quality review for the third SOW. If a potential Severity Level I problem exists (defined below), the case is held in a pending status until a pattern of problems emerges. For all other severity levels, the maximum time frame for completion of the review is 135 days.

Determine source of the problem. All initial case reviews are completed by a nurse reviewer, with potential quality problem cases passed on to a physician advisor. If the physician advisor and the PRO decide that an apparent quality problem does exist, the PRO determines the source of the problem (e.g., individual physician or hospital) and, after an opportunity for discussion with the caregiver in question, assigns a "severity level."

Assign severity levels and weights. Severity levels are a way to categorize quality problems according to the nature of the problem and its potential for causing adverse patient outcomes. The relevant phrase, significant adverse effects, is defined as unnecessarily prolonged treatment, complication, or readmission or patient management that results in anatomical or physiological impairment, disability, or death. Weights (numerical points) assigned to severity levels indicate when PROs must take various corrective steps. The levels (with weights in parentheses) and definitions are as follows:

- *Severity level I* (1): Medical mismanagement without the potential for significant adverse effects on the patient;[8]
- *Severity level II* (5): Medical mismanagement with the potential for significant adverse effects on the patient; and
- *Severity level III* (25): Medical mismanagement with significant adverse effects on the patient.

Conduct profile analyses. The purpose of profiling as part of the QIP is to identify areas for focused review or other corrective action. The PRO is required to produce several types of profiles of physicians, providers, and quality problems on a quarterly basis, as a means of tracking problems and determining whether various thresholds for mandatory interventions (see below) have been exceeded.

Quality interventions. When a PRO identifies and eventually confirms that a quality problem exists, then it develops a corrective action plan using a variety of interventions. These include:

1. *Notification.* The PRO sends a notice that it has made a final determination of a confirmed quality problem to the practitioner or provider. This notice must describe the quality problem, what the appropriate action should have been, the severity level, and what interventions will be taken.
2. *Education.* These include telephone and in-person discussions with the responsible parties, suggested literature reading, continuing medical education (CME) courses, and self-education courses.
3. *Intensification.* The PRO may increase its scrutiny of the provider's or practitioner's cases through 100-percent retrospective review or intensified review of just certain types of cases (a focused subsample).
4. *Other interventions.* The PRO may take other steps, such as concurrent or pre-discharge review; prior approval or pre-admission review; and referral to hospital committees (e.g., infection control, tissue, or quality assurance committees).
5. *Coordination with licensing and accreditation bodies.* The PRO must disclose confidential information to state and federal licensing bodies upon request when such information is required by those entities to carry out their legal functions, and the PRO may do so even without a request (e.g., when a practitioner or provider has reached a weighted score of 25 points in one quarter).
6. *Sanction* plans (discussed below).

The PRO must use certain thresholds, called weighted triggers, to decide what intervention it should use. The interventions and weighted triggers (points per quarter) are as follows: notification, 1 (or 5 per bi-quarter); education, 10; intensification, 15; other interventions, 20; coordination with licensing bodies, 25; and sanctions, 25. The PRO has some flexibility to take interventions before a threshold is reached (such as a weighted severity score of 25) or to apply lower-weighted interventions in special circumstances. The PRO also has some discretion not to invoke coordination and sanctions interventions, although it must consider them and document why it did not take such action.

Sanctions

PRO, OIG, and DHHS Responsibilities

The Secretary of DHHS, not the PROs, holds the authority to impose sanctions on Medicare providers. The Secretary has delegated that authority to the OIG. The PROs' power is in making sanction recommendations to the OIG in either of two instances: (1) cases of "substantial violation" of a practitioner's or provider's Medicare obligations "in a substantial number of cases" (Figure 6.2A), and (2) single cases of a "gross and flagrant" violation (Figure 6.2B). A substantial violation in a substantial number of cases is a pattern of care that is inappropriate, unnecessary, does not meet recognized professional standards of care, or is not supported by sufficient documentation. Gross and flagrant violation means a violation of an obligation (in one or more cases) that represents an imminent danger to a Medicare beneficiary's health, safety, or well-being or that places a beneficiary at an unnecessarily high risk.

No regulations define the criteria to be used by a PRO in making a determination whether a practitioner or provider has violated a Medicare obligation. The preamble to the PRO regulations states that PROs must apply professionally developed standards of care, diagnosis, and treatment based on typical patterns of practice in their geographic areas (*Federal Register*, 1985). The PRO *Manual* also contains some material on the elements of a sanctionable offense.

For cases in which the PRO determines that the provider or physician has failed to comply substantially with a Medicare obligation in a substantial number of cases, it sends the practitioner or provider an initial sanction notice.[9] This notice gives the recipient 20 days to respond to the notification with additional information or to request a meeting with the PRO. If, after considering the additional information, the PRO confirms its original finding, it develops a corrective plan of action. If the practitioner or provider fails to comply with that plan, the PRO sends a second sanction notice. In such cases, the provider or practitioner has a second opportunity

FIGURE 6.2A   Overview of PRO/HHS Sanction Process for Substantial Violations[a]

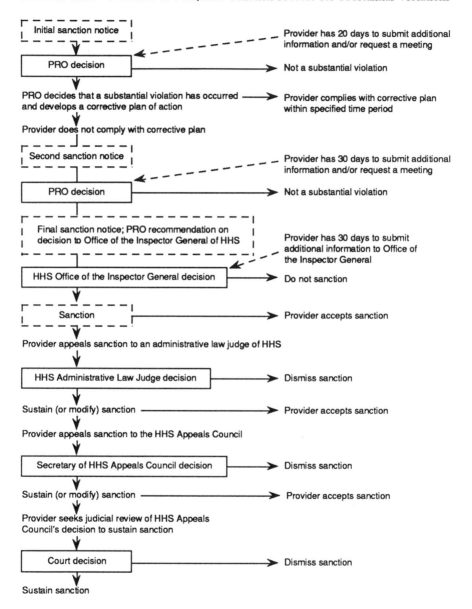

[a]A substantial violation is a pattern of care over a substantial number of cases that is inappropriate, unnecessary, does not meet recognized patterns of care, or is not supported by the documentation of care required by the PRO.

SOURCE: Adapted with permission from OTA, 1988.

FIGURE 6.2B   Overview of PRO/HHS Sanction Process for Gross and Flagrant Violations[a]

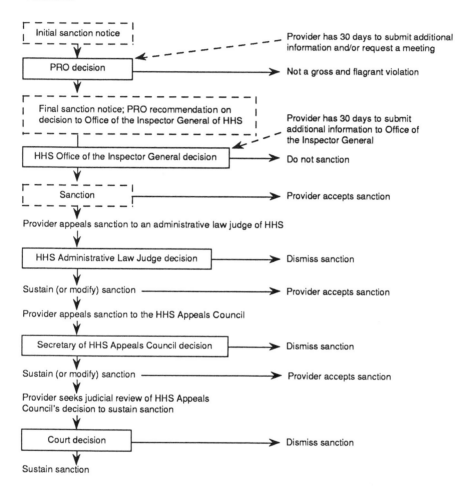

[a]A gross and flagrant violation is a violation that has occurred in one or more instances and presents an imminent danger to the health, safety, or well-being of a Medicare benificiary.

SOURCE: Adapted with permission from OTA, 1988.

to submit additional information or discuss the problem with the PRO (within 30 days of the second notice).

If the concern is not resolved, the procedures at this point follow the pattern for "gross and flagrant" violations. Several specific procedures direct how the PRO should forward its recommendation to the OIG and how it should notify the individual or organization that is has done so, what the recommended sanction is, and how further information can be forwarded directly to the OIG (again within 30 days). The PRO must also give the practitioner or provider a copy of the material it used in reaching its decision. At this point, the responsible sanctioning party is the OIG, not the PRO.

The OIG must determine whether the PRO followed appropriate procedures, whether a violation occurred, whether the provider has "demonstrated an unwillingness or lack of ability substantially to comply with statutory obligations" (known as the "willing and able" provision), and ultimately whether it agrees with the PRO recommendation (OIG, 1988b). In these determinations, the OIG is expected to consider the type and severity of the offense, the previous sanction record, previous problems that Medicare may have had with the individual or institution, and the availability of alternative medical resources in the community. The OIG can sustain the PRO recommendation, alter it, or reject it.

If the OIG does not accept the PRO's recommendation, the sanctioning process stops. If, however, a PRO recommends exclusion and the OIG does not act on that recommendation within 120 days, the exclusion automatically goes into effect until a final determination is made. To date, the OIG has met the statutory deadline in all cases.

If the OIG does accept the PRO's recommendation, it must give notice that the sanction is to be imposed, effective 15 days after the notice is received by the practitioner or provider. The OIG notifies the public by placing a notice in a newspaper of general circulation in the individual's or institution's locality.[10] It also informs state Medicaid fraud control units and state licensing bodies, hospitals and other facilities where the practitioner has privileges, medical societies, carriers, FIs, and health maintenance organizations (HMOs).

Sanctioned providers or practitioners may appeal the OIG decision to an administrative law judge (ALJ), who conducts a separate hearing starting essentially from scratch. If practitioners or providers are dissatisfied with the outcome of their hearing, they can request review by the Department's Appeals Council and then still seek judicial review of the decision at the level of a federal district court.

If the OIG proceeds successfully with these steps, the Secretary, through the OIG, can apply two kinds of formal sanctions: (1) exclusion from the Medicare program (for one or more years) and (2) monetary sanctions (which at present cannot exceed the cost of the services rendered). Excluded hospitals and providers must petition to be reinstated in the Medicare program, and they can receive (with a few exceptions) no payment for services rendered or items provided during the exclusion period.

Historical Record of Interventions and Sanctions

The most frequent PRO intervention appears to be the formal letter of notification. By contrast, intensified review, formal education or similar programs, and sanction recommendations are used much less often, although during the second SOW more than 53 percent of hospitals were under intensified review for at least one quarter (HCFA, 1989c). PROs differ markedly in the rates at which they invoke various interventions. For instance, GAO (1988b) cites the following two ranges for letters of notification: zero to as frequently as 111 times per 1,000 "new" physicians, and zero to 396 times per 1,000 "repeat" physicians.

PRO activity. Tables 6.6 a, b, and c summarize intervention activity tabulated by HCFA for the second SOW, the most recent aggregate information. Of the more than 6.6 million completed reviews (mainly for the second SOW), PROs denied payment in over 4 percent of cases; the range across PROs was 1.2 percent to 25.5 percent. For about 33 percent of these denials the practitioner or provider requested a reconsideration (range, 0.6 percent to 69.6 percent). Of those reconsiderations, the denials were reversed in 44 percent (range, 15.1 percent to 100 percent); that is, the original decision was upheld in 56 percent of the cases (Table 6.6a).

Through early 1989, the PROs had identified more than 87,000 physicians with some level of quality problem (Table 6.6b). Over 81,400 of those problems had been resolved, presumably through the more than 70,000 quality interventions carried out (HCFA, 1989c). HCFA data compiled from the start of the program through June 1989 shows that 43 PROs had sent a total of 1,065 first notices; the vast majority were to physicians rather than hospitals. More notices to physicians were for gross and flagrant violations than for substantial violations; the opposite was true for hospitals.

They had also recommended a total of 119 sanctions to the OIG (Table 6.6c), the vast majority (80) for gross and flagrant violations by physicians. Many of the sanction cases date from earlier years of the program. The relatively lower numbers of sanction recommendations in more recent times has generated some debate and has been attributed to three factors: (1) revisions in procedures (prompted by the AMA) that give practitioners the right to counsel during discussions with PROs of possible sanctions, (2) the OIG directives that discouraged use of monetary fines as an alternative to exclusion, and (3) possibly the high reversal rate of the ALJs, who had

TABLE 6.6a Quality Intervention Activities of Peer Review Organizations (PROs) Through June 1989: Reconsiderations

Type of Action	Number	Percent of Completed Reviews	Percent of Denials	Percent of Reconsiderations Requested
Completed reviews	6,655,505			
Payment denials	278,294	4.2		
Reconsiderations requested	91,268	1.4	32.8	
Reconsiderations upheld	51,252	0.8	18.4	56.2

SOURCE: HCFA, 1989d.

TABLE 6.6b Quality Intervention Activities of PROs Through February 1989: Quality Interventions for Physicians

Category	Number of Cases	
	Newly identified	Repeat cases
Physicians with quality problems	87,075	20,598
Physicians with quality problems resolved	81,440	19,888
Quality interventions taken	70,321	26,871

SOURCE: HCFA, 1989c.

TABLE 6.6c Quality Intervention Activities of PROs Through June 1989: Sanctions

Category of Activity	Number of	
	Physicians	Providers
First notices sent	907	158
Substantial violations	335	109
Gross and flagrant violations	572	49
Second notices sent[a]	68	17
Cases referred to the		
Office of Inspector General	109	10
Substantial violations	29	1
Gross and flagrant violations	80	9

[a]Second notices are sent only in cases of substantial violations.

SOURCE: HCFA, 1989d.

upheld only 8 of 18 sanctions on appeal during this period (McIlrath, 1989). In addition to these points, the growing confusion and tension caused by mixed signals from HCFA and the OIG concerning the relative emphasis to place on an educational and disciplinary approach to PRO implementation may have played a role in the sanction-recommendation picture.

OIG activity. From FY 1986 through September, 1989, the OIG reported it had received 197 referrals (150 gross and flagrant, 46 substantial, and 1 lack of documentation) (unpublished data made available to the study). Of these, 79 cases (40 percent) were rejected. Of the remainder, two cases were closed because the physician died, three physicians retired before exclusion, and three cases were pending. A total of 110 sanctions had been imposed (56 percent). Of the latter, 83 were exclusions (82 physicians; 1 facility) and 27 were monetary penalties (25 physicians; 2 facilities). In short, the OIG accepts about three in five sanction recommendations from PROs, a figure that has been fairly constant across the years. Of cases rejected, about two in five are because the case did not meet regulatory requirements, about two in five because the practitioner could show he or she was willing and able to improve, and one in five for adequate medical evidence. Of the sanctions imposed, the great majority are exclusions from the program.

Other Required Activities

Beneficiary Relations

PROs are required to act on behalf of Medicare beneficiaries in four ways not directly related to the technical quality of care rendered by providers or physicians. First, they must monitor hospitals' distribution to Medicare patients of the *Important Message from Medicare*; this pamphlet describes patients' rights to appeal denials of hospital care. Second, they must monitor how well hospitals issue notices of noncoverage when the hospitals themselves determine that the patient's care is not (or will not be) covered because it is not medically necessary, is not delivered in the appropriate setting, or is custodial.

Third, PROs must conduct at least five specific types of community education and outreach activities. The required tasks are quite broad. They include: maintaining a toll-free hotline; responding to written inquiries; conducting education programs, seminars, and workshops to inform beneficiaries about PRO review, PPS, and their appeal rights; developing and disseminating informational materials (e.g., brochures, slides, tapes) about those same topics; and coordinating with concerned beneficiary and provider groups. They must also have at least one consumer representative on the PRO board.

Finally, PROs must investigate all written complaints from beneficiaries about the quality of care rendered by hospitals (inpatient or outpatient), SNFs, HHAs, ASCs, HMOs, and CMPs. Here, the focus is on overuse of care or care that does not meet professionally recognized standards because PROs are barred from reviewing complaints involving underuse.

Community Outreach

The PROs must conduct programs to inform beneficiaries about Medicare PRO review and PPS, more specifically about the purpose of the PROs and PPS, types of PRO review, and their right to appeal a PRO determination. The PROs are also expected to devise ways to explain how they ensure the quality of care and respond to complaints from beneficiaries.

Provider Relations

The PRO program continues to stress "peer review"; in PRO terms, this is taken to mean physician advisors who practice in a setting similar to that of the reviewed physicians and/or who were trained in the appropriate discipline. It also calls for an "interaction plan" to enhance the relationships between the PROs and providers, physicians, and other practitioners. That plan must describe how physicians will be given opportunities to discuss problems or proposed denials and how the PRO will carry out educational efforts. The outreach activities for practitioners and institutional providers are similar to those required for beneficiaries (seminars; informational material; etc.).

The PRO is also required to publish and disseminate (at least annually) a report that describes its findings about care that does not meet Medicare obligations (i.e., necessary, appropriate, and of acceptable professional standards). This task mirrors the requirement that DHHS should submit to the Congress an annual report on the administration, impact, and cost of the program; such reports have not been published to date, however.

Data Acquisition, Sharing, and Reporting

Rules governing PRO data acquisition, sharing, and disclosure are complex and open to different interpretations. PROs can obtain any records and information pertaining to health care services rendered to Medicare beneficiaries that are in the possession of any practitioner or provider in the PRO area. Often a quality problem may be adequately handled for Medicare patients only by addressing it for all patients; if authorized by the practitioner or provider, PROs can gain access to non-Medicare patient records.[11]

Generally, information or records acquired by a PRO are confidential[12] and not subject to disclosure. PROs are granted by statute a flat exemption from requirements of the Freedom of Information Act. In some circumstances, PROs are required to disclose certain confidential information to appropriate agencies (for instance, when the PRO believes that not to do so would pose a risk to public health or in fraud and abuse situations).

Summary hospital-specific information that does not identity patients or physicians (such as average length of stay or death rates) is usually not considered confidential and thus can be released. PROs must, however, notify a hospital when it intends to disclose information about that institution (other than certain routine reports) and give the institution a copy of the information to be released and an opportunity to submit comments. Release of patient-identifying and physician-identifying information is limited to that required for PRO review or for other statutorily required reasons; one effect of this restriction is that hospitals might not be informed about physicians whose practice patterns are being examined by the PRO for quality-of-care reasons.

PROs are required to exchange information with FIs and carriers, with other PROs, and with other public or private review organizations. For instance, they must contact state medical licensing boards to exchange data about quality review efforts and to establish mechanisms by which the state medical boards can send to the PRO the names of physicians against whom the board has taken disciplinary action. The PRO is then required to review all of that practitioner's cases (except for services provided in the physician's office) for the three months following notification by the board. PRO responsibility to provide information to state agencies on physicians who are involved in quality interventions (corrective action plans) or in sanction proceedings is less clear but certainly is contemplated. PROs are not at present required to submit information about physician sanction recommendations to the National Practitioner Data Bank (which is being established through the Health Care Quality Improvement Act of 1986 (P.L. 99-660) (*Federal Register*, 1989b).

Costs

The annual PRO program budgets (excluding internal expenditures of HCFA) have risen markedly in absolute terms in the late 1980s, although in earlier years they did not keep pace with the funding levels of the PSRO program (see Table 6.7). Overall, the budget now approximates $300 million a year (estimated for FY 1989), up from $157 million for the first round of PRO contracts.[13] The Congressional Research Service (CRS) cited a figure of $187.5 million for FY 1987 and a proposed level of $176 million for FY 1988 (Cislowski, 1987); a budget of $330 million is estimated for FY 1991.

TABLE 6.7 Medicare Program, Professional Standards Review Organization (PSRO) Program, and Peer Review Organization (PRO) Program Expenditures: Selected Fiscal Years

| | Type of Expenditure | | | | |
Fiscal Year	Medicare Expenditure (in billions)	PSRO Program Budgets (in millions)	PSRO Expenditures as a Percentage of Medicare Expenditures	PRO Program Budgets (in millions)	PRO Expenditures as a Percentage of Medicare Expenditures
1973	$9.5	$4.3	0.45		
1981	42.5	173.7	0.4		
1987	81.6			$187.5	0.2
1989	98.5[a]			300	0.3
1991	130.0[a]			330	0.3

[a]Proposed

SOURCES: Medicare expenditures: Committee on Ways and Means, 1989, Table 15. PSRO budgets: HCFA, 1980. PRO Budgets: Cislowski, 1987; HCFA, unpublished estimates, 1989.

PRO budgets are based on negotiated costs for "simple," "complex," and ambulatory reviews, for fixed administrative costs and some start-up costs (largely accounting system updates), for photocopy and postage costs, and for costs of CHAMPUS review for those PROs doing such review. According to data from negotiated three-year contracts, per-review costs average $17.03 for simple review (range, roughly $13 to $32), $33.29 for complex review (range, nearly $27 to over $48), and $9.16 for ambulatory review (range, $4 to almost $15) (unpublished HCFA data, 4/11/89).

In FY 1987, Part A Medicare benefits amounted to $50.8 billion and Part B outlays to $30.8 billion (for a total of $81.6 billion) (Committee on Ways and Means, 1989). Two different figures have been cited for FY 1987 PRO outlays: $187.5 million by the CRS and $155 million (for just inpatient review) by the General Accounting Office (GAO, 1988a). Taking the higher (total) figure, PRO expenditures as a percent of Medicare outlays that year still amounted to only about 0.2 percent of all outlays (Table 6.7); focusing on just inpatient care, PRO expenditures approximated 0.3 percent of expenditures.

Table 6.7 shows estimated PRO budgets and Medicare outlays for FY 1989 and FY 1991; an intermediate estimate for FY 1990 puts expenditures at better than $112 billion and the PRO budget at $290 million. In all cases, PRO program budgets as a percentage of Medicare outlays 0.3 percent.

In proportion to total Medicare expenditures, these amounts for program are lower than those for the PSRO program (see Table 6.7). Even if the $11 million or so intended for pilot projects (see below) were added in to the estimates above for the PRO program, its expenditures would not exceed those of the PSRO program as a percentage of expected Medicare outlays.

Given the expanded responsibilities of the PROs compared with the PSROs, the markedly changing environment of health care for the elderly, and the greater perception of threats to high quality care in the future, some view this level of funding as parsimonious. Furthermore, even if the $300 million per year were adequate for all the varied activities presently required of the PROs, the need for future congressional or executive branch assignments to be adequately budgeted should be clear.

Quality Review in Medicare HMOs and CMPs[14]

As of April 1989, one million Medicare beneficiaries were enrolled in 133 risk contracts held by health maintenance organizations (HMOs) and competitive medical plans (CMPs); that figure accounts for about 3 percent of the Medicare population. The history of quality review for the care rendered to such beneficiaries by HMOs and CMPs is both complex and significant, the latter chiefly because it ushered in efforts (a) to design a way to reduce required review for providers having an adequate quality assurance plan of their own, (b) to review "episodes" of care, and (c) to review ambulatory care provided in physicians' offices.

Before COBRA 1985, no specific *legislative* requirements existed for the review of services provided to Medicare beneficiaries enrolled in risk-contract HMOs and CMPs. Because of continuing concern about possible underuse in risk-contract programs, COBRA 1985 mandated "comparable review" of care rendered in HMOs and CMPs for services given after January 1, 1987; it did not provide for pilot projects or staged implementation. The "comparable review" language was interpreted to mean that the number of cases reviewed must be at the same level as was occurring under PPS in the fee-for-service system; this in turn implied a substantial volume of medical record review.

To stimulate competition among review organizations, OBRA 1986 allowed review of HMO and CMP services by entities other than PROs (namely, Quality Review Organizations or QROs). At the outset, one QRO was awarded the review contracts for the states of Illinois, Kansas, and Missouri.[15] All remaining HMO and CMP review was done by PROs for plans in their own states, except for California Medical Review, Inc., which was awarded the review for Arizona and Hawaii.

Limited, Basic, and Intensified Review

HMO and CMP review has three possible levels: limited, basic, and intensified (see Table 6.8). *Basic* review is the core approach to HMO and CMP review. *Limited* review is intended to reduce the volume of active

TABLE 6.8 Summary of Activities for Health Maintenance Organization (HMO) and Competitive Medical Plan (CMP) Review, by Requirements for Limited, Basic, and Intensified Review

Type of Review	Sample Size for		
	Limited	Basic	Intensified
Thirteen sentinel conditions[a]	50% RS[b] (of only 4 conditions)	50% RS	100%
Hospital admissions	3% RS	3% RS	6% RS
Transfers[c]	100%	100%	100%
Readmissions within less than 31 days	25% RS	50% RS	100%
Nontrauma deaths in all care settings	5% RS	10% RS	100%

[a]These conditions, which are defined by ICD-9-CM codes, include: diabetic complications (ketoacidosis, hyperosmolar coma, other coma, and hypoglycemic coma); acute appendicitis with generalized peritonitis or peritoneal abscess; hypertensive problems (several categories, including occlusion and stenosis of precerebral arteries and transient cerebral ischemia); gastrointestinal catastrophes (acute, chronic, or unspecified gastric ulcer with hemorrhage without obstruction; chronic duodenal ulcer with hemorrhage without obstruction; unspecified intestinal obstruction); gangrene of the extremity; operations for breast malignancy (including certain biopsies and unilateral radical mastectomy); malignant neoplasm of the genitourinary organ; adverse drug reactions (several categories, mainly poisoning by specific pharmacologic agents); other cellulitis and abscess; malignant neoplasm of colon; hypokalemia; septicemia; and pulmonary embolus.
[b]RS means random sample.
[c]Transfer category eliminated 8/89.

SOURCE: HCFA, 1988.

PRO review relative to that of basic review, mainly by requiring smaller sample sizes. *Intensified* review has the same general meaning as in fee-for-service settings; that is, it is invoked when a threshold for a quality problem is reached, and sample sizes are larger (usually 100 percent of relevant cases). The three levels are not a continuum, because for plans on limited review, quality problems that reach specified thresholds trigger intensified, not basic, review.

For all three levels, medical record review is now required for five main areas of care (Table 6.9). First are hospital admissions for certain "sentinel" conditions such as serious complications of diabetes, certain malignancies, and adverse drug reactions. For these, both pre- and post-hospitalization ambulatory care is reviewed against criteria developed by the PRO. Second is a random sample of inpatient admissions. Third are samples of readmissions within specified time periods. Fourth are nontrauma deaths in all health care settings. A fifth area is focused review of ambulatory care, for which PROs were given six months to develop a methodology. Finally, beneficiary complaints are also monitored, and PROs must do community outreach activities for risk-contract enrollees similar to those for fee-for-service beneficiaries.

Limited review is available only to those HMOs and CMPs that request it and then pass a review of their internal quality assurance program. It has two basic components. First, if the PRO judges the plan's written quality assurance program to be adequate,[16] it re-reviews a subsample of cases already reviewed by the plan to validate the plan's judgments; this is done when the plan is first assessed and on a quarterly basis thereafter. The purpose is to monitor the plan's internal program, not to provide a generalized statement about the quality of care provided. If patterns of problems are apparent, the PRO would monitor the plan's corrective actions. Second, the PRO will conduct the types of reviews noted just above.

Plans not opting for or not eligible for limited review are placed on *basic review*. This focuses on the same five areas (and community outreach) described above but requires larger samples. *Not* included in basic review is the extra quarterly review of charts to validate decisions made by plans on limited review.[17]

Under *intensified review*, the sample of cases reviewed is larger (up to 100 percent of cases). Limited review plans move to intensified review in one of two instances: first, for cases in the subsample validation review, if the PRO finds that 5 percent or 6 cases in a quarter have a problem that the HMO or CMP did not detect and, second, if 5 percent or 6 cases of all other cases reviewed are found to have problems related to standards of quality, appropriateness of care, or access. Basic plans move to intensified review only in the latter instance. Plans placed in intensified review remain in this status for six months before the status is reviewed.

TABLE 6.9 Topics to be Covered in Health Maintenance Organization (HMO) and Competitive Medical Plan (CMP) Review, by Type of Review

Type of Review	Main Topics
Thirteen sentinel conditions	Inpatient care
	Quality (including generic screens)
	Timing of care
	Premature discharge
	Appropriateness
	Ambulatory care and post-hospital care[a]
	Quality
	Access to care
	Appropriateness
Hospital admissions	Quality (including generic screens and discharge review)
	Underutilization
	Appropriateness
Transfers[b]	Quality (including generic screens)
	Appropriateness of transfer (including medical stability of patient)
Readmissions within less than 31 days	Inpatient
	Quality (including generic screens)
	Post-hospital care
	Quality
	Care between admissions
Nontrauma deaths in all settings	Inpatient care
	Quality (including generic screens)
	Underutilization
	Premature discharge
	Appropriateness
	Ambulatory care and post-hospital care
	Quality (underutilization)
	Access to care
	Appropriateness
Focused review of ambulatory care	Quality (underutilization)
	Access to care
	Appropriateness

[a]For post-hospital care review, the numbers of conditions to be reviewed differ by level of review. For HMOs and CMPs on limited review, PROs must review at least two of the following conditions: diabetic complications, gangrene of the extremity, adverse drug reactions, cellulitis and abscesses, hypokalemia, septicemia, and pulmonary embolus. For those plans on basic review and intensified review, PROs must review these seven conditions.

[b]Review of transfers eliminated 8/89.

SOURCE: Exhibit C-I, HCFA, 1988.

Episodes and Ambulatory Review

By and large, the process for reviewing care rendered to Medicare beneficiaries in risk-contract HMOs and CMPs is similar to that followed for traditional fee-for-service settings (e.g., use of generic screens, assignment of severity levels, physician or plan notification, and the like). The main difference is that HCFA has tried to implement an "episode of care" approach through review of "complex" cases. A "complex case" is one in which services being reviewed were provided in more than one setting or involve more than one hospital stay; for example, cases selected under the 13 sentinel conditions would normally be classified as complex.[18] For complex cases, PROs are expected to review the care rendered in all relevant settings (ambulatory, hospital, and post-acute).

Arguably the most significant step was the requirement for ambulatory review. This left to each PRO the responsibility for developing a focused review methodology and establishing clinical screening criteria to be used in reviewing the care rendered in the office setting for the 13 sentinel conditions. Because the HMO industry, the PRO community, and HCFA agreed that the possibility of dozens of different approaches to ambulatory review was not an attractive proposition, these groups agreed that an industry-PRO Task Force would be established to develop model methods to recommend to the PRO community. As of mid-1989, experience with the set of instruments developed was limited, but the process of collaboratively developing acceptable tools for such an effort was considered valuable.

Other Initiatives

HCFA has embarked on several efforts to improve its ability to review and assure quality of care for the Medicare program. Among those considered most important by the agency are the Uniform Clinical Data Set, improvements in inpatient and ambulatory review through pilot projects, small area analysis, and remedial medical education efforts[19] in conjunction with state medical societies and others (Morford, 1989b). The first three activities, plus one relating to the hospital/post-acute care interface, are briefly described below.

Uniform Clinical Data Set

HCFA began in 1987 a complex project to develop a data set, known as the Uniform Clinical Data Set (UCDS), for use by the PROs and the wider research community. It was intended to contain far more detailed clinical data than was heretofore available in the HCFA data files. The genesis of the UCDS was the recognition that PRO judgments about the necessity, appropriateness, and timeliness of care vary appreciably and are too subjective.

One objective of the UCDS, therefore, was to put in place a mechanism to make PRO review more objective, systematic, and efficient through the application of a uniform set of electronically applied decision rules (computer algorithms) for screening cases. The second purpose of the UCDS is to permit the development of more and better epidemiologic information about the effectiveness of medical practices. This would give PROs, among others, a broader and stronger basis for decisions about quality, appropriateness, and medical necessity of care than is available from billing data alone. More broadly, HCFA hopes to be able to set national and individual PRO goals to improve quality of care and to measure PROs' success in reaching those goals (Morford, 1989a). Finally, the agency plans to make the UCDS data available for intramural and extramural analysis.

The basic operating premise of the UCDS is that relevant clinical data will be abstracted from medical records of all inpatient admissions reviewed by the PROs for whatever reason. The total number of data elements available on the UCDS is about 1600, although not every data element is relevant for every case. The contents of the UCDS fall into 10 major categories: I. Patient identifying information, II. Patient history and physical examination findings, III. Laboratory findings, IV. Imaging and other diagnostic test findings, V. Endoscopic procedures, VI. Operative episodes, VII. Treatment interventions, VIII. Medication therapy in hospital, IX. Recovery phase, and X. Patient discharge status and discharge planning.

Medical record data will be gathered by PRO abstractors either on-site or at a central office; data will be entered via desktop or laptop computers. At present, data abstraction requires about one hour per case, but that time requirement is expected to decrease as software is improved and experience gained. Detailed guidelines describe the data to be acquired.

Quality-of-care algorithms have been developed to screen cases for potential quality problems automatically; nurse reviewers will have more organized, objective, clinical information with which to flag instances of potential quality deficiencies for more in-depth review, and physician advisors will have better organized information on which to base their quality-review decisions. The computer algorithms fall into several categories: surgery (12 specific procedures), disease-specific algorithms (12 conditions), organ system algorithms (10 systems), generic quality screens (six classes of problems), and discharge screens.

As of April, 1989, the project was in a small pilot-test phase. Field testing of the whole approach, including use of algorithms to assist in the selection of cases for physician review, is expected to begin during the winter of 1989-1990. An assessment and recommendation about whether to go forward with this approach as an integral part of the PRO quality review task is expected late in 1990.

Pilot Projects for PROs

HCFA and the PRO community are embarking on a series of pilot projects designed to begin several review activities called for in legislation over the last few years. The two primary topics of these efforts are reduced (or alternative) hospital review and review of care given in noninstitutional settings, specifically physician offices and post-acute (HHA and SNF) settings. The reduced hospital review pilots may be constructed around use of the UCDS by hospitals themselves; the entire proposal for this pilot has been opposed by some groups because it appears to be too close to "delegated review" of the sort discussed earlier with respect to the PSRO program (Vibbert, 1989e).

Approximately $9 to $11 million in Medicare Trust Fund monies will be set aside over three years to fund new pilot programs. Only PROs will be eligible for funding (through contract modifications), although they can and will subcontract with each other and with outside research and academic groups for relevant expertise. Two formal requests for contract modification proposals (for noninstitutional and alternative hospital review methods) were released in May and July 1989, and several PROs have submitted proposals. One pilot project on noninstitutional review began on December 1, 1989. The emphasis is on ambulatory (office-based) care, and the project will evaluate the practicality and usefulness of techniques to evaluate care in this setting.

Small Area Variations

Perhaps the most ambitious PRO project currently underway is a small area analysis of variation in utilization and outcomes of hospital care, which is being conducted by the American Medical Review Research Center (AMRRC, 1989). The project began in October 1987 and is expected to continue until June 1990. This project will compare rates of use of hospital services in 1984-1986 in approximately 4,800 hospital market areas. Using these data, project investigators will (a) develop and disseminate information on use and outcomes of hospital care; (b) engage 12 PROs in a complex pilot education program to review, interpret, and feed back information to physicians on identified practice patterns;[20] (c) improve the use of small area analysis methods as an operational tool for PROs; and (d) examine various intervention strategies (such as physician study groups) to determine how they might best be applied in both the public and the private sectors. The physician study group phase will include five surgical conditions (coronary artery bypass graft, cardiac catheterization, carotid endarterectomy, male reproductive organ operations, and small and large bowel operations) and five medical diagnoses (chronic obstructive pulmonary disease, pneumonia, bronchitis and asthma, acute myocardial infarction, and diabetes).

Uniform Needs Assessment

OBRA 86 mandated the development of a "uniform needs assessment instrument" to evaluate the needs of patients for post-acute care such as HHA and other health-related long-term-care services. This instrument would be used by discharge planners, hospitals, nursing facilities, HHAs, and other providers, as well as by FIs, to make decisions about post-discharge needs and payment.

HCFA (specifically the Office of Survey and Certification of HSQB) has pursued instrument development with the assistance of an advisory panel. An extensive effort was made to solicit review and comment on the final draft of the instrument in preparation for its final approval and proposed field testing for reliability, validity, and administrative feasibility. HCFA plans to develop a users' manual and a standard training process in its use.

Monitoring and Evaluating PROs

PROMPTS-2

The PROMPTS-2 system focuses on whether individual PROs have fulfilled their contractual obligations. Specific attention is given to timeliness and accuracy of medical review, responsiveness to beneficiary and provider inquiries, personnel requirements, report generation, and cost effectiveness. This review is required twice during a contract cycle and is completed by HCFA Regional Office (RO) staff.

PROMPTS-2 does not generate information on the types of quality problems the PROs detect (or fail to detect). The process largely duplicates the SuperPRO effort, although on a considerably smaller scale. Questions have also been raised about inconsistency across ROs, the expertise of their medical reviewers, and the validity of their decisions, as well as about the ability of data so generated adequately to discriminate among PROs (OIG, 1989). A new PROMPTS is being developed to ensure consistency among regions.

SuperPRO

SuperPRO (a contract activity performed by SysteMetrics) conducts one aspect of performance evaluation of individual PROs by reviewing a sample of hospital records previously examined by each PRO and making an independent decision about necessity, appropriateness, and quality of care. The main objectives of SuperPRO have been (a) to validate the determination made by the PROs, specifically on admission review, discharge review, and DRG validation; (b) to validate the medical review criteria being used by nonphysician reviewers for admission review; (c) to verify that nonphysicians are properly applying the PRO's criteria for referring cases to physicians for review; and (d) to identify quality issues that should have been addressed by the PRO.

Cases identified by the SuperPRO as having quality problems are reported to the PRO, which can further review the case, appeal the judgment of the SuperPRO, and provide additional information in its rebuttal. Approximately 25 percent of PRO appeals lead to reversals of decisions in favor of the PRO.[21] HCFA then attempts to compare SuperPRO findings with PRO findings to determine whether either the PRO program or individual PRO performance needs improvement or modification.

SuperPRO cannot provide information about the incidence of quality problems in the Medicare population because it only re-reviews cases already reviewed by the PRO; neither does it address how the PRO selects cases or whether cases not reviewed by the PRO should have been. Comparisons of PRO and SuperPRO information about the prevalence of quality problems cannot be exact because the review methods (particularly the level of information from the attending physicians or hospitals) are not the same. Generally, SuperPRO data cannot be used to assess a specific PRO's performance, and the value of SuperPRO review compared with that of PROMPTS-2 has been questioned (OIG, 1989). Until mid-1989, SuperPRO reports were considered "advisory" and did not affect payment of claims for Medicare services.

A new competitive contract for the SuperPRO was issued in mid-1989 and awarded to the previous SuperPRO contractor, SysteMetrics. It had several significant changes from the earlier SuperPRO effort (HCFA, 1989a). First, HCFA (not the PROs) will select the random sample of cases, now to be 600 per month per six-month cycle in the following allocations: inpatient admissions (217); HMO cases (195); and ambulatory surgery cases (188). Second, if the PRO disagrees with the SuperPRO decision and sends a rebuttal, the SuperPRO will do a review that may include "local" criteria. HCFA intends that the PROs and SuperPRO should be on a "level playing field" and that the SuperPRO should use the same information that the PRO originally had in making quality judgments—that is, the material reviewed by SuperPRO in making its decision is the information the PRO obtained from the hospital or physician in reaching its final decision. Nevertheless, the SuperPRO still will not seek additional input from the hospital or physician whose care is under question. (This is the point at which PRO and SuperPRO procedures differ and conceivably "bias" the evaluation against the PROs.) Third, HCFA will now use SuperPRO results as a formal (not advisory) part of its evaluation of PROs, and thus the PRO rebuttal process has been strengthened.

Because disputes between PROs and the SuperPRO are likely, HCFA has decided to implement a nationwide "physician consultant contract" by which they can be adjudicated (Vibbert, 1989c); another option is to ask the HCFA Regional Offices to resolve differences between SuperPRO and the PROs (OIG, 1989). Given the serious questions that have been raised about SuperPRO performance and usefulness, these moves must be regarded with some skepticism.

AMPRA 1989 Impact Survey

Neither of these evaluation activities provides any concrete sense of "how well" PROs are doing either individually or collectively in improving the quality of care rendered under Medicare. PRO evaluators give great attention to compliance with contract specifications, have a much more complex program to assess, and face essentially the same difficulties as did the evaluators of the PSRO program.

To help overcome this paucity of "real life" information about impact on quality and what PROs are doing to accomplish this goal, the American Medical Peer Review Association (AMPRA) begin in mid-1989 the first of several contemplated surveys on PRO impact. Topics of the survey include each PRO's general impressions of the impact of PPS on quality of care, the impact of PRO review on rates of hospital utilization and on quality issues, and the impact of DRG validation; it also asks each PRO to describe its educational focus, to give its views on how to improve PRO review methods, to document the level of involvement in private review activities, and to supplement the survey with commentary on PRO effectiveness. Results from these surveys were expected in fall of 1989.

CONTROVERSIAL OR PROBLEMATIC ASPECTS OF THE PRO PROGRAM

Several experts and sources of information for this study have pointed to various problems with the current PRO program. Some of these problems apply generally to the program's review methods, to its administrative and sanctions approaches, or to legal or financial constraints. Others relate to the efforts to move the fee-for-service (and PPS-) oriented review activities to the prepaid group practice (HMO and CMP) settings. This section briefly summarizes these problematic aspects of the PRO program; they are discussed more fully in Volume II, Chapter 8.

Generic Screens

Inpatient Generic Screens

The initial experience with inpatient generic screens has come under considerable scrutiny and criticism.[22] Issues include extreme variation across PROs and poor yield of true quality problems.

Data compiled by HCFA through June 1989 reflect wide variation across PROs in the incidence of screen failures and confirmed quality problems; depending on the specific screen, screen failures among cases reviewed ranged from 0.2 percent to over 38 percent, and confirmed problems from 0.0 percent to 100 percent (Table 6.10). Similar variations were documented by the GAO (1988a) and by the OIG (1988a). GAO (1988b) noted that the PROs themselves rate generic screens behind nurse judgments and profiling and tied with intensified review in terms of their effectiveness in identifying cases with possible quality of care problems.

One drawback of these rate calculations is that the percentages of confirmed problems are based on a denominator of referred screen failures, not of the universe of cases reviewed. Thus, PROs that look quite different on the two measures may actually be detecting fairly similar rates of problems.[23] The more fundamental question, therefore, is what fraction of all charts reviewed actually reflects a true quality problem.

TABLE 6.10 Range of Generic Screen Failures and Confirmed Problems (in Percentages), by Type of Screen

Generic Screen	Range of Screen Failures (Percent)	Confirmed Problems (Percent)
Adequacy of discharge planning	0.2 - 19.1	2.1 - 100.0
Medical stability of patient at discharge	1.4 - 38.6	0.1 - 68.5
Deaths	0.4 - 5.8	0.0 - 37.1
Nosocomial infections	1.1 - 20.4	0.4 - 95.7[a]
Unscheduled return to surgery	0.2 - 2.6	0.0 - 66.7
Trauma suffered in hospital	1.0 - 24.1	2.2 - 65.8

[a]One PRO reported numbers that yielded a figure of 106.7 percent.

SOURCE: HCFA, 1989d.

Table 6.11 gives the average rates of screen failures and confirmed problems among screen failures compiled by HCFA through June 1989, which document the large differences across the different generic screens, based on more than 6.3 million cases reviewed. The first two columns clearly reflect the highly dissimilar rates of failures and confirmed problems as a percentage of screen failures. The third column of Table 6.11 gives the percentages of confirmed problems among all cases reviewed. It shows the very low yield of confirmed problems as a percentage of cases reviewed. Thus, the screens appear to be of some, but only modest, success; the most productive screens relate to adequacy of discharge planning and nosocomial infections.

Generic screens are applied to cases targeted for review for many reasons. The 3-percent sample could be said to represent the universe of Medicare admissions, and the lower panel of Table 6.11 reports the percentages of actual quality failures and confirmed problems for just that sample. If those figures are compared with the data relating to all reviewed cases (the upper panel of Table 6.11), the yield from the random sample is roughly the same than from all sources of reviewed cases, for every generic screen except medical stability at discharge. The latter includes, of course, the randomly selected cases, cases selected for expected quality problems, and other cases picked for review that do not relate presumptively to quality problems (e.g., those required for review by virtue of being one of the 12 Medicare Code Editor principal diagnoses). How useful the screens are for the last type of cases is unknown.

Another, and perhaps more pressing, issue is *why* PROs differ so dramatically in the rate of referrals and confirmed problems. The process is supposed to be quite standardized (through interpretative guidelines), but it clearly can differ very much from PRO to PRO (ProPAC, 1989). For instance, training for nurse reviewers and physician advisors, the use of specialists, and consultation with attending physicians are not standardized.

Another facet of the differences across PROs is that of quality problems never detected (and hence never addressed) in any formal way. One study estimated that as many problems were present among cases not flagged by screens (e.g., in about 5 percent of the cases reviewed) as were identified by the screens (ProPAC, 1989). Reasons for this may include the fact that nurse reviewers differ in how narrowly or expansively they interpret the screens and guidelines. Moreover, because of the required case selection specified in their contracts and the close relationship of the budgets to those required types of review, PROs may choose not to select "extra" providers, physicians, or problems for review even though they may suspect substandard care, although recently HCFA has begun to pay for such review.

Furthermore, PROs differ in the collection of cases to which they apply generic screens both because they have hospitals and physicians on 100-

percent intensified review for different reasons and because they have different mixes of hospital transfers to other types of units. Finally, some cases are targeted for review precisely because a quality problem is considered more likely (e.g., day or cost outliers; the first of a pair of admissions within 31 days; and most cases on intensified review). The question here becomes the *marginal* productivity of the screens given that there is already reason to believe a quality problem might be present.

The PRO community initially argued for this type of review tool to be used nationally, and a majority of PRO officials and HCFA staff believe they have been at least moderately effective (OIG, 1988a; GAO, 1988b). Nevertheless, generic screens as applied so far have not been entirely successful in efficiently identifying quality problems, and generic screen data

TABLE 6.11 Percentage of Cases Failing Generic Screens and with Confirmed Problems, by Generic Screening and Universe of Cases

Generic Screen and Universe of Cases	Percent Failing Screen Review	Percent Confirmed Problems Among Failures	Percent Confirmed Problems Among Reviewed Cases
All cases[a]			
Adequacy of discharge planning	3.05	71.27	2.18
Medical stability of patient at discharge	12.47	10.60	1.32
Deaths	1.49	7.50	0.11
Nosocomial infections	7.84	35.67	2.80
Unscheduled return to surgery	0.99	7.56	0.08
Trauma suffered in hospital	4.92	20.82	1.03
Cases in the 3-percent sample[b]			
Adequacy of discharge planning	2.93	79.52	2.33
Medical stability of patient at discharge	12.87	10.76	1.39
Deaths	1.24	8.45	0.11
Nosocomial infections	6.53	31.84	2.08
Unscheduled return to surgery	0.62	7.07	0.04
Trauma suffered in hospital	4.05	21.46	0.87

[a]Number of all cases reviewed: 6,309,839.
[b]Number of cases reviewed in 3-percent sample: 705,983.

SOURCE: HCFA, 1989d.

cannot be used to project "national rates of occurrence" of the various problems identified through the screens (HCFA, 1989b).

Various difficulties remain. Their application is highly labor-intensive. Apparently they still yield considerable false-positives, regardless of the relaxation of the requirement that nurse reviewers must refer failures for physician review, and they have a nontrivial false-negative rate as well. Revisions to the generic screens for the third SOW are essentially untried as of this date. Furthermore, some PROs have found that their own additional screens do as good a job or better than the HCFA screens.[24] Finally, there are numerous reasons why PROs can legitimately differ in the rate of cases detected by the screens, making conclusions about the uniformity of this tool difficult to draw.

Thus, standard, well-known generic quality screens may allow HCFA and the public to track quality problems at least at a state level (depending on how much should be assumed about the reliability and validity of these, or any, generic screens). Less certain is whether they can or should be used to compare PROs' performance. In short, whether generic screens are a strong and reliable tool on which to base a considerable part of the Medicare quality assurance effort seems problematic, unless and until they receive closer examination and refinement.

Related Approaches

This experience with inpatient generic screens underscores the need for rigorous pilot-testing of similar instruments designed for application in nonhospital settings, where there is vastly less experience with them. Perhaps more importantly, it argues for considerable testing and review of the computerized screening algorithms now being developed for the UCDS, which are intended to supplant the present generic screen approach. Reasons for caution are that the UCDS approach is so radically different from what the PROs have used so far and that the cost of implementing such an extensive data collection effort is likely to be high.

Home Health Agency Review

PROs that had begun HHA review during the site visits for this study noted two significant problems. First, selecting an appropriate sample for this task requires that hospitals bill for the two admissions in a reasonably timely way. At least one PRO noted, however, that some hospitals bill for two admissions more than 31 days apart (which would not constitute a reviewable readmission) and only much later bill for the admission that occured within 31 days of the first admission. This practice severely complicates the identification of 31-day readmissions and hence of cases that would constitute the potential pool of HHA care. A related sampling problem is simply that the pool of HHA cases for readmissions only is itself small and whether it is representative of all HHA care is unknown.

Second, at least one PRO noted that the HHA sector is undergoing great growth and change, including the emergence and disappearance of "fly-by-night" agencies. Agencies might be out of business by the time the PRO knew what cases of HHA intervening care had fallen into its sample. Review in that case probably would be impossible and certainly would be moot.

Pre-procedure Review

Whether PROs should be doing pre-procedure authorizations is part of a complicated issue concerning what entities should be doing physician review. It has generated considerable debate for the Physician Payment Review Commission (PPRC, 1989). The debate concerns two issues. First, which entities (carriers, FIs, and or PROs) should conduct prior authorization of procedures? Carriers and FIs have a history of prepayment review of physician services more extensive than that of PROs.

Second, is this primarily an exercise in utilization and cost control or in quality assurance? It may never be possible to draw a firm distinction between prior authorization activities that serve a quality assurance function and those that are more purely intended to control use. To the extent that the latter purpose is preeminent, however, it could be claimed to detract from an emphasis on quality intended by Congress for the PROs.

Physician Review for Quality of Care

A related issue concerns the appropriate locus of responsibility for reviewing services, particularly ambulatory services. PROs, FIs and carriers have overlapping, or possibly conflicting, responsibilities. They operate in different ways, with different data bases and different rules, such as when (before or after hearings) they can deny payment and what information about review criteria and screen thresholds must be made public. They also collectively leave a big gap. According to PPRC (1989), none of these entities has specific responsibility for reviewing most Part B services for *quality of care*. Carriers have authority to deny payment and initiate sanctions for substandard, unnecessary, or inappropriate care. PROs, however, are charged with reviewing office-based (ambulatory) care, which they do not yet do (although one pilot project on office-based care has begun). In short, the picture of what agencies have what authority to review outpatient care for quality of care and to take action in the face of instances of poor care remains clouded.

PPRC (1989) made four recommendations concerning Part B carrier and PRO utilization and quality review. First, HCFA should establish procedures to encourage input from carriers and PROs in designing utilization and quality criteria, in developing physician profiling methods, and investigating physicians suspected or providing inappropriate or substandard care or billing inappropriately. Second, HCFA, carriers, and PROs should work together to delineate future roles of PROs in doing ambulatory care review. Third, PROs and carriers should consult with appropriate medical organizations when developing review criteria (over and above what they are required to do now). Fourth, HCFA should designate a single entity to support research, demonstrations, evaluations, and technical assistance for all three entities doing utilization and quality review.

Peer Review

Despite the historical emphasis on peer review in federal programs and on this specific emphasis in the PRO SOW, physicians and hospitals heard from during this study during widely contended that PRO reviewers are not "peers." The points in contention concern rural practitioners and providers, specialists anywhere not reviewed by members of their own specialty, physicians fully in private practice reviewed by physicians only partly still in practice (e.g., because they are semi-retired), physicians for whom the relatively low reimbursements for PRO review are an important portion of their income, and physicians in prepaid group practice settings reviewed by those in fee-for-service settings.

Several issues arise concerning review of care rendered in the TEFRA risk-contract HMOs and CMPs. Most basically, physicians in fee-for-service practice are believed to be poorly placed (and historically to be ill-disposed) to judge the care in HMOs on a "peer basis"; the premises underlying prepaid practice and the resulting styles of practice are simply too different. There is some concern that using "local standards of care" may perpetuate existing practice patterns and vitiate the potential of prepaid systems for innovation and improved service to the Medicare population. Conflicts of interest can arise in several instances: when only fee-for-service physicians review prepaid group care, when HMO or CMP physicians review care rendered by a plan from which they may receive financial benefit, and when they review care from a competing plan. The PROs are expected to develop mechanisms for addressing these possible situations.

PROs we visited acknowledged the problems concerning rural areas and specialists but generally defended their record of using peers. They cited budget constraints as playing a large role in these problems; among these were not being able to maintain regional offices in rural areas and not being able to reimburse reviewers at competitive levels. The emerging debate about "quality denial letters" discussed elsewhere in this chapter is expected to add to the problems of recruiting specialists and, especially, subspecialists.

Sanctions

Retention and Strengthening of Sanction Authority

The role of PROs in the sanctioning process, and the role of sanctions in the quality assurance efforts of the PROs, have both been misunderstood over the course of the program. PROs can only recommend sanctions to the OIG, not impose or enforce them. Although their recommendations are the driving force behind the sanction process, they may have little influence over the outcomes of sanction efforts that are carried through the entire set of legal procedures.

Nevertheless, PROs are virtually uniform in their view that having the sanction-recommendation capability is an indispensable tool in their dealings with providers and practitioners whose performance is unacceptable, as evidenced by statements on study site visits, testimony from the PRO community, and other information (GAO, 1988b). PROs would not be willing to relinquish the sanctioning authority they now have in favor of simply greater educational or persuasive interventions, even if that step seemed to place them in a more "positive" light vis-a-vis the provider community. In view of the difficulties of the PSRO program, which did not have all the regulatory powers of the PRO program, weakening them for the PRO program does not seem to be an attractive option.

Correcting other problems of the entire sanctioning process, however, does appear to offer ways to strengthen the government's ability to protect the quality of care delivered to Medicare beneficiaries (Jost, 1988). Several issues have been debated over the past year or two, and developments toward the end of 1989 may solve some of the more knotty problems, including monetary penalties, the "unwilling and unable" provisions, and adequacy of notice to practitioners and providers.

Three different groups (the OIG, the GAO, and the Administrative Conference of the United States [ACUS]) have all recommended that the monetary penalty option be strengthened. Options include, for instance, allowing the PROs to recommend a "substantial" fine of, for instance, up to $10,000 per violation of Medicare obligations (Vibbert, 1989c; OIG, 1988b) or enacting legislation that sets a fixed upper limit to monetary policies in place of the present cost-based limit (GAO, 1988b). The requirement that providers or practitioners be found "unable or unwilling" to meet their Medicare obligations (in addition to finding that they have not in fact complied with those obligations) has caused unending confusion and frustration with the sanction process. The problems were sufficiently apparent and persuasive toward the end of 1988 that the OIG recommended that DHHS submit a legislative proposal to the effect that failure to comply with patient care obligations was sufficient basis for sanctioning (OIG, 1988b). The ACUS has endorsed a recommendation to remove the "unwilling and unable" requirement before sanctioning and to build in protections concerning due process (Vibbert, 1989c),[25] suggestions that seem worth pursuing.

The concept of not meeting "professionally recognized standards of care" has evidently been confusing to some parties (from PROs through ALJs). This creates difficulties for PROs in documenting the sanctionable infraction. PROs have in some cases issued vague charges and in other instances raised new issues at sanction meetings that were not reflected in the original notice (Jost, 1988). A possible result has been a high rate of reversals of OIG sanction actions by ALJs (10 of 18 cases by one recent count) (Vibbert, 1989b). In an effort to correct this problem, HCFA has issued model notice letters for PROs to use, but additional steps would probably be needed.

Denials for Substandard Quality of Care

COBRA and OBRA 87 allow PROs to deny Medicare payment for substandard quality; a draft proposed rule to implement these requirements was published in January 1989 (*Federal Register,* 1989a). It required payment to be denied when substandard care resulted in actual, significant adverse effects on the beneficiary (defined very broadly) or placed the beneficiary in imminent danger of health, safety, or well-being (i.e., put the beneficiary in a situation that constituted a gross and flagrant violation).

To protect the concept of peer review, the proposed rule specified that physician reviewers engaged in initial denial determinations of substandard quality be specialists in the same field as the attending or consulting physician whose care is under question. This requirement would be relaxed when meeting it would compromise the effectiveness or efficiency of PRO activities.

The proposed rule further provided that hospitals will be held financially liable even if they did not contribute directly to the substandard care rendered by the physician; thus, any denial of physician payment on these grounds would also result in a denial of reimbursement to the hospital. Furthermore, physicians may not charge patients for the care denied for these reasons and, if they have done so, must refund those payments to the beneficiary.

The proposal then specified that the PRO shall notify the patient when such payment has been denied on the basis of substandard care. The key paragraphs would read: ". . . Our determination [concerning denial of Medicare payment of a hospital admission or physician services provided in connection with that admission] is based on a review of your medical records, which indicates that the quality of services you received does not meet professionally recognized standards of health care. Denial decisions are made by the PRO physician. Your attending physician and hospital were given an opportunity to discuss your case with the PRO before the denial decision was made . . ." (*Federal Register*, 1989a). In the initial proposal, the letter would have been sent *before* providers were able to exercise their rights to appeal (i.e., to have the case reconsidered), rather than after a final determination had been made, although in this instance the initial denial determination was supposed to be made by a physician in the same specialty as the physician whose payment is questioned.

The entire quality denial process prompted much debate. Among the concerns was the lack of protection for physicians if they cannot invoke their full due process rights to reconsideration before their patients are notified of such denials and the expected increased difficulties in recruiting the specialists that will be needed to participate in these reviews and decisions. The ACUS has recommended that HHS proceed expeditiously to implement PRO authority for quality denials but with appeals *before* patient notification (Vibbert, 1989c).

Other criticisms centered on the effect of the "quality denial letter" on patients and physicians (and the patient-physician relationship), the impetus such letters might provide for increased malpractice suits filed by beneficiaries, and the impact of higher litigation on PRO activities. Yet other controversies focused on how much specific information the PRO should have to put in the letter to the beneficiary; some want to keep the letters general but specify that care was substandard, others want more specificity about what was discovered that led to that decision, and yet others want the letters to say only that care did not meet Medicare payment guidelines (and not refer to the denial as a quality denial) (Vibbert, 1989b).

OBRA 1989, passed in late November 1989 (after the main part of this study had been completed), addressed some of these issues (Congressional Record, House, November 21, 1989, p. 9380). First, it protected the physician or institutional provider from unwarranted notices to patients. Specifically, it provided that the PRO should not notify beneficiaries until after the PRO had notified practitioners or providers of its determination about the quality problem and their right to a reconsideration; if the practitioner or provider requests such a reconsideration, then one would be conducted before any notices to beneficiaries. Second, it softened the wording of the beneficiary notice, by saying that the letter need only state: "In the judgment of the peer review organization, the medical care received was not acceptable under the Medicare program. The reasons for the denial have been discussed with your physician and hospital" (p. 9380).

Administrative Procedures

The authority for PRO activities resides in several legislative acts, a broad array of regulations, guidelines, and directives, and various quasi-regulatory documents. The practice of relying on *Manual* transmittals, contracts, and other less formal instructions, instead of promulgating regulations through "public notice and comment" rulemaking as required by the Administrative Procedure Act (APA), has raised serious questions (Jost, 1988). Arguably, HCFA has opened the door to accusations that it is attempting to govern the PRO program through "a continual and confusing stream of instructions [that has] severely hampered their [the PROs'] ability to carry out their mandate" (Jost, 1988) and earned the hostility of those governed by the program. Some experts argue that sound policy reasons support using the more cumbersome process (Jost, 1988). It promotes public participation and fairness to parties who will be affected by the rules; it also forces the agencies to consider their proposals with greater care and to express them clearly.

Legal suits and legislation in the last few years have clarified the situation somewhat, apparently in favor of somewhat more rigorous rulemaking and public procedures.[26] Nevertheless, the question of public access to, understanding of, and ability to comment on the myriad rules governing the PRO program remains important. One approach to resolving it might be to appoint a "national advisory council" similar to the one that existed during the PSRO program.

Other or additional options also exist. These include: publishing PRO SOWs and any changes or modifications made during the contract cycle for an abbreviated period for comments; publishing final provisions at least 30 days before their effective date; making PRO contracts, interpretive rules, statements of policy, and guidelines of general applicability available in places of easy public access; and publishing updated lists of these materials every three months. The ACUS argues for even more formal rulemaking procedures ". . . except when the agency has 'good cause' to believe the process is 'impracticable, unnecessary, or contrary to the public interest'" (Vibbert, 1989c). The national PRO trade association favors the appointment of a "National Peer Review Council" comprising representatives from Congress, HCFA, PROs, providers, Medicare beneficiaries, and academic research. One major assignment would be to develop performance indicators for the PRO program as a whole (Vibbert, 1989e).

Evaluation

Considerable criticism can be leveled at how the PRO program itself is evaluated, especially in terms of its impact on the quality of care. Virtually no reliable or comprehensive examination of PRO program impact has been undertaken by DHHS. The several careful external examinations by, for instance, the OIG and GAO have tended to focus on specific operational aspects, such as the usefulness of generic screens or structural aspects of PROs. The same assessment can be made of how HCFA evaluates individual PRO performance; existing tools such as PROMPTS-2, although in transition to improved efficiency, have not been especially successful at providing a coordinated approach to evaluation. The OIG in particular has been critical of HCFA's ability to assess efforts at PRO performance evaluation (OIG, 1989). When combined with the lack of public oversight and accountability, these evaluation issues appear to have high priority for attention and correction.

Issues in HMO and CMP Review

Records and Case Selection

For HMOs and CMPs, cases for inpatient review are selected on the basis of claims submitted to FIs. This approach does not work well because of insufficient reporting of HMO and CMP admissions (because hospitals have no incentive to bill for such admissions). Thus, it produces a very inadequate "universe" of inpatient claims from which to select the relevant samples. Although efforts have been made to force hospitals to prepare and submit these bills to the FIs, HCFA still estimates that only about half are being submitted (O'Kane, 1989). HCFA has designed measures to overcome this inadequate pool of cases that rely on random sampling procedures; because HMOs and CMPs will differ in the proportion of their total hospitalizations subject to this form of random sampling, an additional source of variability has been added to review in the risk-contract segment of the Medicare program.

Obstacles to acquiring medical charts are also considerable. Obtaining hospital charts is not appreciably more difficult for the prepaid group practice sector than for the fee-for-service sector, although both systems contend that low reimbursement of copying costs ($0.049 per page) and lack of reimbursement for administrative costs have been problems.[27] For outpatient records, however, the problems can be extreme, when records for one plan must be retrieved from numerous health centers. Although the problem is manageable for most group- and staff-model HMOs and even for group network models, it presents IPA-model HMOs with extraordinarily complex logistics, since large plans of this sort may have hundreds of physicians practicing in individual offices. HCFA has indicated it would support legislation to allow HMOs to be reimbursed for administrative costs of retrieving such records, which should alleviate the problem to some degree.

Limited Review

One of the more contentious issues in HMO and CMP review has been the limited success of so-called limited review (only 11 of 133 risk contractors currently). Several factors seems to have been at work. First, PROs were unfamiliar with the notion of reviewing an HMO's own quality assurance plan, and HMOs may have been reluctant to put themselves in the position of having their internal programs subjected to an unpredictable and uneven evaluation process. Second, PROs are expected to review all care rendered in a case that falls into the limited review sample even if, in the HMO's own program, only selected parts of that care had been subjected to review; the HMO thus became liable for a failure relating to care it had never reviewed as part of a quality assurance plan that the PRO had found acceptable. Third, the main argument for limited review was that it reduced the number of cases subject to review; in practice, however, HMOs subject to limited review can end up having as many cases reviewed as if they were on basic review. Finally, in theory the HMO under limited review can run more of a risk than the HMO under basic review of being subjected to intensified review because of the quarterly PRO review of the "validation subsample" (that is, the cases that the HMO was investigating as part of its own plan).

Ambulatory Care Review

With respect to ambulatory review, the interesting question is how physicians will respond to review of the care they provide in their own offices. Given the lack of experience and the absence of proven tools for ambulatory review, implementing fee-for-service office-based review incrementally is arguably a good strategy for the Medicare quality assurance program; the expected PRO pilot projects are a step in the right direction. This differential between the fee-for-service and the prepaid group practice sectors does, however, place the HMO community in a position that they can understandably regard as unfair. HMO physicians' resistance to being reviewed when their fee-for-service counterparts are not might add to the incentive for plans to withdraw from the risk-contract program.

Accountability

Who is responsible for quality problems is a question that arises in any health care delivery system, but it is especially salient in the complex world of prepaid group practice arrangements. For instance, for HMOs that do not own their own hospitals, that contract for certain types of care (e.g., subspecialty care), or that cover their members on a fee-for-service or contractual basis for out-of-plan care, the issue of whether they are accountable for care well beyond their ability to oversee or control becomes very complicated. When an HMO's patients are widely dispersed across hospitals and other providers, the HMO can find itself held responsible by the PRO program for quality problems without any authority or ability to monitor or control the performance of those providers. Legal precedent and rulings concerning whether entities that employ physicians and other professionals are held to different standards than those that only contract with physicians (essentially the distinction between group and staff models on the one hand and IPA-type models on the other) further complicate this picture.

Other Issues Relating to HMO and CMP Review

PROs differ dramatically in the proportions of quality problems they find in HMOs; one accounting showed a range of 1.8 percent in one state to upwards of 30 percent in three states (O'Kane, 1989). Variations of that magnitude call into question more than the true quality of the care being rendered. They raise red flags about whether HMOs operating in several states are being subjected to the "same" review (because the PRO in each state is responsible for the state-specific portion of the HMO risk-contract care[28] and about the validity of inferences drawn from comparisons of HMOs with each other and with the fee-for-service system. The question of valid comparisons is especially problematic for states with only a single risk contractor, because information about numbers of cases reviewed and numbers and percentages of quality problems cannot be protected from public disclosure. For an HMO with an "unblemished" record, this obviously poses no problems, but for an HMO with anything less, the risk to its competitive position (vis-a-vis other HMOs in the state) could be considerable.

CONCLUSIONS ABOUT THE PRO PROGRAM

The most important conclusions drawn by the committee from this description and review of the PRO program, in the context of this study's long-term goals for Medicare quality assurance, are the following. First, the program is sufficiently well-established that it should be improved and built on, not dismantled. It is costly in financial and psychological terms to dismantle an existing program and to create a new one. Moreover, the existing program has procedures and organizational relationships (some dating from the PSRO program) that should be brought to bear for any future Medicare quality assurance program. The cadre of experienced professionals in PROs across the nation is a particularly valuable asset for any future quality assurance program for Medicare.

Second, Congress has invested the PRO program with responsibility for

the quality of care of an appropriate range of health services, but defini-
tional, operational, and strategic problems remain. We noted in Chapter 1
and elsewhere the importance of defining quality of care as a means of
directing the efforts of a quality assurance program, and we have further
emphasized the importance of health outcomes in that definition. Neither
of those concepts is yet specifically tackled as part of the present PRO
program.

Third, the program should be focused much more single-mindedly on
quality review and quality assurance, less on direct cost and utilization
control, and even less on activities of at best peripheral utility to improving
the quality of health care. Some current program activities, such as review
of hospital notices of denial and the *Important Message to Beneficiaries* or
aspects of beneficiary and community outreach, warrant explicit assessment
and re-consideration in terms of their contribution to improving quality and
in terms of whether they should be conducted "locally" or through a different national effort. Some activities might be conducted by other agents.
For instance, the carriers might profile physician claims to detect aberrant
patterns of practice, leaving "on-site" review of quality of care that requires
clinical judgment to the quality assurance program. Beneficiary communications and outreach materials might be developed and disseminated at the
federal level.

Fourth, a more forceful emphasis on quality is especially important because the PRO program is not now in a good position to focus on important
health outcomes, especially as broadly envisioned as in this report. It is
also not well positioned to focus on populations (outside the small HMO
and CMP enrollee population). Transforming the Medicare quality assurance program into one as heavily oriented toward patient well-being and
population outcomes as intended by this committee will require considerable resources, sophisticated planning, and concentrated effort within the
PRO and professional communities. Activities that do not obviously serve
this central quality assurance purpose should be eliminated, downgraded, or
moved to other agencies. For instance, one might envision much greater
responsibility for claims analyses for FIs and carriers, with timely and substantial sharing of information on problem practitioners and providers to the
Medicare quality assurance program. That program would, in turn, have
much greater responsibility for the clinical aspects of quality review and
assurance methods and for longitudinal patient outcomes.

Fifth, some rethinking of the methods for doing nonhospital review is
warranted. Reviewing "intervening care" for the HHA and SNF settings
does not make much sense in either a conceptual or a statistical sense, and
it has proven technically troublesome and unproductive; a considerable
overhaul of post-acute review would be in order. In addition, the mismatch
between the fee-for-service and the prepaid group practice sectors in ambu-

latory care review (both scope and methods) seems unfair and possibly counterproductive. Limitations of and uncertainties about the implementation of the HMO-CMP ambulatory care effort suggest that ending the present approaches and conducting pilot projects in both sectors to develop appropriate methods might be desirable.

Sixth, the system of legislation, regulations, interpretative guidelines, transmittals, and so forth that comprise the rules governing the program has less public oversight and input than desirable. Moreover, the great complexity, confusion, and lack of uniformity in the program prompts questions as to how well agency planning, implementation, and oversight has served the congressional purposes for the program or the Medicare beneficiaries' needs. The program needs to have a more open or public mechanism for program planning, oversight, evaluation, and accountability.

Seventh, this committee has strongly endorsed a move to finding ways to emphasize positive achievements, to recognize good (and "excellent") performance, and to reward providers and practitioners when they provide good quality care and mount successful quality assurance program. It has also emphasized that the Medicare quality assurance program should be able to identify and deal with poor performance. For the latter objective, a "quality intervention plan" with several types of interventions and sanctions has been developed. Although the new QIP procedures (especially sanctions) warrant some changes, generally it might be seen as a reasonable starting point for the regulatory aspects of the MPAQ.

The program has little or no experience, however, with the former goal, namely recognizing and rewarding good performance. One strategy is to reduce the level of external review for good performers (and perhaps concomitantly to increase the level of internal review). The acceptance of and results of limited review in the HMO and CMP plans to date suggest that that approach does not provide a satisfactory model. Although delegation in the old PSRO sense may not be an attractive plan and is actively opposed by some in the peer review and provider communities, some form of delegation clearly has to be contemplated. This is tantamount to saying that relying on hospitals to conduct chart review, with external oversight from PROs, deserves careful consideration and testing.

Virtually no information is available on more radical ideas, such as rewarding good performance with public acknowledgement or financial payments, certainly not in the PRO program. Thus, much attention will have to be given to achieving the related goals of meaningfully recognizing the provision of good quality care (or of maintaining a good internal quality assurance program) and reducing the level and intensity of external review. Greater public and expert inputs into and oversight of such efforts are desirable.

Eighth, it is unclear that the present approach to "peer review" provides the PROs with state-of-the-art professional knowledge or the highest levels of specialist expertise. Several factors militate against involvement of busy private practice specialists in PRO review, such as the low reimbursements for review activities (especially relative to what is paid by HCFA Regional Offices or other review entities), distaste for the "quality denial letter," and knowledge of the frustrations inherent in certain PRO processes (such as review of high volumes of false-positive generic screen failures and the cumbersome sanctioning process). Lack of understanding of the need for specialist participation in developing and promulgating procedure-specific practice guidelines and prior-authorization criteria, and consequent lack of acceptance of the guidelines and criteria that PROs do develop, may also play a role. Finally, despite two decades of inspired leadership in the medical community in the quality assurance and peer review movement, many physicians remain suspicious of and hostile to PRO activities, continuing to perceive it at one and the same time as intrusive, arbitrary, and punitive—*and* fundamentally irrelevant to improving quality of care.

Ninth, PROs individually and the program more generally do a poor job of documenting their impact on quality of care. They are therefore not in a good position either to defend their own record or to judge and comment on how well other organizations are doing. These issues call for much improved evaluation criteria and procedures, so that documented improvements in quality of care become significant parts of the scope of work on which PROs would be evaluated. This in turn argues for an in-depth review of past and impending SuperPRO efforts, of the contemplated "physician consultant" program, of the role of the Regional Offices, and similar evaluation schemes. A thorough review of the contracting mechanism itself and a re-consideration of the potential advantages of using the grant rather than the contracting mechanism is also in order, especially to the extent that the quality assurance agent should be focusing on "local" in addition to "national" problems.

Tenth, two issues about PRO financing are important. The PRO program has been assigned a vast array of quality of care, utilization review, PPS implementation, and other responsibilities for the Medicare program. To meet these assignments, it has a budget that remains well under one-half of 1 percent of Medicare expenditures. This level of funding is no greater, proportionally, than it was for the PSRO program nearly a decade ago, yet the peer review program assignments have been appreciably expanded (not entirely for quality-of-care concerns, however). We view this overall investment in a program intended to monitor and improve the quality of care for the elderly as likely to be too low ever to accomplish the expected tasks adequately. We are also concerned that the mechanism of funding individual PROs through extraordinarily detailed contracts and contract modifications is too limiting; it seems to foster evaluations of contract performance rather than impact on quality of care and to constrain innovation and flexibility to meet local conditions and problems.

SUMMARY

Since nearly the beginning of the Medicare program, the federal government has tried to ensure that services reimbursed through the program are medically necessary, appropriate, and of a quality that meets professionally established standards. The two main efforts in this arena were the PSRO and then the PRO program.

These programs share some characteristics: They have adopted purposes and methods reflecting the expected incentives of the prevailing financing mechanisms of Medicare. They have been oriented more toward controlling utilization and costs than toward improving quality of care. Both attempted to preserve "local" and "peer" review. They have concentrated on inpatient care. Both programs have been funded at a rather anemic level (more or less one-half of 1 percent of Medicare expenditures). Both programs have produced a good deal of variability in review criteria, findings, and statistics, despite considerable detailed prescription (especially for the PROs) of their operations. Finally, neither program has been able satisfactorily to demonstrate an impact on quality of care for the elderly, in large part because their emphasis has been on cost and utilization control.

The programs also differ in important ways: the PRO program has been fully operational far longer than the PSRO program was, and it has responsibilities related to implementation of Medicare's PPS that the PSRO program could not have had. The PSRO program probably had more public oversight of its activities than the PRO program has had. The PSRO program was more local than the PRO program (e.g., 195 PSRO areas versus 54 PRO contracts today). PSROs were funded through grants, whereas PROs are awarded competitively bid contracts. Partly as a consequence of these two factors, the PSRO program was probably more flexible and responsive to local utilization and quality problems than the PRO program can be. The PSRO program attempted to implement a form of "delegated review" so as to reduce intrusive external efforts; the PRO program has been precluded from any form of delegated review, partly because of the perceived weakness of delegation as it was managed during the PSRO days. Finally, the PSRO program was subjected to more rigorous evaluation than the PRO program has been to date.

Apart from these comparisons, the PRO program has some strengths that should be acknowledged. Most important may be that PROs have a committed and experienced group of physicians, nurse reviewers, and administrators with considerable expertise in the tasks needed to be accomplished by any present or future Medicare quality assurance program. Much of this cadre of quality assurance experts came initially out of the PSRO and earlier peer review efforts. In addition, PROs can operate on the basis of better Medicare data sets than were available during PSRO days, and they have a considerable advantage in computer technology compared to the earlier program.

The PRO program also has some limitations that would constrain its ability to fulfill the goals and objectives of a Medicare quality assurance program as envisioned by this committee and detailed in Chapter 12. These include its presently inadequate ability to address or to affect health outcomes for the elderly, the relative paucity of public oversight or accountability, and the enormous burden of conducting activities that are not demonstrably related to improving the quality of care or that involve tasks (such as public outreach) for which PROs do not have a comparative advantage. Other problems include the fuzzy legal status of sanctioning authority (for both PROs and the OIG), regulations that forbid or constrain innovation (such as alternative approaches to in-hospital chart review), and continuing difficulties with data sharing and data release. In designing a strategy for quality review and assurance for Medicare that will put in place a program to assure quality of care as it was defined in Chapter 1, this committee will thus attempt to build on the known capabilities of PROs and offset the perceived weaknesses. That program and the strategy for implementing it are discussed in Chapter 12.

NOTES

1. For more complete discussions of approaches to quality measurement and assurance other than those mounted by the Medicare program, see Chapter 9 and Volume II, Chapter 6. Chapter 5 and Volume II, Chapter 7, discuss Medicare Conditions of Participation more fully. Volume II, Chapter 8 provides a more complete description of the PRO program; later sections of this chapter rely heavily on lengthy excerpts and tables from that volume.
2. Profiling can also be used to identify patterns of problems with the quality of care other than those related specifically to use of services, such as failures on generic screens or unexpected patient deaths. This is one application of profiling found in the present PRO program.
3. The HCFA evaluation cautioned strenuously against drawing inferences from these data, which are *per discharge,* about costs *per review,* because the PSRO program compiled no comprehensive information on the number of reviews that were conducted by hospitals or by PSROs.
4. Waiver of liability meant that unless a hospital "knew or could reasonably have been expected to know" that the care it was providing was unnecessary, the costs of that care would still be reimbursed and the hospital was not financially liable. Only if the hospital's waiver was revoked would it become financially at risk for days of care or services provided to a beneficiary, but revocation was rarely, if ever, accomplished because the necessary regulations were not promulgated.

5. The PRO for Washington State also reviews Alaska and Idaho. The following PROs review in two states: West Virginia for Delaware; Maryland for the District of Columbia; Hawaii for Guam/American Samoa; Indiana for Kentucky; Rhode Island for Maine; Iowa for Nebraska; New Hampshire for Vermont; and Montana for Wyoming.

6. HCFA put PROs into one of four categories. Two of those categories (28 states in all) were to be awarded full three-year contracts; the remaining categories (26 states and territories) were to be awarded either six or twelve-month extensions of their existing two-year contracts. As of summer 1989, four PRO contracts had not been awarded.

7. The 11 conditions are cholecystectomy, major joint replacement, coronary artery bypass graft, percutaneous transluminal coronary angioplasty, laminectomy, complex peripheral revascularization, hysterectomy, bunionectomy, inguinal hernia repair, prostatectomy, and pacemaker insertion. A PRO can also select a procedure not on this list if it can document why it should be subjected to 100 percent pre-admission review in the state.

8. Comments to study site visitors from PRO officials indicated that many Severity Level I cases ultimately turn out not to be quality problems as defined, because they are related to poor documentation. The "quality problem" is not confirmed when the target physician or provider provides sufficient additional information.

9. HCFA prescribes the format and wording of these letters (apart from the specifics of the case at hand). Presumably for legal reasons, they are very formal in tone and must contain the following information: (1) the Medicare obligations involved; (2) description of the activity resulting in the violation; (3) the authority and responsibility of the PRO to report violations of obligations; (4) a suggested method and time period for correcting the problem (at the discretion of the PRO); (5) an invitation to submit additional information or discuss the problem with the PRO within 20 days of the notice; and (6) a summary of the information used by the PRO in reaching a determination.

10. As part of a case involving the American Medical Association (AMA) *(A.M.A. v. Bowen)* settled three years ago, the OIG committed itself to seek a regulatory alternative to the practice of newspaper notices, one that would permit sanctioned physicians to inform their Medicare patients personally that Medicare would no longer pay for the physicians' services. The OIG drafted a proposed regulation that would require a physician to notify all his or her patients, not just those covered by Medicare. No regulations had been issued, however, as of mid-1989.

11. The preamble to certain PRO regulations notes that quality problems that affect Medicare patients usually affect all patients, particularly in the context of acute care. Consistently throughout this study, respondents at site visits confirmed this observation. Especially in hospitals and prepaid systems, our respondents noted that most quality problems tended to be with "systems" that cut across units and patient age groups. Moreover, facilities and groups with well-established internal quality assurance systems deliberately did not single out "the elderly" or "Medicare patients" for specific quality assurance attention (except insofar as they needed to meet PRO demands for records and similar requirements), believing that a more efficient and ultimately more successful approach

to quality improvement would involve the entire institution, its entire staff, and its entire patient census.

12. Regulations classify "confidential information" as follows: (a) information that explicitly or implicitly identifies an individual patient, practitioner, or reviewer; (b) sanction reports and recommendations; (c) quality review studies that identify patients, practitioners, or institutions; and/or (d) PRO deliberations. "Implicitly identifies" means that the data are sufficiently unique or the numbers so small that identification of an individual patient, practitioner, or reviewer would be easy.

13. Because PRO budgets are tightly tied to the number of expected reviews, their individual budgets range vary widely. For instance, of the PROs awarded full three-year contracts for the third SOW, the California PRO was awarded nearly $82,838,000—the largest in the country and a record for the PRO program (Vibbert, 1989a)—and the PRO for Wyoming was awarded $1,210,000. Other PROs were awarded extensions of existing contracts for six or 12 months. Of these, the largest award, for 12 months, was to Texas (just over $16.1 million) and the smallest award, also for 12 months, was to American Samoa and Guam ($24,120) (HCFA, unpublished data made available to the study, April 1989).

14. Material for this section is based in part on a paper prepared for this study, "PRO Review of Medicare Health Maintenance Organizations and Competitive Medical Plans," by Margaret E. O'Kane, Director of Quality Assurance, Group Health Association, Washington, D.C., May 1989 (O'Kane, 1989). The history of PRO review efforts for HMOs and CMPs is recounted in more detail in Volume II, Chapter 8.

15. As of December 1989, Quality Quest is the QRO only for Missouri. The Illinois PRO (Crescent Counties Medical Foundation) is the QRO for Illinois. The QRO contract for Kansas had not yet been awarded.

16. HCFA defined *de novo* a set of "areas of focus" by which HMO/CMP internal programs would be evaluated, rather than using existing models developed by the National Committee on Quality Assurance (an HMO industry group), the Joint Commission, and similar groups. The HCFA areas were: whether the plan reviews individual cases of patient care; whether it includes physician review of medical records; whether physicians make final decisions on quality issues; whether review includes all settings; whether the plan uses reasonable sampling methods to select cases for review; and whether the plan has been operating long enough for it to be able to demonstrate actual performance. The industry widely regarded these as rather old-fashioned and lacking in an understanding of what HMO and CMP QA plans actually do.

17. For plans on limited review, the total number of cases selected for the random validation subsample plus the total number selected for the remaining reasons for review cannot exceed the number that would have been reviewed under the basic plan.

18. By contrast, a "simple" case is one in which services being reviewed were provided in only one setting and during only one admission (if inpatient)—for instance, those in the 3-percent inpatient sample.

19. Volume II, Chapter 6 discusses several PROs' remedial education efforts.

20. The 12 PROs involved in the educational component of the project, known as Medical Assessment Program (MAP) pilots, are located in the following states:

Arizona, Arkansas, Colorado, Connecticut, Illinois, North Carolina, Ohio, Pennsylvania, Texas, Utah, Virginia, and Washington. It is intended that all PROs receive data, technical training in small area analysis methods, and necessary computer software.

21. Data provided by HCFA reviewer of draft report. Also see GAO (1988a).

22. Recall that the screens are (1) adequacy of discharge planning; (2) medical stability of patient at discharge; (3) deaths; (4) nosocomial infections; (5) unscheduled return to surgery; and (6) trauma suffered in the hospital.

23. Take, for instance, the OIG calculations on data from 12 PROs for Screen 1 on adequacy of discharge planning. According to their data, PRO D failed 0.2 percent of 24,382 cases screened and confirmed problems in 100 percent of failures, whereas PRO F failed 0.6 percent of 80,624 cases and confirmed problems in only 40.5 percent. Both, however, detected confirmed problems in 0.2 percent of cases reviewed (see OIG, 1988b).

24. For instance, the Peer Review Organization of Washington reported during a site visit that some of its specially developed screens identify more failures and/or confirmed problems than do the HCFA screens.

25. Countering these moves are recommendations from the Commerce Committee of the U.S. House of Representatives to expand the time during which a physician can claim to be willing and able to change poor practice patterns, extend special appeal rights to most physicians (instead of just those in rural areas), and cap the monetary fines at just $2,500 (Vibbert, 1989d). As of mid-1989, the question of whether the PRO sanctioning capability would be strengthened or weakened was still open.

26. However, the course of one suit *(Amer. Hosp. Assn. v. Bowen)* seems to have left HCFA with considerable latitude, because the final court of appeals ruling held that the contracting process, issuance of the SOWs, and *Manual* transmittals were all covered by exceptions to the APA.

27. The issue of reimbursing hospitals for costs incurred in photocopying medical records has been especially contentious since 1985. A recent court order requires that HCFA reimburse hospitals retroactively for costs incurred in photocopying; the American Hospital Association argues in favor of a reimbursement at a level of $0.12-per-page (Vibbert, 1989f).

28. Multi-state HMOs visited during this study differed in their views on this issue. At least one felt very strongly that it wished to deal with only a single PRO because it was experiencing considerable, unexplainable variation in review from the different PROs in the different states in which it operated. By contrast, at least one other plan found PRO review sufficiently benign that differences across PROs were either not noticeable or not a problem.

REFERENCES

AAPSRO (American Association of Professional Standards Review Organizations Task Force). *PSRO Impact on Medical Care Services: 1980.* Vols. I and II. Report of the 1980 Ad Hoc Task Force on Impact. Potomac, Md.: The Association, 1981.

AMRRC (American Medical Review Research Center). SMAA PRO Pilots are Progressing Well: An Update. *AMRRC Update,* pp. 1-2, March-July 1989.

Blum, J.D., Gertman, P.M., and Rabinow J. *PSROs and the Law.* Germantown, Md.: Aspen Systems Corporation, 1977.

Blumstein, J.F. Inflation and Quality: The Case of PSROs. Pp. 245-295 in *Health— The Victim or Cause of Inflation?* Zubkoff, M., ed. New York: Prodist (for the Milbank Memorial Fund), 1976.

CBO (Congressional Budget Office). *The Effect of PSROs on Health Care Costs: Current Findings and Future Evaluations* Washington, D.C.: Congress of the United States, Congressional Budget Office, June 1979.

CBO. *The Impact of PSROs on Health-Care Costs: Update of CBO's 1979 Evaluation.* Washington, D.C.: Congress of the United States, Congressional Budget Office, January 1981.

Chassin, M.R. and McCue, S.M. A Randomized Trial of Medical Quality Assurance: Improving Physicians' Use of Pelvimetry. *Journal of the American Medical Association* 256:1012-1016, 1986.

Cislowski, J.A. The Peer Review Organization Program. Washington, D.C.: Congressional Research Service, U.S. Library of Congress, October 23, 1987.

Committee on Ways and Means. *Background Material and Data on Programs Within the Jurisdiction of the Committee on Ways and Means. 1989 edition.* Committee Print WMCP 101-4, March 15, 1989. Washington, D.C.: Government Printing Office, 1989.

Egdahl, R.H. Foundations for Medical Care. *New England Journal of Medicine* 288:491-498, 1973.

Federal Register, Vol. 50, pp. 15364-15389, April 17, 1985.

Federal Register, Vol. 54, pp. 1956-1967, January 18, 1989a.

Federal Register, Vol. 54, pp. 42722-42734, October 17, 1989b.

GAO (General Accounting Office). *Problems with Evaluating the Cost Effectiveness of Professional Standards Review Organizations.* HRD-79-52. Washington, D.C.: General Accounting Office, July 1979.

GAO. *Medicare Improving Quality of Care Assessment and Assurance.* PEMD-88-10. Washington, D.C.: General Accounting Office, May 1988a.

GAO. *Medicare PROs Extreme Variation in Organizational Structure and Activities.* PEMD-89-7FS. Washington, D.C.: General Accounting Office, November 1988b.

Goran, M.J., Roberts, J.S., Kellogg, M.A., et al. The PSRO Hospital Review System. *Medical Care* 13:1-33 (Supplement), 1975.

Harrington, D.C. Ambulatory Medical Care Data: 20 The San Joaquin Foundation Peer Review System. *Medical Care* 11:185-189 (Supplement), 1973.

HCFA (Health Care Financing Administration). *Professional Standards Review Organization 1979 Program Evaluation.* Health Care Financing Research Report. HCFA Pub. No. 03041. Baltimore, Md.: Department of Health and Human Services, May, 1980.

HCFA. 1988–1990 PRO Scope of Work. Baltimore, Md.: Health Care Financing Administration, Department of Health and Human Services, 1988.

HCFA. Request for proposal for the SuperPRO contract, Attachment II. Baltimore, Md.: Health Care Financing Administration, Department of Health and Human Services, 1989a.

HCFA. Technical Notes. Peer Review Organization Data Summary dated May 1989. Baltimore, Md.: Office of Peer Review, Health Standards and Quality Bureau, Health Care Financing Administration, 1989b.

HCFA. Utilization and Quality Control Peer Review Organizations Second Scope of Work. Executive Data Summary. Report through March 1989. Report dated 7/5/89. Baltimore, Md. Health Care Financing Administration, 1989c.

HCFA. Peer Review Organization Data Summary. May 1989 (includes June 1989 data). Baltimore, Md.: Office of Peer Review, Health Standards and Quality Bureau. Health Care Financing Administration, 1989d.

Jost, T. *Administrative Law Issues Involving the Medicare Utilization and Quality Control Peer Review Organization (PRO) Programs: Analysis and Recommendations.* Report to the Administratrive Conference of the United States. Washington, D.C.: Administrative Conference, November 8, 1988 (reprinted in *Ohio State Law Journal* 50(1), 1989).

Kane, R.A., Kane, R.L., Kleffel, D., et al. *The PSRO and the Nursing Home: Vol. I, An Assessment of PSRO Long-term Care Review.* R-2459/1-HCFA. Santa Monica, Calif.: The Rand Corporation, August 1979.

Lohr, K.N. *Peer Review Organizations: Quality Assurance in Medicare.* P-7125. Santa Monica, Calif.: The Rand Corporation, July 1985.

Lohr, K.N., Brook, R.H., and Kaufman, M.A. Quality of Care in the New Mexico Medicaid Program (1971-1975): The Effect of the New Mexico Experimental Medical Care Review Organization on the Use of Antibiotics for Common Infectious Diseases. *Medical Care* 18:1-128 (January Supplement), 1980.

Lohr, K.N., Winkler, J.D. and Brook, R.H. *Peer Review and Technology Assessment in Medicine.* R-2820-OTA. Santa Monica, Calif.: The Rand Corporation, August 1981.

McIlrath, S. Receding Tide of Physician Sanctions by Medicare PROs Triggers Debate. *AMA News* 3:57, April 21, 1989.

Morford, T.G., Director, Health Standards and Qualtity Bureau, HCFA. Testimony before the U.S. House of Representatives' Committee on Government Operations, Subcommittee on Human Resources and Intergovernmental Relations, April 4, 1989a.

Morford, T.G. UpDate. Federal Efforts to Improve Peer Review Organizations. *Health Affairs* 8(2):175-178, Summer 1989b.

OIG (Office of Inspector General, Department of Health and Human Services). *The Utiliztion and Quality Control Peer Review Organziation (PRO) Program Quality Review Activities.* Washington, D.C.: Office of Inspector General, Office of Analysis and Inspections, August 1988a.

OIG. *The Utilization and Quality Control Peer Review Organization (PRO) Program Sanction Activities.* Washington, D.C.: Office of Inspector General, Office of Analysis and Inspections, October 1988b.

OIG. *The Utilization and Quality Control Peer Review Organization (PRO) Program. An Exploration of Program Effectiveness.* Washington, D.C.: Office of Inspector General, Office of Analysis and Inspections, January 1989.

O'Kane, M.E. PRO Review of Medicare Health Maintenance Organziations and Competitive Medical Plans. Paper prepared for the Institute of Medicine Study to Design a Strategy for Quality Review and Assurance in Medicare, May 1989.

OTA (Office of Technology Assessment). *The Quality of Medical Care: Information for Consumers*. OTA-H-386. Washington, D.C.: U.S. Government Printing Office, 1988.

PPRC (Physician Payment Review Commission). *Annual Report to Congress, 1989*. Washington, D.C.: Physician Payment Review Commission, April 1989.

ProPAC (Prospective Payment Assessment Commission). *Medicare Prospective Payment and the American Health Care System. Report to the Congress. June 1989*. Washington, D.C.: Prospective Payment Assessment Commission, 1989.

Vibbert, S., ed. Watchdog Criticizes HHS IG Over PRO Monetary Sanctions. *Medical Utilization Review* 17(7):1, April 4, 1989a.

Vibbert, S., ed. PROs Denied 2 Percent of 1986-1988 Medicare Cases. *Medical Utilization Review* 17(9):1, May 2, 1989b.

Vibbert, S., ed. Regulatory Activity. Legal Panel Backs PRO Reform Package. *Medical Utilization Review* 17(13):5-6, June 27, 1989c.

Vibbert, S., ed. PRO Sanctions Fight Moves to Senate. *Medical Utilization Review* 17(15):1-2, August 8, 1989d.

Vibbert, S., ed. HSQB Softpedals Controversial Pilot. *Medical Utilization Review* 17(18):3-4, September 21, 1989e.

Vibbert, S., ed. Hospitals Gain Class Action Status in Federal Suit over PRO Photocopying. *Medical Utilization Review* 17(21):1, November 2, 1989f.

7

Quality Problems and the Burdens of Harm

INTRODUCTION

Good health care requires the technical proficiency and means to deliver services correctly and the cognitive and communication skills necessary to elicit and evaluate needed information and then decide which mix of available services is most likely to achieve desired health outcomes for particular patients. When these requirements are not met patients are at risk.

Choices among methods to prevent, detect, and correct quality problems should be based on (1) how well they do at detecting different types of problems such as overuse versus underuse of care, and (2) what relative burden of harm is imposed by these different problems. This burden can be quantified in terms of incidence, distribution across populations, and degree of impact on patient outcomes (such as functional status and survival). Other things being equal, if we knew that problems of overuse caused twice as much harm as those of underuse, we would devote twice as much of our quality assurance resources to those specific techniques designed to discover and correct overuse problems.

Importance of Poor Technical and Interpersonal Quality

We use the term "technical quality" to refer generally to the ways health care is delivered by individuals and organizations, such as whether correct diagnoses are made, appropriate medications prescribed, or surgical procedures performed skillfully. It includes not only practitioner knowledge and manual or technical skills, but also interpersonal skills—listening, answering questions, giving information, and eliciting and including patient preferences in decision making. Poor interpersonal skills can deny patients the information they need to make informed choices, care for themselves, or adhere to treatment plans. Those problems, as well as poor organization and coordination of various aspects of patient care, can lead to harm ranging from discomfort or distrust to disfigurement or death.

The classic approaches to quality assurance, including risk management and infection control, focus on poor technical quality, particularly problems of skill, performance, and system functioning. Within hospitals, such methods of problem detection as surgical review, morbidity and mortality conferences, incident reporting, and review for adverse occurrences have this focus.

Problems with poor technical quality may involve one or more "outlier" practitioners whose skills are inadequate, or they may involve broader weaknesses in a system. Practitioners or institutions that are outliers in one area cannot be presumed to be outliers in all areas of practice. For instance, the hospital-specific mortality data released by the Health Care Financing Administration (HCFA) identified very few hospitals that were high-mortality outliers across several different diagnoses and very few that were outliers across several years (see Chassin et al., 1989). Moreover, "good" practitioners or providers cannot be assumed to be uniformly good (Palmer, 1988). In any case, methods for dealing with outliers may differ from those appropriate for responding to problems with average performance.

Importance of Overuse in Quality of Care

Some problems with quality of health care can be classified under the term overuse. Overuse is the provision of services whose likelihood of harm to the patient outweighs the likelihood of benefit. Benefits include increased life expectancy, relief of pain, reduction in anxiety, or improved functional capacity. Harms include the morbidity and mortality that accompany the provision of service (such as a surgical procedure). They also include other, less commonly measured adverse effects such as the anxiety of anticipating and undergoing a procedure, time lost from work, and time spent in rehabilitation.

Excessive diagnostic services may have direct negative side effects and may also, if falsely positive, lead to other more invasive and hence more risky examinations and treatments. A case in point is the patient who has an unnecessary exercise stress test that is falsely positive and who as a result undergoes coronary angiography (Graboys, 1989).

Excessive use of medications such as antibiotics (Foxman et al., 1987) exposes patients and the population in general to unjustified side effects, for example the proliferation of antibiotic-resistant organisms. When patients are hospitalized unnecessarily, they risk falls, medication errors, and hospital-acquired infections.

In addition, resources are limited, and overuse of some services may preclude others from getting needed care. Use of the intensive care unit by a patient who does not need it, for instance, may delay or prevent care for another patient who does need it. Overuse of services adds to the cost of care for the individual and for society. The study committee's concern with overuse as a quality issue focuses on whether the services provide a net expected benefit to a patient, not whether those resources might have produced more benefits if applied elsewhere.

Importance of Underuse in Quality of Care

Underuse is the lack of provision of services whose expected benefits outweigh their expected risks to the patient. In less technical terms, underuse is a missed opportunity, for instance, the omission of a preventive service such as mammography screening of older women that carries a small risk but greatly enhances the likelihood of survival if it speeds detection of an operable tumor. Harms can be a foregone cure, a condition not improved, or a symptom not ameliorated. Again, the study committee's focus is on the net benefits and risks to the patient, not the relative costs and benefits for society.

Differentiating Problems of Poor Technical Quality, Overuse, and Underuse

Often it is quite apparent whether a problem stems from poor technical quality, overuse, or underuse. Problems of poor technical quality are most easily differentiated from overuse when a clear intervention, such as a surgical procedure or prescribing decision, is involved. The decision to intervene may itself be appropriate (not overuse), but the execution (technical quality) is improper. For instance, an outmoded technique is used, the wrong dose of medications prescribed, an instrument misread, or a test result ignored.

In other situations, such as in long-term management of chronic conditions, distinguishing poor technical quality, overuse, or underuse may be much more difficult. A physician who suspects essential hypertension could, for example, explore the problem over a series of patient visits, laboratory tests, and trials of medication. Incorrect choices in the process of diagnosis and treatment could result in delayed diagnosis (underuse by insufficient testing), incorrect medication (poor technical quality), or unnecessary or potentially harmful tests (overuse). Iatrogenic illness or complications arising from medical treatment result from side effects of unnecessary medications or drug interactions (overuse), infection because hospital procedures are not followed (underuse), or preventable complications of a procedure such as hemorrhage following careless surgical technique (poor technical quality).

Similarly, failure to obtain informed consent for services might be viewed as underuse of the informed consent procedure, overuse of services that the informed patient would have foregone, or poor interpersonal care because the patient's preferences were not elicited. These examples suggest that classifying problems may sometimes be rather arbitrary.

Underuse of services can be conceptually linked to overuse in that both are concerned with the *appropriate* use of services as opposed to the technical competence in providing them. Underuse and overuse may also coexist. For instance, some admissions might be regarded as overuse of hospital care because of underuse of nonhospital nursing care. A quality assurance technique that detects the former may not detect the latter. Whether the hospital care or lack of nursing care is avoidable or governed by external factors such as geography or availability of nursing staff is an issue for any quality assurance program.

To the extent that both overuse and underuse of services arise from lack of physician knowledge of the natural history of the patient's condition, of the patient's preferences, or of the probabilities of various outcomes of diagnostic tests and therapy, they may represent the *same* problem; regulatory and financial mechanisms are not likely to be effective. Other interventions, such as better dissemination and use of available medical knowledge or continuing medical education, may be more useful.

Sources of Information About Burdens of Harm

Ideally, before we design a quality assurance program for the elderly, we should understand the relative burdens of harm created by poor technical quality, overuse, and underuse. This knowledge would permit us to build specific mechanisms tailored to the efficient identification and effective amelioration of these quality problems. Unfortunately, our knowledge in this area is meager. Physicians and other practitioners frequently complain that current programs require much effort but often overlook or fail to address what they consider to be serious problems.

We have attempted to assess the burden of harm imposed on the elderly by the three major categories of quality problems. To do this the committee used four sources of information. First, we commissioned two background papers—one from a medical perspective (Rubenstein et al., 1989) and one from a nursing perspective (Lang and Kraegel, 1989)—to examine the state of health care for the elderly as it has been documented in the research literature. A third commissioned paper concerned home health care (Hawes and Kane, 1989). Second, during public hearings, we asked respondents whether they could estimate how widespread quality problems were and whether those were problems primarily of overuse, underuse, or poor technical quality (see Chapter 2 in Volume II). Third, we raised these same questions in the focus groups held among elderly individuals and among practicing physicians and during our extensive site visits around the country (Chapters 3 and 4 in Volume II). Finally, we used published studies and available data on disciplinary and malpractice actions.

The following examination of the burden of harm necessarily emphasizes problems. It should not imply that health care in this country is generally of dubious quality. Participants in the beneficiary focus group were generally satisfied with their primary physicians and the medical care they received. Many commented positively on the Medicare program itself, asserting that adequate health care would be a financial burden without the assistance of Medicare. They viewed medical care in the United States as very good and as one of the best medical systems in the world. Other positive aspects of medical care frequently mentioned were scientific advances, the level of medical technology, increased efficacy of medications and pharmaceuticals, and a high skill level among providers of care.

EVIDENCE OF PROBLEMS IN TECHNICAL QUALITY OF CARE

We reviewed both direct and inferential evidence to assess the frequency and severity of poor technical quality of care. Sources of such evidence include the literature on clinical and health services research, national data on malpractice compensation, and disciplinary actions by state boards of medical examiners. For evidence specific to the elderly, we considered sanctions recommended by Medicare Peer Review Organizations (PROs) and imposed by the Department of Health and Human Services (DHHS) (see Chapter 6) and the results of the committee's public hearings, site visits, and focus groups.

General Evidence of Poor Technical Quality

Malpractice Data

Malpractice data are often assumed to be a good source of information concerning poor technical performance of physicians or other providers. Although a review of these data by the Office of Technology Assessment (OTA, 1988) throws that assumption into considerable question, we report some of the better known work, because it provides a sense of the more egregious problems with technical quality of care.

A Pennsylvania study, which was commissioned by the Pennsylvania Medical Society and Pennsylvania Trial Lawyers Association, showed that 1 percent of Pennsylvania physicians (228) were responsible for 25 percent of the malpractice loss payments by the Pennsylvania Medical Professional Liability Catastrophe Loss Fund (Wolfe, 1986). Of this 1 percent, nearly half had three or more loss claims over a 10-year period. Similarly, in Michigan, 2.5 percent of physicians accounted for almost 20 percent of all claims, and just under 20 percent of physicians accounted for over 70 percent of all claims (Wolfe, 1986). In Florida, the Orlando *Sentinel* reported that 3 percent of doctors were responsible for almost half of all malpractice claims paid in the state between 1975 and 1984 (cited in Wolfe, 1986).

In 1987, there were 6.7 professional liability claims per 100 physicians (Slora and Gonzales, 1988). About 37 percent of physicians have had a malpractice claim filed against them at some time during their practicing career. The mere filing of a claim provides no information, however, about whether malpractice occurred.

In the most comprehensive analysis to date, the General Accounting Office reported on claims closed in 1984 (GAO, 1987).[1] Fifty-seven percent were dismissed without a verdict, settlement, or any compensation going to the claimant. Seventy-one percent of the providers sued were physicians; 21 percent were hospitals, and the remainder involved other facilities, nurses, dentists, and others. Forty-two percent of the physicians had previous malpractice claims filed against them. The three most frequent allegations, surgical error, failure to diagnose, and treatment errors, accounted for 69 percent of all malpractice claims reviewed.

The data on principal allegations in closed claims files are not differentiated by overuse, underuse, and poor technical quality, although they might be so categorized by imputation. For instance, the nearly 18,700 allegations of surgical errors accounted for 25 percent of the claims, and almost 90 percent of these could be classified as poor technical quality (retained foreign bodies, improper positioning, or wrong body part) and 8 percent as overuse (unnecessary surgery and failure to obtain consent for surgery).

For claims of diagnostic errors (about one quarter of all allegations), 38 percent could be linked to poor technical quality (misdiagnosis, improper performance of diagnostic test), 1 percent overuse (failure to obtain consent), and 60 percent to underuse (failure to diagnose, or delay in diagnosis).

Allegations of treatment errors constituted nearly 20 percent of all allegations. Of these, 75 percent can be classified as poor technical quality (improper performance, improper choice of treatment) and 21 percent for underuse (failure to render treatment, delay in treatment). Data provided by one of the nation's largest underwriters of malpractice liability insurance, St. Paul Fire and Marine Insurance Company, reflect similar experience. *The St. Paul's 1988 Annual Report to Policyholders* (1987) cited 15.4 claims per 100 physician policyholders. Major allegations involved surgical errors (29 percent of claims, mainly related to complications), failure to diagnose

(28 percent, mainly related to cancer), improper treatment (27 percent, mainly birth-related), and anesthesia errors (3.5 percent). Other types of allegations accounted for 12 percent of claims. Of the total, 67 percent referred to the hospital, 32 percent to the physician's office or clinic, and 1 percent to a surgicenter.

Data on claims filed or closed cannot be used to estimate the prevalence of quality problems in medical care in the United States for several reasons. Patients may not know that malpractice has occurred; patients may know but may choose not to make a claim; or they may act, but legitimate claims may be rejected. These reasons can be labelled "false negatives," that is, the absence of a successful claim despite actual malpractice. Among successful claims, on the other hand, may be some false-positives. For example, a claim may be settled even though it lacks merit, or for strategic reasons a malpractice complaint may include practitioners who were only tangentially involved in the patient's care. Such false-positives mean that claims closed with compensation cannot give even a minimum estimate of poor quality.

Research Evidence

Although more than a decade old, the California Medical Insurance Feasibility (CMIF) Study (Mills, 1977) remains the most comprehensive estimate of the incidence of "potentially compensable events" (an injury worthy of seeking legal recourse) occurring in short-stay acute hospitals. This study, which reviewed records of about 21,000 discharged patients, found that 4.65 percent of admissions resulted in some potentially compensable event (PCE), defined as a "disability (temporary or permanent) caused by health care management (including acts of commission and omission by health providers)." Seventeen percent of these were judged to have involved legal liability. By applying these figures to the 38.8 million patients hospitalized in the United States in 1983, Wolfe (1986) estimated that there were 310,400 people injured (or killed) as a result of negligent behavior.

Comparing the frequency of PCEs in the CMIF data with data on insurance claims led investigators to believe that only about 1 valid claim in 10 was brought at that time. Since claims frequency has doubled since the 1974 data were gathered, Danzon (1985) estimates that today only one in five actionable claims are brought and that poor care resulting in temporary or permanent disability or death occurs in 1 percent of hospital admissions.[2]

A prospective study by Couch and his colleagues (1981) looked at the frequency of surgical mishaps (adverse outcomes because of error) in the field of general surgery. They identified 36 mishaps in a review of 5,612 admissions (0.6 percent) and described five sources of physician error: overestimation of surgical skills, unwarranted urgency in performing major surgical procedures, urge for perfection beyond the patient's needs, uncritical performance of vogue therapies, and insufficient restraint and deliberation in patient care. The last four problems might be considered to result from overuse rather than poor skills. When Wolfe (1986) applied this rate of mishaps to all surgical admissions in the United States, he estimated 136,000 injuries to surgical patients caused by doctor error.

Steele and his colleagues (1981) reviewed the care of 815 consecutively admitted elderly patients to a medical service of a university hospital and found that 36 percent suffered some form of adverse complications attributable to medical management. About 9 percent of the 815 had a major event that was life-threatening or disabling, and in 2 percent of the cases the patient died. The most frequent complications involved drug reactions, complications of cardiac catheterization, and falls. The authors cautioned that the teaching hospital where the study was done might have had a higher proportion of seriously ill patients who might have been more difficult to treat. Other studies reviewed by McPhee et al. (1982) point to avoidable and sometimes severe reactions resulting from polypharmacy, transfusion reactions, and nosocomial (hospital-acquired) infections.

Hospitals using Medical Management Analysis (MMA), a system of standardized reporting of adverse occurrences, are reported to identify "adverse patient occurrences" (APOs) in about 18 to 20 percent of patient hospital records (Craddick and Bader, 1983). Adverse patient occurrences are defined as "any untoward patient event which, under optimal conditions, is not a natural consequence of the patient's disease or procedure" (Craddick and Bader, 1983, p. 7). A study of surgeons who had been recommended by peers as "good" surgeons revealed that some 23 percent of charts showed one or more APOs. These records were then further reviewed by their peers to determine whether management had been acceptable, questionable, or a breach of the standard of care. Questionable management was defined as "those instances in which the peer reviewer might have managed the case differently, but the subject physician's management was within the range of variation of standard practice" (Craddick and Bader, 1983). The reviewers identified questionable management for 12 percent of the APOs involving 4 percent of the patients and no cases that suggested that the standard of care was breached. The percentage of APOs per surgeon ranged from 18 percent to 31 percent and was correlated with the complexity of the surgery (Craddick and Bader, 1983).

Dubois and Brook (1988) reported that among 182 deaths reviewed independently by at least three physicians, 14 percent were probably or definitely preventable. Reasons varied by type of admission and included errors in management and or diagnosis.

Research studies in which medical practice as recorded in the medical chart is compared with standards set by peers and experts virtually always demonstrate substantial deficiencies. In fact, differences among providers and among practice settings are usually smaller than those between average and "ideal" practice, even when practitioners have set their own standards. For instance, a review of antibiotic use in a community hospital by Jogerst and Dippe (1981) found substantial misuse. Only 72 percent of therapeutic uses and only 36 percent of prophylactic uses were appropriate, according to standards developed by the physicians in the hospital under study.

Disciplinary Actions by State Medical Boards

Reports on disciplinary actions by state medical boards can provide information about the prevalence of medical incompetence. The Federation of State Licensing Boards (FSLB) reported that in 1986, 2,302 disciplinary actions were taken against the country's approximately 500,000 practicing physicians, an overall rate of 4.6 per 1,000 physicians.[3] The rate of disciplinary actions by medical boards varied by state and territory from 0 to 15 per 1,000 practicing physician. This variation probably reflects state differences in laws, attitudes toward regulation, and board willingness to engage in disciplinary activities (OTA, 1988).

Disciplinary actions covered by the above figures are revocation of license, suspension, probation, and reprimand. The State boards may also take milder actions. One example is a letter agreement in which no harm is alleged and the physician acknowledges a problem (such as impairment) and agrees to enter a program for impaired physicians; other informal actions include letters of concern and recommendations for continuing education.

The Public Citizen Health Research Group (Public Citizen) compared 1987 FSLB data on serious disciplinary actions to previous years (Wolfe, 1989). Disciplinary actions rose for three consecutive years and in 1987 reached 2.78 serious disciplinary actions for every 1,000 United States doctors.[4] The lowest ranking state had 0.45 serious actions per 1,000 physician. The highest ranking state had 8.58, a 19-fold difference. Although there is no evidence that the proportion of poor practitioners is evenly distributed among the states, Public Citizen estimates that if all states had the highest rate the overall rate of disciplinary actions would have been three times higher.

Wolfe (1989) also cited a Tufts University study that found that physician-owned insurance companies terminated coverage of 6.6 per thousand physician policyholders in 1985 because of "negligence-prone behavior." They restricted the scope of covered practice or imposed other sanctions on an additional 7 per 1,000 policyholders because of substandard care. Public

Citizen noted that the combined rate of 13.6 terminations or other sanctions per 1,000 is almost five times the 1987 rate of serious disciplinary actions by state licensing boards.

The most common violation, and the one accounting for one-half of disciplinary actions, is inappropriate prescription writing, often for controlled substances. The second major category of violation is substance abuse (drugs or alcohol, or both). A report from the Office of Inspector General (OIG, 1986) points out that this second category is expanding both in absolute and proportionate terms. Inappropriate prescription writing and substance abuse together account for three-quarters or more of all disciplinary actions. Other kinds of violations acted on by the state medical boards, such as professional misconduct, fraud, economic violations, or felony conviction, are not directly related to technical competence. Derbyshire (1984) has hypothesized that 10 percent of physicians are professionally "incompetent" to practice, based on his experience on a state board of medical examiners and as past President of the FSLB.[5]

Evidence of Poor Technical Quality for the Elderly

PRO Sanctions and Corrective Actions

Sanctions imposed by DHHS on the basis of recommendations by PROs are a potential source of data about the rate of poor quality care for Medicare beneficiaries. As of September, 1989, the OIG reported that since the start of the PRO program it had received 197 referrals for possible sanctions, had imposed 110 sanctions, rejected 79, and had 8 cases pending or moot because of the physicians' death or retirement (unpublished data). Sanction data should be considered, at best, a very minimal measure of the rate of poor quality care because most of those sanctioned are cited for multiple violations, because PROs undertake many more corrective actions than sanction recommendations, and because of the extensive due process accorded physicians during the sanctioning process, including the "willing or able" requirement for physician exclusion (see Chapter 6).

The number of corrective action plans together with sanction recommendations might provide a more reasonable estimate of the number of physicians with recognized quality-of-care problems. During the second PRO Scope of Work (a two-year period from 1986 to 1988), PROs identified more than 82,600 physicians with quality problems among the estimated 300,000 physicians who bill Medicare. It resolved 75,200 cases and instituted nearly 65,750 interventions (HCFA, 1989).

When asked during the public hearing whether the number of sanctions could be used to estimate the prevalence of physicians that one "would not send a neighbor to," a representative of the California PRO replied that this description would apply to perhaps 6 to 8 percent of the 50,000 physicians in the state. However, during a 19-month contract period the California PRO had sent first notices of sanction to only 137 physicians and forwarded just 14 recommendations for sanction to the OIG, a very small fraction of the almost 50,000 physicians practicing in that state. The medical director of another PRO estimated that about 5 percent (200) of 3,800 practicing physicians in his state account for 95 percent of the quality problems with perhaps 60 physicians accounting for approximately 80 percent of the quality problems. Quality problems were instances detected by PRO quality screens and confirmed after review by a PRO physician and possibly other specialists. To further hinder the estimation problem, more than one respondent during our site visits pointed out that PRO review includes hospital care only. They estimated that far more physicians with poor skills evade detection than are detected during PRO review, because they do not have hospital privileges or do not claim reimbursement from Medicare.

SuperPRO data (relating to re-review of charts initially reviewed by Medicare PRO physicians) were discussed in Chapter 6, and will be only briefly recapped here. According to a GAO report (1988a), the SuperPRO found that between 2.0 and 8.5 percent of hospital admissions had a quality problem, but this figure is based on a nonrandom selection of 17 percent of claims paid.[6]

Clinical Research Evidence on Quality of Care for the Elderly

In their reviews of the literature, both Rubenstein et al. (1989) and Lang and Kraegel (1989) examined the research evidence of poor technical quality of care for the elderly. Both papers cited extensive evidence of deficient treatment for conditions such as breast cancer, psychiatric disorders and confusion, pneumonia, urinary tract infection, incontinence, pressure sores, and malnutrition. They also reported patient management deficiencies in drug therapy, functional disability, and monitoring of fluids. Their review suggested the need for quality standards for ethical aspects of care and for rehabilitation and supported indications that higher nurse staffing ratios might reduce patient falls, improve the mental status of cognitively impaired elderly, strengthen hospital discharge planning, and provide more structured teaching for self-care.

Beneficiary Complaints

Data on beneficiary complaints about poor quality care are sketchy. The numbers of complaints and the percentages of confirmed quality problems vary greatly by PRO. During the second year of the second Scope of Work (roughly 1988), the rate of complaints per 100,000 beneficiaries ranged from 0 in several PROs to 108 in one PRO. Of those PROs receiving any complaints, the median percentage of problems confirmed by the PRO was 4 percent (range, zero to 100 percent) (GAO, 1988b). It is not clear whether the low reporting rate reflects an absence of quality problems, failure by the patient or family members to recognize quality problems, a lack of understanding about how to lodge a complaint, or some combination of reasons.

Evidence About Quality Problems in Home Health Care

Leader (1986, in Hawes and Kane, 1989) reports the results from a 1985 HCFA survey of Medicare-certified home health care providers in New Jersey and Region 2 (New York, the Virgin Islands, and Puerto Rico). The survey showed widespread and serious deficiencies in compliance with current standards of patient care (Hawes and Kane, 1989). For example

• coordination of patient services: 40 percent of New Jersey certified providers and 22 percent of Region 2 providers were deficient;
• plan of treatment: 60 percent of New Jersey providers and 25 percent of Region 2 agencies failed to meet the standard;
• conformance with physician orders: 70 percent of agencies in New Jersey and 26 percent of Region 2 providers were deficient; and
• clinical record review: 48 percent of New Jersey Medicare-certified agencies and 24 percent of Region 2 agencies were deficient.

A pilot study of posthospital community care for almost 300 elderly patients conducted by Mathematica Policy Research Center specified minimum adequate care for 40 conditions (e.g., instruction before discharge, visit to practitioner by the third day, or number of visits expected in a two-week period) (Phillips et al., 1989). An average of 4.3 guidelines applied to any one patient. The researchers looked for adverse outcomes that might result from failure to comply with the minimum guidelines. Of patients sampled to represent a high risk group, 69 percent received care that did not meet the minimal guidelines and 24 percent experienced adverse outcomes such as unscheduled physician or emergency room visits, or rehospitalization for dehydration or malnutrition. Of those classified as lower risk, 52 percent had care that did not meet guidelines, and 12 percent suffered adverse outcomes. The data were not reweighted to reflect the population as a whole.

The National League of Nursing, an accreditation group for agencies providing home health aides, undertook a study in 1987 to assess aides' skills (Hawes and Kane, 1989). They found widespread deficiencies among 265 home nursing aides in knowledge of such skills as responding if a patient stops breathing (30 percent were deficient), caring properly for a diabetic patient (45 percent), safely helping a stroke victim to walk (40 percent), and properly monitoring a patient's fluid intake (46 percent). These findings support an argument made by the American Bar Association (1986) that aides are poorly trained or untrained, are frequently hired by subcontractors, and are often not supervised by home health agency personnel. In addressing these disturbing findings, Hawes and Kane (1989) point out that little is known about the overall quality of home health, but they argue that the available information gives cause for concern. It indicates that improved measures of quality are needed, especially considering the growing demand for services, the apparent increase in patient acuity, and the pressure to contain costs.

Public Testimony

During public testimony for the study, 20 witnesses stated that they believed that lower quality care is provided in some geographic locations such as inner cities and some rural areas. Policy experts were divided about whether there should be different quality standards for underserved areas or areas with few resources.

Numerous witnesses also asserted that the health care system is not responsive to the uniqueness of the elderly population and argued for a more humane relationship between the elderly patient and the clinician. Other comments focused on the fragmentation of the health care system, the increase in subspecialty practices, and the decrease in the role of the primary physician.

Several witnesses distinguished quality of care from quality of service. For the latter, they expressed the need for increased continuity of care among delivery settings and among various providers within a given setting. They cited case management as a means to achieve this. Continuity concerns were mentioned by one in four of all respondents.

About one in six respondents were concerned about a current or emerging decline in the humane aspects of health care. As Martha Holstein of the American Society on Aging expressed it during the hearing in San Francisco,

> Quality of care becomes a fine line between attending to their [the elderly] objective needs while respecting their subjective selves. It is an honoring of limits. This honoring—and the provision of supports necessary for protecting autonomy despite limits—may be, for the old and the very old, as important a goal of medicine as curing what can be cured... Quality rests not only in what is done to and for the older person but also in the quality of the relationship—the respect for persons and what it takes to enhance personhood despite increasing frailty.

EVIDENCE OF OVERUSE

Several powerful factors are thought to promote the intensive use—and overuse—of physician-determined services in the United States (Eisenberg, 1979). First is a cultural and professional "imperative." In the face of uncertainty, physicians (and their patients) will generally opt to intervene rather than to wait (Wennberg et al., 1982; Wennberg, 1984; Eddy, 1984; Eddy and Billings, 1988; Eisenberg, 1986). This has been described by Eddy (1984) as a philosophy of "when in doubt, do." Kassirer (1989), in reference to diagnostic testing, speaks of an "inordinate zeal for certainty." Uncertainty may arise because the true benefits and costs of various actions have not been researched; if researched, the results may not be known to the physician; or even if known, they may apply only to particular subsets of patients rather than to all patients needing care. Second, even when diagnosis or prognosis is relatively certain, people in this country may prefer action rather than resignation in the face of debility and declining health. Health care practitioners demonstrate their concern for the patient or the patient's family by ordering a test or writing a prescription as well as (or instead of) providing supportive care.

A third factor is the development of new technologies that promise earlier or more accurate diagnosis, less invasive or less risky diagnostic tests, or more definitive therapies. They are produced, publicized, and actively promoted to physicians, and even to patients, through extensive marketing in advance of thorough technology assessment or rigorous evaluation (McPhee et al., 1987). In this respect, some overuse may be a response to patient demand and some to the eagerness of physicians to use the most recently available technologies.

Fourth, financial gain may be a powerful incentive for the practitioner who is paid a fee for individual services, a fee that may reward the use of office and other outpatient diagnostic tests and procedures (Schroeder and Showstack, 1978). An OIG (1989a) study, for instance, reported a higher frequency of referral of patients for diagnostic tests by doctors with a financial interest in the referral laboratory than by doctors without such an interest.

Fifth, an often stated pressure leading to overuse is the fear of malpractice exposure. A physician might be sued for not having performed the definitive test to rule out an unlikely diagnosis, but he or she is unlikely to lose a suit for having done more than was required. Weisman et al. (1989) documented such practices in a survey of Maryland physicians conducted in 1985. In surveys of defensive medical practices conducted by the AMA during 1983 and 1984, 70 percent of the physicians responding said they engaged in defensive medicine before 1984, and 42 percent said they had increased their defensive medical practices above past levels (Slora and

Gonzalez, 1988). Along with increased documentation, spending more time with patients, and providing more information to patients about risks and benefits of procedures, defensive behavior included ordering additional laboratory tests, speciality consultations, x-rays, and follow-up visits.

Many other factors may also lead to overuse. They include peer pressure, convenience for either the physicians or the patients, curiosity, "irrational and ossified habits," practice style, and a human tendency to avoid the difficult calculations necessary to determine the likelihood of various outcomes of testing and how they would affect decisions about care (Moskowitz et al., 1988; Kassirer, 1989).

General Evidence of Overuse

Strong evidence of overuse is available from several sources. McPhee et al. (1982) summarized a considerable body of evidence of overuse of radiological and surgical procedures, pharmaceuticals, and hospital length of stay. Schroeder (1987) reviewed multiple sources of evidence: small area and international comparisons; hospital admission and length of stay by members of health maintenance organizations (HMOs) in comparison to traditional hospital insurance; retrospective views of care by senior clinicians; uses of diagnostic data for clinical management; and the results of natural experiments at various institutions.

Overuse of services has been documented for a wide range of services, including various procedures, diagnostic tests, and hospital inpatient care (Brook and Lohr, 1986). Work from The RAND Corporation is among the most widely cited as documenting overuse of services through retrospective review of records using criteria developed by expert panels (Park et al., 1986).[7] In their review of almost 5,000 hospital patient records of Medicare patients in three large geographic areas, Chassin et al. (1986, 1987) reported that, based on information available to the physician before the procedure was done, 17 percent of upper gastrointestinal (UGI) endoscopies were inappropriate and 11 percent were equivocal. For coronary angiography, 17 percent of procedures were judged inappropriate and another 9 percent equivocal (Chassin et al., 1987). Review of records of patients receiving carotid endarterectomies indicated that 32 percent were inappropriate and 32 percent equivocal (Winslow et al., 1988b). Other estimates of inappropriate surgery include coronary artery bypass surgery, 14 percent (Winslow et al. 1988a); cardiac pacemaker implantation, 20 percent (Greenspan et al., 1988); and carotid endarterectomy, 13 percent (Merrick et al., 1986).[8] In a monograph prepared for the American Association of Retired Persons, Brown et al. (1989) estimated similar ranges of overuse for electrocardiograms, cataract removal and lens insertion, colonoscopy and sigmoidoscopy, prostatectomy, and hip arthroplasty, but noted that appropriateness studies are not presently available. Fewer data are available on other major medical and surgical procedures or on common diagnostic and x-ray procedures to estimate the level of overuse. Because, however, diagnostic technologies are widely believed among medical experts to be overused (Moloney and Rogers, 1979), the medical profession has developed guidelines for common diagnostic tests (Sox, 1987).

Small Area Analysis

Small area analysis, in which rates of use are standardized for a specific, defined population at risk, has demonstrated large geographic variations in the use of surgical procedures and medical admissions in similar patient populations (Wennberg and Gittelsohn, 1973, 1975). The literature on variations in health services utilization analyzed at the level of the state, province, hospital service area, city, demographic subpopulations, and nation shows large variations in discharge rates, average lengths of stay, patient days of care, and expenditures for a long list of surgical procedures at every geographical level studied (Paul-Shaheen et al., 1987). For example, Chassin et al. (1986) noted an 11-fold difference in hip arthroplasty and a four-fold difference in rates of carotid endarterectomy. As another case in point, citizens of Boston have half the rate of coronary artery bypass surgery and twice the rate of carotid endarterectomies as those in New Haven, despite the similar demographic characteristics of the two cities (Wennberg et al., 1987).

Even larger differences in use rates are found among different countries. Rates of many surgical procedures and other interventions in the United States greatly exceed the rates in Canada, the United Kingdom, Scandinavia, and Europe (Bunker, 1983; McPherson et al., 1982). For instance, the rate of coronary artery bypass surgery ranged from 19 operations per million population in France to 483 in the United States in 1978 (Banta and Kemp, 1980). The rate in the United States now probably exceeds 1,000 per million (McPhee et al., 1987). Hysterectomy is performed three times as often in the United States as in England and Wales, and prostatectomy 2.5 times as often (McPherson et al., 1982).

Variations in health services utilization may be linked to health system characteristics such as the supply of hospital beds or number of surgeons and to individual factors such as the socioeconomic and health status of the population. Wennberg and Gittelsohn (1982) have argued persuasively that much of the observed variation lies with the physicians' style of practice— a "surgical signature" that varies by procedure and indicates the surgeon's relative propensity to use a given surgical intervention. This propensity reflects personality, training, and cultural differences. In addition, Wennberg and others assert that large variations in practice patterns reflect current levels of uncertainty about the effectiveness of a procedure.

Surgical procedures with high variations suggest, but do not prove, overuse. The variations flag practices warranting further investigation. In their study evaluating the appropriateness of procedures in areas of high and low use, Chassin et al. (1987) found small but statistically significant differences in rates of appropriateness between high- and low-use areas. Nevertheless, the proportion of inappropriate, as opposed to equivocal or appropriate, use was considerable in both kinds of areas. Similarly, Siu et al. (1986) found large variations in the rate of inappropriate hospitalization (varying from 10 to 35 percent), but areas with low admission rates did not necessarily have low proportions of inappropriate admissions. This suggests that any policy to reduce unexplained variation on the assumption that the services are marginally indicated or discretionary would have an unpredictable effect on the quality of care (Wennberg, 1987).

Evidence of Overuse for the Elderly

Evidence of overuse of services for the elderly is accumulating rapidly. Many of the reports cited above relate in whole or in part to services used by Medicare beneficiaries (for example, the RAND studies used Medicare Part B data).

The OIG (1988b) reported on a review of a random sample of 7,050 Medicare patients discharged from 239 hospitals between October 1984 and March 1985. Physician and nurse reviewers assessed the appropriateness of admissions using the patient's condition on admission, during the stay, and at the time of discharge. Nurse reviewers used the Appropriateness Evaluation Protocol (Gertman and Restuccia, 1981) and referred any problems to physicians for further review. "An admission was considered unnecessary if no reason for admission existed at the time a patient entered a hospital" (OIG, 1988a, p. 3). Major findings included the following

- 10.5 percent of hospital admissions were unnecessary;
- 78 percent of the unnecessary admissions for acute care could have been treated more appropriately in outpatient settings. Other patients were social admissions, belonged in nursing facilities, did not need acute care, or received no acute care services during their hospital stays;
- 14 percent of the hospitals had high rates of unnecessary admissions (i.e., 20 percent or more of their admissions); these hospitals also had twice as many premature discharges and patients with quality-of-care problems;
- 71 percent of the hospitals had 5 percent or more unnecessary admissions; and

• five diagnosis-related groups (DRGs) occurred frequently in the sample as unnecessary admissions: medical back problems (DRG 243); diabetes patients over age 35 (DRG 294); bone cancer (DRG 239); digestive disorders, patients aged 18 to 69 (DRG 183); and upper respiratory tract infections, patients over age 69 (DRG 68). DRG 39 (cataract surgery) was also frequently the reason for an unnecessary admission, but the investigators noted that this surgery has since shifted to the outpatient setting.

Clinical Research Studies on Overuse of Services for the Elderly

Rubenstein et al. (1989) accumulated considerable evidence of overuse of institutional services, in particular, nursing homes used when skilled care was not required. Other evidence cited indicated that geriatric intervention and better discharge planning could reduce hospital length of stay. Some prolonged hospital stays seem to be the result of limited supplies of long-term-care services. Rubenstein et al. (1989) also reviewed literature on overuse of specific interventions such as drugs, surgery, diagnostic tests, and restraints. These studies have shown that some older patients receive unnecessary and often harmful prescription medications and a substantial amount of unneeded surgery.

Lang and Kraegel (1989), in reviewing the nursing literature, found equally broad evidence of overuse of some types of treatment and services among the elderly. They, too, cite overuse of nursing home placement and of hospital admissions (because of a lack of nursing services in other settings) and excessive medication use among patients with dementia and cardiac problems.

Public Hearings, Focus Groups, and Site Visits

In the study's public testimony, only about one in ten of our respondents expressed a concern about overuse. During site visits and physician focus groups, however, physicians repeatedly noted their impressions of overuse among colleagues, especially in the areas of medications, procedures, and aggressiveness of therapy. Almost all the physician participants in focus groups stated that overuse was a common occurrence in the health care system and that it was more pervasive than underuse of services, but they found it very difficult to estimate the amount of overuse.[9] Some groups felt that approximately 10 percent of all services provided could be categorized as overuse; another group estimated 20 to 30 percent. All groups cautioned that these estimates vary by individual provider, institution, and geographic area. The focus groups of Medicare beneficiaries did not express concern about overuse of services other than their perception of getting too many prescriptions (Chapter 3 in Volume II summarizes the findings of the focus groups).

EVIDENCE OF UNDERUSE

Less is known about the magnitude or types of underuse than of overuse, because it is difficult to measure an event that should have occurred but did not. Underuse of services has two principal sources: (1) underuse by virtue of lack of access to services and (2) underuse because patients are not offered (or do not accept) available services that are likely to be beneficial to them.

Access

Access barriers are most often viewed in financial terms. They include the obstacles posed by lack of insurance coverage and by copayments and deductibles that deter use.[10] For the Medicare beneficiary, lack of coverage for needed services (e.g., preventive services, dentures, glasses, or special shoes for diabetics) is an access barrier. The most often cited category of underuse of services is for ambulatory care, specifically preventive care (e.g., cancer screening, vaccination, and immunization). The value of preventive care for elderly is supported by a study conducted by Hermanson et al. (1988) showing that elderly smokers with coronary artery disease who ceased smoking had a lower risk of myocardial infarction and death than did continuing smokers. Home care and preventive care (virtually none of the latter being covered services) are widely regarded as underused elderly services.

Barriers to care may also be geographical, physical, or psychological. Beneficiary frailty and lack of transportation can preclude travel, even in urban or suburban areas. Unavailability of needed expertise and services in remote rural areas are equally obvious access barriers. Other possible obstacles to care are more directly related to Medicare. For instance, decisions by physicians not to accept Medicare patients may create an access barrier for patients; decisions not to accept assignment may impose the same obstacle for at least some Medicare beneficiaries. The complexity of the Medicare program itself may be an access barrier if patients (or their physicians) do not understand what services are covered or how to obtain care through Medicare. Beneficiaries for whom English is not the primary language are at particular risk from this access barrier.

Rules governing the frequency with which services covered by Medicare will be reimbursed in an ambulatory or institutional setting can also affect access, and there has been concern that the prospective payment system (PPS) for hospitals may lead to premature discharge and that capitation payment for HMOs may lead to undercare. Finally, differing decisions by fiscal intermediaries (FIs), carriers, and Medicare PROs concerning covered benefits or pre-admission and pre-procedure approvals can cause confusion and, perhaps, underuse of services for beneficiaries in some parts of the country. Studies that evaluate underutilization of health care tend to be descriptive surveys of utilization patterns and unmet needs. These studies can provide data for assessing health service needs and for identifying areas of maldistribution or inequity in delivery of care for the elderly population (Rubenstein et al., 1989).

Underdiagnosis and Undertreatment

In medical care, underuse of services not related to direct access barriers may be classified as either underdiagnosis or undertreatment. Underdiagnosis (or lack of case finding) in the elderly has been studied for such conditions as depression, substance abuse, urinary incontinence, and confusional states. It may be attributed in some part to practitioners simply not identifying with medical problems they have not experienced or not treating certain categories of patients (the poor, women, racial and ethnic minorities) as thoroughly as others. Undertreatment includes, for example, lack of timely and appropriately vigorous medical therapies, follow-up, adequate nursing care, discharge planning, and home health visits. Malpractice suits frequently allege underdiagnosis and undertreatment (e.g., missed diagnosis, or lack of follow-up of abnormal x-ray or test).

Often underuse is only inferred. For instance, descriptive studies, surveys of utilization patterns, or controlled trials that demonstrate improved outcomes from a service that is not generally provided may support inferences about underuse. In addition, care may be found insufficient when individuals are hospitalized for complications of conditions that can (and should) be successfully managed in the outpatient setting or long-term-care facility or when they are hospitalized for the first time at excessively advanced stages of disease. Furthermore, care may be insufficient when patients receive services from primary care physicians that would be more appropriately given by specialists.

In cases discussed above, generalizing to the entire population of elderly might provide an estimate of the "room for improvement" in the overall level of care (often by improving access) rather than in the care provided by organizations or specific providers. However, where providers have an incentive to conserve resources, evidence of possible underprovision of services may need to be sought directly.

Methods to detect underuse related to access barriers are not the same as those used to detect underuse related to underdiagnosis or undertreatment. To measure underuse of services because of access barriers, population data are needed (e.g., all persons eligible for care, not just those using care). That is, when compared to population norms or to rates for other subgroups, rates of use in one group may suggest underuse. Conversely, underuse for patients already receiving services (underdiagnosis or undertreatment) may be detected by the usual methods of quality assessment. These tend to be based less on population-based evidence than on adverse occurrences or evidence from samples of patients. Underuse by specific subgroups can be identified by purposive sampling.

Evidence of Underuse Among the Elderly

Medicare Data

Continued concern about the effects of Medicare's PPS has prompted greater attention to the possibility of premature hospital discharge, which is a type of underuse among the elderly. An OIG review of over 7,000 hospital admissions by Medicare patients between October 1984 and March 1985 concluded that only 0.8 percent of discharges were premature (OIG, 1988b). Premature discharges were characterized by inadequate treatment and incomplete therapies; occurred most often in small, rural, nonteaching facilities; and were often associated with quality-of-care problems during the hospital stay.

PROs have been directed to review hospital readmissions as a screen for possible premature discharge as well as other problems in quality that may have led to readmission within 31 days. The Medicare Prospective Payment Assessment Commission (ProPAC, 1989) reviewed data on patterns of readmission from Medicare claims files from 1984 to 1986 but found no evidence in readmission statistics to indicate significant quality problems related to premature discharge. In their review of generic screen failures based on a 3-percent random sample of Medicare discharges, PROs confirmed that patients were not stable at the time of discharge in less than 1 percent (0.87 per 100) of the records reviewed (ProPAC, 1989).

One area where declining length of stay has been thought to provide evidence that quality of care has been jeopardized is in care of patients with hip fracture. Fitzgerald et al. (1988) found that since implementation of PPS and declining lengths of stay, hospitals have reduced the amount of rehabilitative care given and have discharged more patients to nursing homes (an increase from 38 to 60 percent); in addition, the number of patients remaining in nursing homes after one year rose from 9 to 33 percent. HMO patients in that study were also discharged to nursing homes at a higher rate than before PPS, but only 16 percent of HMO patients were still in nursing homes after a year, compared to 35 percent of other patients. Russell (1989) regards this finding as indicative of differences in nursing home care management rather than an underuse effect of PPS. If so, the data do not permit differentiating such patterns as underuse or poor technical quality.

The OIG study cited earlier also sought to identify the incidence of poor care, defined as "medical care *clearly* failing to meet professionally recognized standards under any circumstances in any locale" (OIG, 1989b, p. 1). After data were adjusted for hospital size to reflect the population of Medicare patients in all hospitals, the proportion receiving poor quality care was estimated to be 5.5 percent. Eighty percent of the reasons for poor quality care involved the omission of necessary services, for instance, failure to order or provide appropriate tests and services either at all or in a timely manner. Many hospitals with high rates of poor quality care also had high rates of unnecessary admissions and premature discharges. Six DRGs were frequently associated with poor quality care: DRG 14 (strokes, except transient ischemic attack); DRG 15 (transient ischemic attacks); DRG 87 (pulmonary edema and respiratory failure); DRG 89 (simple pneumonia and pleurisy, patients over age 69); DRG 141 (fainting, patients over age 69); and DRG 320 (kidney and urinary tract infections patients over age 69) (OIG, 1989b).

In response to a legislative emphasis on quality, the PROs have been reviewing cases failing generic screens. ProPAC reported that a generic screen-based study of 3,250 records found 162 quality problems (5.0 percent). Indication of underuse might be found in these researchers' estimate that an additional 5.3 percent of records had problems (not detectable in the generic screens) that involved "insufficient attention to medical problems, rather than problems with the care that was provided" (ProPAC, 1989, p. 34).

PRO review of "sentinel admissions" by patients enrolled in risk-contract prepaid group practices is oriented to possibly insufficient ambulatory care (see Chapter 6), but no findings have yet been reported.

Other Research Evidence of Underuse of Services for the Elderly

With respect to underuse of services, Rubenstein et al. (1989) cited two articles indicating underuse of emergency services and intensive care units for the elderly. They also documented many different forms of underdiagnosis and undertreatment in their review of the clinical literature. Physicians spend less time with the elderly and diagnose a smaller proportion of older patients' medical problems. When diagnostic assessments made by geriatricians are compared with those by patients' primary care or hospital physicians, all 11 studies they reviewed showed less complete diagnostic services for the elderly. Diagnoses often missed by primary care physicians include: treatable incontinence, curable infections, gait disorders, and metabolic problems. Similar findings were reported in six studies of nursing home patients, in six studies of elderly patients in general medical clinics, and in five of six studies of elderly patients later diagnosed with cancer. In all these settings, it appeared that underdiagnosis was prevalent among elderly patients, and, in those studies that made the comparison, less common among comparable groups of younger patients.

Rubenstein and his colleagues also reviewed studies of undertreatment of older patients in hospital settings, nursing homes, and general outpatient settings. Studies in all settings found a high prevalence of treatable conditions for which treatment was less adequate for older compared to younger patients. Problems included underprovision of rehabilitation in both hospital and nursing home settings, a need for more acute care in nursing homes, deficiencies in disease-specific care including underuse of mental health services for depression, delayed and less aggressive treatment for cancer patients, and underprovision of acute care and rehabilitation for older versus younger stroke patients.

In short, Rubenstein and his colleagues saw major gaps in the health care delivered to the elderly. They also pointed out that because they reviewed only published studies of patients already receiving care, their estimates probably understated problems of underuse in the community.

In their review of the nursing literature for areas of underuse of those nursing interventions that maintain or restore function, Lang and Kraegel (1989) emphasized evaluation of the functional status of the elderly and the impact of loss of function and increased dependency for those with chronic disease. They reported evidence of underuse of home-care nursing services because some elderly do not know that services are available or because services are prematurely terminated. Older females have differentially fewer home visits than males despite greater functional impairment and fewer available caretakers.

Public Hearings, Focus Groups, and Site Visits

During the public hearings, focus groups, and site visits, the study committee heard frequently about lack of Medicare coverage for long-term care, preventive services, and primary care. Cost barriers were reported to result in implicit rationing based on class, sex, and ability to pay. Underuse was also linked to isolation (economic, social, transportation, and housing).

Nearly one-half of all public testimony respondents expressed concern that the quality of health care would decrease as a result of cost-containment measures. Premature discharges, utilization review, financial factors for underuse, and health care decisions being made by the "wrong people" (e.g., staff of FIs, PROs, and third-party payers) are examples of the cost-containment concerns mentioned.

More than one-third of public hearing respondents believed that the quality of care for the elderly is less than optimal because of deficiencies in Medicare coverage of health-related services that encourage independent living for those with certain chronic conditions. These include custodial, homemaker, and other services. Other respondents stressed that the Medicare reimbursement system does not take into account the health needs of the elderly that relate to quality of life. The public hearing testimony did not elicit specific information about underdiagnosis or undertreatment of patients who were already using the system.

Elderly participants in focus group mentioned interpersonal issues in care more than problems of access or undertreatment. Issues mentioned included the amount of time and interest devoted to them by providers (especially in contrast to younger patients), the amount of nursing care and the quality of attention in the nursing home. They did express concern about PPS leading to premature discharge.

During the site visits, our contacts raised numerous concerns about underuse. These included failure to diagnose (particularly acute pneumonia, myocardial infarction, and meningitis) and inadequate follow-up of positive diagnostic findings. Other points raised were the lack of preventive services (influenza vaccination and cancer screening), inadequate mental health care, and lack of home care services.

Findings to date do not indicate that Medicare PPS has had demonstrable negative effects on quality of care or the health of the elderly population (e.g., in terms of higher mortality rates). Nevertheless, the hearings, focus groups, and site visits show that patient and provider groups remain apprehensive about the future.

SUMMARY

Evidence of overuse of health care services is substantial; virtually all factors of a fee-for-service system promote it. Information on underuse is more sketchy and inferential; incentives of capitation are a source of concern. Underuse is hard to detect through available surveillance systems. One background paper for this study concluded that, for the elderly, underuse is more prevalent than overuse, but no estimate could be made of the actual burden of harm (frequency and severity). Finally, setting- and disease-specific examples of poor technical quality can be found in many arenas, although they do not translate easily into national estimates of levels of quality of care.

Little information is available on national estimates of prevalence of quality problems, and no data document the burden of harm by problem, by disease category, by setting, or by population group such as the elderly. This lack of data is not surprising, for several reasons. Compiling data on national quality problems has not been seen as Medicare's responsibility; no current monitoring system can provide such data; and provider groups do not view their internal quality assurance programs as needing to contribute to national estimates of quality problems.

Nevertheless, there is good reason to believe that problems exist in all three areas, of different magnitudes in different settings. For this reason, the study committee believes it prudent, indeed necessary, that a Medicare quality assurance program develop and use appropriate measures to track all three types of problems and to find ways to estimate the burden of harm better, so that differential emphasis on improvement can be placed where most needed.

NOTES

1. The investigators sampled 25 insurers from a pool of 102 insurers that in 1984 closed an estimated 73,500 claims involving about 103,300 health care providers. They then analyzed a sample of 2,781 claims for types of allegations, which include claims closed with and without compensation.
2. The final report of the Harvard Medical Practice Study, which is expected to be published early in 1990, has been designed to investigate the incidence during hospitalization of injuries resulting from medical intervention and the proportion of these injuries that are due to substandard care (Hiatt et al., 1989).
3. The 1986 figure was based on numbers of all duplicated disciplinary actions reported to the Federation of State Licensing Boards for 1986, divided by numbers of practicing physicians reported by the American Medical Association (AMA, 1986) using the sum of nonfederal office-based practitioners and full-time hospital-based (nonresident) physician staff.
4. The figure is lower than the 1986 data quoted above because it includes only "serious actions"—revocations, suspensions, and probations—and does not include reprimands (or remedial education).
5. The terms professional incompetence, professional malfeasance, moral turpitude, and repeated malpractice are not used with consistency or precision in state legislation. Derbyshire (1984) defines professional incompetence as the "inability of a physician to care for patients satisfactorily because of such failings as faulty judgment, unreliability, unavailability, and professional obsolescence" (p. 136B). He intends this definition to include impairment from substance abuse, but it is not clear whether inappropriate prescription writing or moral turpitude are intended to be or are, in practice, widely included in the term incompetence. Nor is it clear whether incompetence can be established by one incident or requires a pattern of behavior. Thus, comparisons of various estimates of "rates of incompetence" are probably not valid.
6. One might expect the SuperPRO sample to have a higher rate of quality problems than a true random sample of claims. The SuperPRO reviews randomly selected cases reviewed by each PRO, but the PRO pool of cases is not a random selection of all hospital admissions. In addition to the "3 percent random sample" nearly five times as many cases are selected either because there is reason to believe a quality problem exists for that case or for reasons unrelated to poor technical quality per se, but perhaps related to overuse of services or to coding problems. Generally speaking, however, because of the nonrandom nature of PRO cases, the SuperPRO estimates cannot be used to estimate either the incidence of poor quality care in the 83 percent of claims not

reviewed or the number of inappropriate admissions. Of the 1,187 cases identified (and re-reviewed) by the SuperPRO, they found

- 58 cases where the potential for patient risk was of a serious nature (4.9 percent);
- 3 cases where actual reversible or minor harm was done to the patient (0.25 percent); and
- 9 cases where irreversible or significant harm was done to the patient (0.76 percent).

7. Retrospective review of appropriateness depends on the information that is recorded in the medical record. Factors relevant to the treatment decision might
not have been documented.

8. Many of these studies were done in the early 1980s; rates of inappropriate use
may have changed since then. Furthermore, such rates may vary among different populations. For instance, Chassin et al. (1987) found one-third of carotid
endarterectomies to be inappropriate in each of three large geographic areas in
1981. Merrick et al. (1986) found that only 13 percent of procedures among 95
patients in California Veterans Administration Medical Centers were "clearly
inappropriate." Physicians in the United Kingdom and in the United States
reviewed the same cases of coronary artery bypass surgery. U.K. physicians
judged 35 percent of cases and U.S. physicians 13 percent of cases to be inappropriate, a difference that was interpreted as indicating substantial cultural differences (Brook et al., 1988).

9. When asked about the distribution of overuse, underuse, or poor technical quality, most study respondents found it difficult to make estimates. Issues of
underuse were most frequently expressed as access and benefits problems.
Concerns expressed about continuity, fragmentation, and shared decision making, which occurred with some frequency, did not fall easily into any of our
three categories; we generally viewed them as reflecting poor technical quality.

10. The most extensive evidence of the effect of cost-sharing on use of services
comes from The RAND Corporation's decade-long Health Insurance Experiment (HIE). Although the HIE did not include the elderly, its strong results
across all other age groups make clear that even relatively mild levels of copayments and deductibles have marked impacts on use of services (Newhouse et
al., 1981, 1987). The evidence concerning the effect of cost-sharing on adult
health status is less powerful—the main findings indicate that having completely free care significantly improved the health of adults in two areas of
particular importance for the elderly: hypertension and visual acuity (Brook et
al., 1983; Keeler et al., 1985). Cost-sharing may also have had a differential
effect on persons of low income (particularly children). Finally, cost-sharing
was found to be at best only a blunt instrument for curtailing the use of inappropriate services; except for persons of higher income and education, cost-
sharing reduced the use of appropriate and inappropriate ambulatory services to
about the same degree (Lohr et al., 1986).

REFERENCES

American Bar Association. *The Black Box of Home Care Quality* (a report prepared for the Chairman of the Select Committee on Aging, U.S. House of Representatives). Comm. Publ. No. 99-573, Washington, D.C.: Government Printing Office, August 1986.

American Medical Association. *Physician Characteristics and Distribution in the U.S., 1986 Edition.* Chicago, Ill.: American Medical Association, 1986.

Banta, H.D. and Kemp, K.B. *Background Paper No. 4: The Management of Health Care Technology in Ten Countries.* Washington, D.C.: Office of Technology Assessment, 1980.

Brook, R.H. and Lohr, K.N. Will We Need To Ration Effective Health Care? *Issues in Science and Technology* 3:68-77, Fall 1986.

Brook, R.H., Ware, J.E., Jr., Rogers, W.H., et al. Does Free Care Improve Adults' Health? Results from a Randomized Controlled Trial. *New England Journal of Medicine* 309:1426-1434, 1983.

Brook, R.H., Kosecoff, J.B., Park, R.E., et al. Diagnosis and Treatment of Coronary Disease: Comparison of Doctors' Attitudes in the U.S.A. and the U.K. *Lancet* i:750-753, 1988.

Brown, R.E., Sheingold, S.H., and Luce, B.R. *Options of Using Practice Guidelines in Reducing the Volume of Medically Unnecessary Services.* BHARC-013/89/027. Washington, D.C.: Battelle Human Affairs Research Centers, 1989.

Bunker, J.P. Surgical Manpower. A Comparison of Operations and Surgeons in the United States and in England and Wales. *New England Journal of Medicine* 282:135-144, 1983.

Chassin, M.R., Brook, R.H., Park, R.E., et al. Variations in the Use of Medical and Surgical Services by the Medicare Populations. *New England Journal of Medicine* 314:285-290, 1986.

Chassin, M.R., Kosecoff, J., Park, R.E., et al. Does Inappropriate Use Explain Geographic Variations in the Use of Health Care Services? A Study of Three Procedures. *Journal of the American Medical Association* 258:2533-2537, 1987.

Chassin, M.R., Park, R.E., Lohr, K.N., et al. Differences among Hospitals in Medicare Mortality. *Health Services Research* 24:1-31, 1989.

Couch, N.P., Tilney, N.L., Rayer, A.A., et al. The High Cost of Low-Frequency Events—The Anatomy and Economics of Surgical Mishaps. *New England Journal of Medicine* 304:634-637, 1981.

Craddick, J.W. and Bader, B.S. *Medical Management Analysis, A Systematic Approach to Quality Assurance and Risk Management, Vol. I.* Auburn, Calif.: J.W. Craddick, 1983.

Danzon, P.M. *Medical Malpractice: Theory, Evidence, and Public Policy.* Cambridge, Mass.: Harvard University Press, 1985.

Derbyshire, R.C. Medical Discipline in Disarray: Retrospective and Prospective. *Hospital Practice* 19:136A-136P, June 1984.

Dubois, R.W. and Brook, R H. Preventable Deaths: Who, How Often, and Why? *Annals of Internal Medicine* 109:582-589, 1988.

Eddy, D.M. Variations in Physician Practice: The Role of Uncertainty. *Health Affairs* 3:74-89, 1984.

Eddy, D.M. and Billings, J. The Quality of the Medical Evidence. *Health Affairs* 7:20-32, 1988.

Eisenberg, J.M. Sociologic Influences on Decision-Making by Clinicians. *Annals of Internal Medicine* 90:957-964, 1979.

Eisenberg, J.M. *Doctors' Decisions and the Cost of Medical Care.* Ann Arbor, Mich.: Health Administration Press Perspectives, 1986.

Fitzgerald, J.F., Moore, P.S., and Dittus, R.S. The Care of Elderly Patients with Hip Fracture. *New England Journal of Medicine* 319:1393-1397, 1988.

Foxman, B., Valdez, R.B., Lohr, K.N., et al. The Effect of Cost Sharing on the Use of Antibiotics in Ambulatory Care: Results from a Population-Based Randomized Controlled Trial. *Journal of Chronic Diseases* 40:429-437, 1987.

Gertman, P.M. and Restuccia, J. The Appropriateness Evaluation Protocol: A Technique for Assessing Unnecessary Days of Hospital Care. *Medical Care* 19:855-871, 1981.

GAO (General Accounting Office). *Medical Malpractice: Characteristics of Claims Closed in 1984.* HRD-87-55. Washington, D.C.: General Accounting Office, April 1987.

GAO. *Internal Controls: Need to Strengthen Controls Over Payments by Medicare Intermediaries.* HRD-89-8. Washington, D.C.: General Accounting Office, November, 1988a.

GAO. *Medicare PROs. Extreme Variation in Organizational Structure and Activities.* GAO/PEMD-89-7FS. Washington, D.C.: General Accounting Office, November, 1988b.

Graboys, T.B. Conflicts of Interest in the Management of Silent Ischemia. *Journal of the American Medical Association* 261:2116-2117, 1989.

Greenspan, A.M., Kay, H.R., Berger, B.C., et al. Incidence of Unwarranted Implantation of Permanent Cardiac Pacemakers in a Large Medical Population. *New England Journal of Medicine* 318:158-163, 1988.

Hawes, C. and Kane, R.L. Issues Related to Quality Review and Assurance in Health Care. Paper prepared for the Institute of Medicine Study to Design a Strategy for Quality Review and Assurance in Medicare, 1989.

HCFA (Health Care Financing Administration). Utilization and Quality Control Peer Review Organizations Second Scope of Work. Executive Data Summary. Report through February 1989. Report dated 5/30/89. Baltimore, Md.: Health Care Financing Administration, 1989.

Hermanson, B., Omenn, G.S., Kronmal, R.A., et al. Beneficial Six-Year Outcome of Smoking Cessation in Older Men and Women with Coronary Artery Disease. *New England Journal of Medicine* 319:1365-1369, 1988.

Hiatt, H.H., Barnes, B.A., Brennan, T.A., et al. Special Report: A Study of Medical Injury and Medical Malpractice. *New England Journal of Medicine* 320:480-483, 1989.

Jogerst, G.L. and Dippe, S.E. Antibiotic Use Among Medical Specialties. *Journal of the American Medical Association* 245:842-846, 1981.

Kassirer, J.P. Sounding Board. Our Stubborn Quest for Diagnostic Certainty—A Case of Excessive Testing. *New England Journal of Medicine* 320:1489-1491, 1989.

Keeler, E.B., Brook, R.H., Goldberg, G.A., et al. How Free Care Reduced Hypertension in the Health Insurance Experiment. *Journal of the American Medical Association* 254:1926-1931, 1985.

Lang, N. and Kraegel, J.M. Quality of Health Care for Older People in America. Paper prepared for the Institute of Medicine Study to Design a Strategy for Quality Review and Assurance in Medicare, 1989.

Lohr, K.N., Brook, R.H., Kamberg, C.J., et al. Use of Medical Care in the Rand Health Insurance Experiment. Diagnosis- and Service-Specific Analyses in a Randomized Controlled Trial. *Medical Care* 24:S1-S87, September Supplement, 1986.

McPhee, S.J., Myers, L.P., and Schroeder, S.A. The Cost and Risks of Medical Care—An Annotated Bibliography for Clinicians and Educators. *Western Journal of Medicine* 137:145-161, 1982.

McPhee, S.J., Garnick, D.W., and Schroeder, S.A. Cardiac Imaging and Cost-Containment: On a Collision Course. *American Journal of Cardiac Imaging* 1:204-206, 1987.

McPherson, K., Wennberg, J.E., Hovind, O.B., et al. Small Area Variations in the Use of Common Surgical Procedures: An International Comparison of New England, England, and Norway. *New England Journal of Medicine* 307:1310-1314, 1982.

Merrick, N.L., Brook, R.H., Fink, A., et al. Use of Carotid Endarterectomy in Five California Veterans Administration Medical Centers. *Journal of American Medical Association* 258:2531-2535, 1986.

Mills, D.H., ed. California Medical Association and California Hospital Association *Report on the Medical Insurance Feasibility Study*. San Francisco, Calif.: Sutter, 1977.

Moskowitz, A.J., Benjamin, J.K., and Kassirer, J.P. Dealing with Uncertainty, Risks, and Tradeoffs in Clinical Decisions. *Annals of Internal Medicine* 108:435-449, 1988.

Moloney, T.W. and Rogers, D.E. Medical Technology—A Different View of the Contentious Debate over Costs. *New England Journal of Medicine* 301:1413-1419, 1979.

Newhouse, J.E., Manning, W.G., Morris, C.N., et al. Some Interim Results from a Controlled Trial of Cost Sharing in Health Insurance. *New England Journal of Medicine* 305:1501-1507, 1981.

Newhouse, J.P., Manning, W.G., Duan, N., et al. The Findings of the Rand Health Insurance Experiment—A Response to Welch et al. *Medical Care* 25:157-179, 1987.

OIG (Office of Inspector General, Department of Health and Human Services). *Medical Licensure and Discipline: An Overview, Department of Health and Human Services*. P-01-86-0064. Washington, D.C.: Office of Inspector General, Office of Analysis and Inspections, June 1986.

OIG. *National DRG Validation Study: Special Report on Premature Discharges*. OAI-05-88-00740. Washington, D.C.: Office of Inspector General, Office of Analysis and Inspections, February 1988a.

OIG. *National DRG Validation Study: Unnecessary Admissions to Hospitals*. Draft. OAI-09-88-00880. Washington, D.C.: Office of Inspector General, Office of Analysis and Inspections, April 1988b.

OIG. *Financial Arrangement Between Physicians and Health Care Businesses: State Laws and Regulation.* OAI-12-88-0140. Washington, D.C.: Office of Inspector General, Office of Analysis and Inspections, April 1989a.

OIG. *National DRG Validation Study: Quality of Patient Care in Hospitals,* OAI-09-88-00870. Washington, D.C.: Office of Inspector General, Office of Analysis and Inspections, July 1989b.

OTA (Office of Technology Assessment). *The Quality of Medical Care. Information for Consumers.* OTA-H-386. Washington, D.C.: U.S. Government Printing Office, 1988.

Palmer, R.H., Hall, J.A., Hargraves, J.L., et al. Performance on Other Tasks. Paper presented at the Annual Meeting of the American Medical Review Research Center, October 31, 1988.

Park, R.E., Fink, A., Brook, R.H., et al. *Physician Ratings of Appropriate Indications for Six Medical and Surgical Procedures.* R-3280-CWF/HF/PMT/RWJ. Santa Monica, Calif.: The RAND Corporation, 1986.

Paul-Shaheen, P., Clark, J.D., and Williams, D. Small Area Analysis: A Review and Analysis of the North American Literature. *Journal of Health Politics, Policy and Law* 12:741-809, 1987.

Phillips, B.R., Schneider, B.W., Steele, K., et al. A Pilot Study of the Adequacy of Post-Hospital Community Care. Paper presented at the 6th Annual Meeting of the Association for Health Services Research and the Foundation for Health Services Research, Chicago, Ill., June 1989.

ProPAC (Prospective Payment Assessment Commission). *Medicare Prospective Payment and The American Health Care System. Report to the Congress.* Washington, D.C.: Prospective Payment Assessment Commission, June 1989.

Rubenstein, L.Z., Rubenstein, L.V., and Josephson, K.R. Quality of Health Care for Older People in America. Paper prepared for the Institute of Medicine Study to Design a Strategy for Quality Review and Assurance in Medicare, 1989.

Russell, L.B. Effects on the Health of the Elderly. Pp. 47-68 in *Medicare's New Hospital Payment System. Is it Working?* Washington, D.C.: The Brookings Institution, 1989.

Schroeder, S.A. Strategies for Reducing Medical Costs by Changing Physicians' Behavior. *International Journal of Technology Assessment in Health Care* 3:39-50, 1987.

Schroeder, S.A. and Showstack, J.A. Financial Incentives to Perform Medical Procedures and Laboratory Tests: Illustrative Models of Office Practice. *Medical Care* 16:289-298, 1978.

Siu, A.L., Sonnenberg, F.A., Manning, W.G., et al. Inappropriate Use of Hospitals in a Randomized Trial of Health Insurance Plans. *New England Journal of Medicine* 315:1259-1266, 1986.

Slora, E.J. and Gonzalez, M.L. Medical Professional Liability Claims and Premiums, 1985-1987. Pp. 18-22 in *Socioeconomic Characteristics of Medical Practice 1988.* Gonzalez, M.L. and Emmonds, D.W., eds. Chicago, Ill.: American Medical Association Center for Health Policy Research, 1988.

Sox, H.C., ed. *Common Diagnostic Tests: Use and Interpretation.* Philadelphia, Pa.: American College of Physicians, 1987.

Steele, K., Gertman, P.M., Crescenzi, C., et al. Iatrogenic Illness on a General Medical Service at a University Hospital. *New England Journal of Medicine* 304:638-641, 1981.

The St. Paul's 1988 Annual Report to Policyholders. St. Paul, Minn.: The St. Paul Companies, 1987.

Weisman, C.S., Morlock, L.L., Teitelbaum, M.A., et al. Practice Changes in Response to the Malpractice Litigation Climate. Results of a Maryland Physician Survey. *Medical Care* 27:16-24, 1989.

Wennberg, J.E. Dealing with Medical Practice Variations: A Proposal for Action. *Health Affairs* 3:6-32, 1984.

Wennberg, J.E. The Paradox of Appropriate Care. *Journal of the American Medical Association* 258:2568-2569, 1987.

Wennberg, J.E. and Gittelsohn, A. Small Area Variations in Health Care Delivery. *Science* 142:1102-1108, 1973.

Wennberg, J.E. and Gittelsohn, A. Health Care Delivery in Maine I: Patterns of Use of Common Surgical Procedures. *Journal of the Maine Medical Association* 66:123-149, 1975.

Wennberg, J.E. and Gittelsohn, A. Variations in Medical Care among Small Areas. *Scientific American* 246:120-134, 1982.

Wennberg, J.E., Barnes, B.A., and Zubkoff, M. Professional Uncertainty and the Problem of Supplier-Induced Demand. *Social Science and Medicine* 16:811-842, 1982.

Wennberg, J.E., Freeman, J.L, and Culp, W.J. Are Hospital Services Rationed in New Haven or Over-Utilised in Boston? *The Lancet* i:1185-1188, May 23, 1987.

Winslow, C.M., Kosecoff, J.B., Chassin, M., et al. The Appropriateness of Performing Coronary Artery Bypass Surgery. *Journal of the American Medical Association* 260:505-509, 1988a.

Winslow, C.M., Solomon, D.H., Chassin, M.R., et al. The Appropriateness of Carotid Endarterectomy. *New England Journal of Medicine* 318:721-727, 1988b.

Wolfe, S.M. Testimony of Sidney M. Wolfe, M.D. before Civil and Constitutional Rights Subcommittee, House Judiciary Committee, October 8, 1986.

Wolfe, S.M., ed. State Medical Board Doctor Disciplinary Actions: 1987. *The Public Citizen Health Research Group Health Letter* 5:1-4, 1989.

8

Settings of Care and Payment System Issues for Quality Assurance

Both the settings of care and systems of paying for care can profoundly affect quality of care. Differences across settings and payments systems need to be considered in designing and implementing quality assurance programs. For example, organizational structures, personnel, data systems, medical technologies, potential hazards, and patient roles vary substantially from hospital to home care. What is possible within the hospital may be infeasible or unreasonable in other settings. Likewise, different payment systems may involve different data collection capabilities and different incentives for overuse or underuse of care.

The first part of this chapter focuses on sites of care with specific attention to the prevention, detection, and correction of quality problems in hospital, ambulatory care, and home settings. It asks how different characteristics of these settings (other than system of payment) may affect different elements of a quality assurance program. The second part of the chapter looks at fee-for-service and capitated systems for paying practitioners and institutions and considers the special quality of care concerns presented by each system.

SETTINGS

Overview

Patients are seen in various health care settings, each having special characteristics that may contribute to the ease or difficulty of assessing and assuring quality. The hospital sector includes acute short-stay, long-term, specialty, and rehabilitation hospitals. The ambulatory care sector includes a broad arrangement of organizational settings. Office-based practice ranges from solo or small group practices to large multispecialty group practice. Ambulatory care can also be delivered in hospital-based outpatient departments, clinics, and emergency rooms, in hospital-related or independent ambulatory surgical centers, and in freestanding urgent care centers. Finally, community-based long-term care includes home care, adult day care, respite care, and care in hospice and residential nursing homes.

This chapter focused on only one of each category of setting: namely, acute hospital care, office-based care, and home health care. We believe the issues raised by these settings and the lessons to be drawn about quality assurance will adequately reflect the challenges for developing a strategy for quality assurance for Medicare. In particular, we note four key aspects of these settings as they relate to the patient-provider encounter: (1) the clarity of the episode of care (how easily it is defined or identified), (2) the extent of information recorded about the intervention or encounter, (3) the relative emphasis on medical and health versus social (including family and environmental) components, and (4) the extensiveness, complexity, or formality of the organizational structure. The three settings of primary interest in this study differ on these four dimensions (Table 8.1). We discuss these issues in only very broad terms here, and are aware that there is great diversity within setting type. Specific methods of quality assessment and assurance are discussed in greater detail in Chapter 9 and by setting of care in Volume II, Chapter 6.

The clarity of the definition of an episode of illness differs by setting. At one extreme is an inpatient hospital stay, which has a very specific beginning and end. By comparison, an episode of ambulatory care may be quite difficult to define, especially when it involves multiple visits for chronic care. When an episode is difficult to define, it becomes more difficult to identify quality problems as occurring within the episode.

The larger and more complex a setting of care is, the more centralized, formalized, and standardized the patient care records and data systems are likely to be. When reimbursement depends on information on insurance claims (e.g., hospitals for Medicare), the insurance claims are likely to be more detailed. The more these conditions hold, the more records and data systems will support quality assessment methods that depend on retrieval of data from patient care, encounter, or financial records, and the more feasible it will be to feedback information about practice patterns to practitioners. Generally, hospitals will rank high on the extent of information recorded and maintained on patients, and ambulatory and home health care will rank much lower.

Settings also differ in the importance of medical and social components. Services with a high medical or technical content may be more easily evaluated with objective measures, such as blood pressure for hypertension con-

TABLE 8.1 Elements That Distinguish Settings of Care

Setting	Clarity of Episode	Completeness of Recording Interventions	Importance of Medical versus Social Components	Degree of Organizational Structure
Hospital inpatient	High	High	High	High
Ambulatory office-based	Very low	Moderate	Moderate	Low
Home health care	Low	Low	Low	Very low

trol, whereas services with a strong social service component will require patient evaluations.

To the extent that practitioners and facilities are members of a larger organization, they will generally be subject to more formal structures for review of credentials and reappointment, internal peer review, patient care policies and procedures, and documentation of care (Luke and Modrow, 1982; Scott, 1982; Rhee, 1983). Historically, organization and formalization of health care has developed first in the hospital, then in some areas of ambulatory care and home care, and minimally in office-based care. The presence of organizational structures generally provides a focal point for interventions to improve quality.

Although we do not wish to overemphasize these differences among the various settings, they have important implications for the design of quality assessment and assurance systems. For example, one could use claims data to identify people undergoing certain inpatient procedures who then have a reoperation. This information could be fed back to the hospital medical staff for review and appropriate intervention. Such a trigger and response system is hard to translate to a home health setting. On the other hand, home care agencies have relatively stable populations who can be surveyed by mail or phone with relatively simple questionnaires.

To structure our review of quality assurance approaches in various settings, we concentrate on three major needs: preventing problems, detecting problems, and correcting problems. The omission in this discussion of approaches to encouraging better performance (e.g., the continuous improvement model) reflects the scarcity of working models of this approach.

The Hospital

Prevention

The hospital inpatient setting is the most structured of the health care settings. The premise is that meeting specified structural requirements strengthens the ability of an organization to deliver good quality care (or, alternatively, to prevent poor care) (Palmer and Reilly, 1979).

Driven partly by risk management concerns and partly by requirements of the Joint Commission for Accreditation of Healthcare Organizations (the Joint Commission),[1] systems for recommending medical staff for appointment and reappointment and for determining clinical privileges (and hence, for denying such appointments and privileges) are, by and large, well developed and set forth in medical staff bylaws. Similarly, data gathered on practitioner-specific performance for reappointment and privileging are increasingly refined. These structural characteristics are considered among the leading first-line defenses against poor care, because the implications for physicians of losing staff or clinical privileges are considerable.[2] It is important to distinguish, however, between the ability to revoke privileges and the practical feasibility of undertaking such actions.

Hospitals are typically divided into services, each with clinical directors or department chiefs. Each will have policies and procedures in addition to general hospital policies and procedures regarding professional and staff obligations and responsibilities. In recent years, the emphasis on accountability, lines of authority, and similar structural variables within the hospital setting has grown tremendously. Particular stress has been placed on the responsibilities of governing boards, especially since the landmark ruling in *Darling v. Charleston Community Hospital* (1965) that established a hospital's direct corporate liability for medical staff quality problems about which it knows (or should know), even when the physicians are not employed by the hospital.

Policies and procedures designed to protect hospital patients from medication errors, misidentification, and numerous other potentially adverse events have evolved over many years. There are well-developed systems for documenting the course of patient care in medical records, for instance, nurses' notes, attending physician notes, operative notes, admission and discharge summaries, and results and interpretations of clinical tests, procedures, and examinations. Finally, issues of patient adherence to treatment plans are minimal in hospitals as compared with other settings of care; the physical environment is within the organization's control and patient compliance is easier to monitor and ensure.

Detection

Quality assessment efforts have been hindered by the virtual absence of sound clinical evidence of the efficacy of much medical care (Komaroff, 1983; Eddy and Billings, 1988; O'Leary, 1988). Quality assurance programs have had to construct standards for reviewing care based on a combination of the best available information, expert opinion, locally developed consensus of practitioners, and guidelines provided by specialty societies. In recent years, hospitals have adopted systems that track indicators of performance. Using methods of epidemiologic surveillance, they identify patterns of nosocomial infections and other unusual occurrences by practitioner, unit, shift, or procedure (Istre et al., 1985; Lynch and Jackson, 1985; Buehler et al., 1986; Sacks et al., 1988). Incident reporting systems are designed for rapid reporting of problems, although the value of these systems is debated (Craddick and Bader, 1983; GAO, 1987). Occurrence screening (discussed in Chapter 9) is widely used by hospitals to detect adverse events.

Quality measurement in hospitals tends to be driven by the requirements of the Joint Commission. In the past its requirements focused heavily on structure and process—specifying quality assurance activities for the medical staff, nursing service, and so forth. More recently, Joint Commission standards began to emphasize "monitoring and evaluation" of high-volume, high-risk, or problem-prone activities, and hospitals, in turn, have reoriented their quality assessment and assurance activities.

The Joint Commission is now moving toward a considerably more complex focus on patient outcomes and the effective use of patient outcome data in quality assurance efforts (Joint Commission, 1987, 1988). These efforts address specific conditions and physician specialties such as anesthesia and obstetrical care as well as hospital care generically.

The success of problem detection activities in the hospital setting rests heavily on the adequacy of patient records and data systems. In the hospital, the dates of admission and discharge define the episode of care. The individual patient admission is the unit of analysis for quality assessment. Patient care assessments, interventions, and responses are recorded in a single medical record. Although the completeness, legibility, retrievability, and other characteristics of patient records can vary widely across hospitals, Joint Commission standards for medical records as well as the function of these records as a primary legal document both dictate their form and constrain their content. After discharge, the hospital prepares a discharge abstract summarizing the main features of the medical care provided and patient status at the time of discharge.

Admission and discharge diagnoses are routinely assigned based on a standard coding system (ICD-9-CM).[3] A code specifying the diagnosis-related group (DRG) is derived from the ICD-9-CM codes as part of the uniform billing system (UB-82 and for Medicare the HCFA-1500), and considerable research and administrative work have gone into trying to assure the accuracy of diagnostic coding (GAO, 1988). Since the inception of the prospective payment system, which tied reimbursement to DRG (principal diagnosis), the coding has become more precise and (some feel) more accurate, although the most recently reported error rate of 20.8 percent is still fairly high (Hsia et al., 1988). The present coding scheme is not adequate to determine the severity of illness, the reason for death, the sequence of diagnoses, or sometimes even the precise location of a procedure. For example, whether myocardial infarction preceded or followed coronary artery bypass surgery during a given admission will not be detectable from coded data; neither can the specific site of a hip replacement (i.e., right or left hip) be known from such data.

Records of medical and nursing interventions are typically extensive in the hospital chart, but the accuracy of the information may be compromised by concerns about confidentiality, utilization review, and malpractice liability (Burnum, 1989). Bearing in mind that the test data themselves may not be wholly accurate, results of tests available in the record form a relatively comprehensive picture of events occurring during an inpatient episode. Thus, for quality assessment purposes, medical, nursing, and other clinical data are available, although retrieval may entail manual abstracting of voluminous amounts of (sometimes poorly organized) material.

The field of health information systems is growing rapidly. Increasing numbers of community hospitals have clinical-care-based management information systems, and investment in sophisticated software is expected to rise with internal and external demands for information and technical capability, all of which tend to take for granted the suitability of medical record-based information. Feinglass and Salmon (forthcoming, pp. 3-4)) optimistically describe the near horizon in medical informatics:

> The development of advanced telecommunications, fiberoptic cabling and local area networking, new magnetic and optical data storage technologies, new print graphics, optical scanning and video display capabilities, speech recognition and voice synthesis methods, and new structured query languages and integrated operating system software have the potential to revolutionize the practice of medicine and the medical work place.[4] Perhaps within a few years, most major hospitals will have bedside computer terminals, with voice input devices and a host of logical audit functions for interpreting medical staff orders, storing clinical data, and providing uniform standards of quality assurance.

These systems will not solve all problems. Virtually no data on previous ambulatory or inpatient care at other hospitals are available in the hospital record beyond a typically brief admitting history that may omit significant past events and illnesses. Patient satisfaction questionnaires may be distributed at the time of discharge, but are not usually part of the medical record. No information about the outcome of inpatient care is gathered routinely after discharge. Thus, assessment of the quality of care must depend on data collected during what is usually a short hospital stay.

In most moderate and large hospitals, patient care is very visible to peers because of the many practitioners who see both the patient and his or her medical record. Major procedures are generally observed by an array of physicians, nurses, and others, who are expected to use the incident and screening systems to report adverse occurrences. Teaching hospitals have substantial numbers of trainees and systems of supervision and accountability. There are multiple opportunities for consultation and patient care conferences, especially in the teaching hospital. The situation may be quite different in small rural hospitals relying on a handful of physicians.

Ideally, guidelines in the form of expert systems could be contemporaneous with care and help the practitioner in decision making. Some prototype interactive systems now provide computerized clinical reminders (McDonald et al., 1984; Tierney et al., 1986, 1988), predictive value of tests, and warnings of drug-drug interactions or misuse of antibiotics.[5] Implementation of these systems is likely to occur first in the hospital environment.

Correction

Medical data systems tend to be more useful for detecting poor technical quality rather than overuse or underuse. Where data permit the development of performance profiles, results can be distributed to providers and performance followed over time. These data can figure prominently in decisions about clinical and staff privileges, which are the chief means of interventions exercised by hospital officials and directed at physicians who are considered to provide substandard care. Assuming that firm standards of care can be developed and applied for quality assessment, peer pressure from colleagues and pressure from chairpersons of departments and others with clinical authority can be brought to bear on those individuals not performing according to expectations.

Nevertheless, these arrangements can be weak instruments of problem correction, especially in smaller institutions where personal and social ties may be stronger than organizational procedures or leadership or where medical staff are intimidated by legal action from sanctioned practitioners. During site visits for this study, people responsible for hospital quality assurance repeatedly noted extreme difficulties in dealing with problem staff members who threaten costly and personally bruising legal suits. Of particular concern is the recent U.S. Supreme Court decision in *Patrick v. Burget* that opens peer review activities to challenge under antitrust statutes. Although the legal implications of this case are not yet clear, it appears already to have had a chilling effect on some peer review activities (Meyer, 1989), and it has added to the difficulty of recruiting clinical chairpersons who are responsible for annual physician review and reappointments.

Apart from quality problems relating to individual staff is an array of systems and interpersonal problems, including cumbersome or irrational bureaucratic procedures, disputes across medical specialties and medical-nonmedical domains, strong hierarchies, and separate medical and nursing quality assurance systems. These system characteristics may (1) create patient care problems themselves, (2) complicate the correction of problems, or (3) prevent the resolution of disagreements about appropriateness of practice (Flood and Scott, 1978; Shortell and LoGerfo, 1981; Hetherington, 1982). During site visits we heard about routine delays of several weeks in receiving autopsy results; surgical specialists not calling in medicine specialists soon enough; disputes between the departments of medicine and surgery on appropriateness standards for endoscopy; inordinate delays in initiating drug therapy because of pharmacy problems; delayed admissions to the intensive care unit (ICU), an increasing patient:nurse ratio in the ICU resulting in demonstrably increased morbidity; long trips to the hospital for magnetic resonance imaging tests for patients with head injury; and delayed patient discharges because plans for prostheses were not timely and forms were difficult to complete.

Hospitals have been buffeted by major changes in their internal operating environment. Efforts to identify and to correct problems are complicated by the shrinking length of stay, a higher patient acuity level, staffing shortages, rapid turnover of employees, and the increasing use of part-time and hourly workers. Because individual clinicians or managers may find it harder now than previously to recognize patterns of problems, they may need to rely more on formal systems of quality assessment and assurance.

In addition, the hospital is increasingly subject to external, community factors that can dramatically affect how and how well it operates. For example, the urban hospital has been stressed by AIDS, the drug epidemic with its related trauma, premature births, child abuse, lack of long-term care beds, abandonment of elderly dependents, increasing numbers of uninsured patients, and growing numbers of non-English-speaking patients. Hospital efforts are also complicated by the absence of an integrated insurance program for the elderly that covers both acute and long-term care beds. This encourages discontinuity of care and communication gaps across settings of care that affect both the quality and efficiency of care.

Ambulatory Care

Prevention

As noted earlier, ambulatory care settings vary widely, and these variations can affect the systems used to prevent quality problems. For instance, credentialing systems in a health maintenance organization (HMO) may be quite organized and extensive; by contrast, the solo practitioner or small fee-for-service (FFS) group typically is subject only to state medical licensing requirements, and a practice partnership may require board certification in a medical or surgical specialty but no more organized assessment of partners' performance.

Each setting may have different resources devoted to developing patient care systems to prevent problems. For instance, systems for obtaining initial or full partnership privileges in an HMO may be extensive. By contrast, to practice as a solo practitioner the physician need only have a state medical license.

Most ambulatory patient-care arrangements have not been designed to provide a systematic means of preventing or identifying quality problems. Follow-up and coordination are generally uneven; peer review is less intense, if it exists at all. In addition, the patient has a more central role. The health care system is limited in what it can do to prevent problems associated with a patient's personal or work life.

For ongoing review and management, a staff-model HMO may have teams of health professionals who engage in informal and formal peer-review programs and hold patient care conferences on a regular basis. A group-model HMO may contract with a multispecialty group practice that, in turn, has its own quality assurance programs. Both may have administrative and clinical professionals to design ambulatory data systems to track care and follow-up involving test results, specialty referrals, and preventive services. By contrast, independent practice associations (IPAs) or FFS solo and small group practice provide little opportunity for sharing observations and expertise of many practitioners, although some IPA-model HMOs have extensive internal claims systems that allow the monitoring of both ambulatory and inpatient services. Some large FFS multispecialty groups may maintain single patient records for their patients; others have separate records in each department in which the patient is seen.

On the other hand, solo and small practices can have positive aspects. Long-term physician-patient relationships allow a practitioner to understand and appreciate the medical history and social needs of individual patients. Such relationships may compensate for the fragmentation of care and medical records that are common in systems where no single provider has primary responsibility for a patient's care.

Detection

Quality evaluation must begin by examining either a process of care to which standards can be applied or an outcome that can be defined and measured such that the assessors can work back from a measurably unsatisfactory outcome to the relevant poor process of care. Standards of ambulatory practice are less well-defined than standards for inpatient care. For example, the proper use of insulin for diabetics, antibiotics for a sore throat, and diagnostic testing for sickle cell anemia are three common but controversial areas (Komaroff, 1983).

Ambulatory quality assessment depends on monitoring the process of care for those patients who obtain it. This requires some system for identifying those who have received care for specific conditions or problems, which is referred to as case-finding. Case-finding based only on recorded diagnosis (when possible) will not detect missed or incorrect diagnoses, yet identifying early serious disease is a crucial aspect of ambulatory quality. Physician offices generally have neither manual nor computerized case registry systems for case-finding.

Outcomes can also be used for case-finding. For example, recent efforts by Medicare Peer Review Organizations (PROs) and others to screen in HMOs for poor ambulatory care using the criterion of a hospital admission that might have been preventable may help to detect deficiencies in both diagnosis and treatment.

Determining whether a poor outcome results from poor care is, however, very difficult. At least three factors (discussed below) are at work: (1) the difficulty of specifying and measuring outcomes, (2) the difficulty in defining an episode of care, and (3) the incomplete and fragmentary nature of data.

Measuring outcomes. Outcomes of care are hard to specify in ambulatory care and even more difficult to measure. The natural history of conditions (for example, their tendency to be self-limiting in many cases) is seldom well defined, and often we have little solid information on how medical interventions should affect outcomes (Palmer, 1983, 1988; Palmer and Adams, 1988; Lohr, 1988). Furthermore, relying on patterns of outcomes for patients seen by specific physicians is difficult for three reasons. First, most physicians have low volumes of particular types of cases compared to hospitals. Second, case mix probably varies markedly across physicians. Third, patients may well choose physicians because of their interventionist or noninterventionist style. In addition, data systems in ambulatory care generally lack information about outcomes of care other than physiologic measures.

Defining episodes of care. Measurements of the process of care hinge on the ability to define and measure an episode of care.[6] Such definition is occasionally possible, for example, with a series of vaccinations or the diagnosis and complete healing of a fracture. Typically, reviewers must make arbitrary decisions about the beginning and end of an episode and about the relevance of intervening office visits, emergency room visits, or telephone calls involving one or more (known) practitioners. Such arbitrary decision making reflects our lack of understanding of the natural history of most ambulatory conditions. It is difficult to judge whether a series of visits by the same patient for similar problems represents (1) continued appropriate treatment (one episode of care), (2) an independent recurrence (two episodes), or (3) a failure of treatment (one episode). Many efforts at assessment avoid the issue of an episode of care and base the assessment on some other unit of analysis, such as a single-patient contact, completion of a health screening protocol, or a patient's summary assessment of satisfaction with care.

Incomplete and fragmented data systems. Case-by-case review of the process of care using ambulatory records is often seriously compromised by poor organization of data and lack of documentation of key aspects of care in the medical record. The degree of documentation in the medical record is said to vary inversely with the experience of the clinician—the most extensive notes reportedly are written by medical students. Where used the problem-oriented medical record (POMRs) might help a reviewer to evaluate the medical logic of care (such as the relationship between a set of patient complaints and their diagnostic evaluation), but the use of the POMR in its complete format is rare.

In general, clinical data systems in ambulatory care are poorly developed, and billing systems rarely include clinical information. The Uniform Ambulatory Care Data Set, approved in June 1989 by the National Committee on Vital and Health Statistics, includes certain clinical data (DHHS, 1981; Felts, 1989). In addition to patient and provider identifiers, patient demographic descriptors, the date and place of encounter, and itemized charges, recommended encounter information would include: problem; diagnosis or assessment; laboratory, radiology, and surgical services; and the patient's reason for encounter (optional). If this minimal data set is widely adopted, claims data might be suitable for initial screening in ambulatory care for those who have access to and the expertise to analyze these data.

Even beyond the difficulties in assessing care from the review of one chart, patients may independently see multiple providers, with little or no communication or record linkage among them. In the hospital setting, practitioners, patients, and their records are gathered in one place; in the ambulatory setting, patient records are scattered among individual offices and recording practices are correspondingly diverse. Even if a set of physicians is linked in an HMO, the patient may use services outside the plan. Furthermore, patients may receive conflicting advice, and follow all, some, or none of it. Little of the advice or the degree of patient adherence to treatment plans will be part of any one medical record, making it still more difficult to build a complete document of care for the purpose of assessment.

One way to avoid the problems of case-by-case review is to focus on patterns of care using claims data alone. Patterns of care reviewed might include, for instance, the percentage of patients receiving recommended tests or procedures or receiving indicated follow-up care, or the percentage of patients diagnosed as having a certain chronic condition (e.g., hypertension or diabetes) (Steinwachs et al., 1989). This single approach is rarely a good solution unless outpatient claims are known to be complete and reliable (that is, to encompass all relevant services such as visits, screening or diagnostic tests and procedures, and medications) and to be accurate and consistent in coding diagnoses and recording information. In practice, diagnostic coding in ambulatory care is notoriously inaccurate and does not distinguish rule out, recurrent, or chronic conditions; until recently diagnosis did not appear on Medicare Part B claims. In addition, financial barriers to care may cause holes in administrative claims data for care paid for out-of-pocket (because of deductibles or for noncovered services) or by supplementary insurance.

Most ambulatory management information systems are not readily useable for quality assurance purposes because of the dearth of patient-specific clinical or outcome information. For instance, the date, code, and charge for a laboratory test is likely to be recorded, but not whether the test was normal or abnormal. Similarly, the code for a surgical procedure may be recorded but not the outcome.

Substantial efforts have been made to develop and adapt for microcomputer such systems as the Computer Stored Ambulatory Record (COSTAR), The Medical Record (TMR), and the Regenstreif Medical Record, which have both clinical management and quality assurance capability. Feinglass and Salmon (forthcoming) envision that new medical decision analysis programs that use "criteria mapping" and branching logic "tree" programs can overcome many of the barriers to outcome assessment that have made chart audits so laborious and uncertain.

Correction

Correcting quality problems in ambulatory practice is currently extraordinarily hard. Feedback loops are difficult to construct, so practitioners generally lack information about their own practice patterns in relation to practice standards or peer patterns. Data about patterns of care can take a long time to assemble and disseminate. Moreover, depending on the size and organization of an ambulatory practice, formal or informal peer pressure raise the possibility of antitrust allegations. Evaluating the effect of quality assurance interventions entails all the usual obstacles of such evaluation. For example, they may be overtaken by changing community practice patterns, when medical specialty societies change their guidelines for appropriate care of a given problem.[7]

Home Health[8]

Before the 1980s, home care was generally provided by relatives with periodic attention from a visiting nurse who evaluated progress, provided care and instruction, and supervised the home health aide who performed low-technology tasks. In this decade, however, the home health field and the roles of both the formal and informal caregiver have become much more demanding and complex. Reasons include the increasing numbers of patients in need of home care, the fact that more acutely ill patients are being cared for in their homes, and that increasingly, high-technology services are now provided at home. Intravenous and respiratory therapy, parenteral nutrition, and electronic monitoring devices are examples of complex and challenging technologies now used on a routine basis in home care. The demand for services that maintain elderly persons, especially the frail elderly, as independent community residents continues to grow.

In short, the technical and service demands on the home care industry are very broad, creating a correspondingly difficult job for measuring and assuring the quality of that care. There are four separate issues associated with assessing quality in the home care arena: (1) the importance of the family and social environment, (2) the roles of many caregivers, (3) the multiplicity of funding sources and programs, and (4) the lack of integrated financing or record systems that span ambulatory, acute hospital, and home health care.

The outcomes of home care may depend on the patient's and family's ability and willingness to adhere to the process of care specified by the physician, visiting nurse, and other home health providers. The goals of home health care vary considerably with the nature of the clients and the multiplicity of their care needs. Home care services encompass such goals as promoting physical and mental health and functioning, maximizing the ability for self-care, and increasing patient and family knowledge about self-care (Hawes and Kane, 1989). The nurse is the predominant health care professional who provides and supervises home health services.

Formal home care can be provided under several sources of funding in addition to Medicare, including the Social Services Block Grant, the Medicaid program, and the Older Americans Act. The elderly or their families often pay for some forms of home care completely out of pocket. These diverse funding sources result in separate programs and agencies (Riley, 1988). Because the programmatic base of fiscal support is so much broader than for either hospital or ambulatory care, the Medicare program may be less likely to affect the quality of home health care to the degree it affects hospital care. In addition to the difficulties arising from multiple programs, multiple caregivers, such as visiting nurses, homemakers, vendors of durable medical equipment, family members, and friends, make attributing outcomes to a particular caregiver or event obscure.

Lack of integrated financing mechanisms among hospitals, nursing homes, and home health agencies results in fragmented care, itself a threat to quality. It also presents a barrier to a uniform clinical information system that would support better quality assurance. Because the episode of illness does not coincide with the episode of home care, one would prefer quality measures that spanned the ambulatory, inpatient, and home health care settings. Neither the process of home health care nor the outcomes for patients can be neatly separated from acute care (the setting in which most patients begin their course of treatment), from the physician who prescribes home health care, or from the nurses and aides who provide it. To a significant degree, each of those providers is likely to affect both the course of home health care and the patient's outcome. Yet little is known about the relationship between the adequacy of acute hospital care, physician care, and the outcomes of home health care (Hawes and Kane, 1989).

Prevention

Home health agencies and hospitals that sponsor them are recognizing the need for training of aides and nurses, defined skill levels, supervision, emergency back-up procedures, training of family and other informal caregivers, and the development of medical record systems with uniform and comprehensive data to ensure that increasingly dependent and vulnerable patients receive safe and appropriate care.

At the same time, serious and fundamental obstacles deter home care agencies from addressing the structural aspects of quality. These barriers include the national nursing and therapist shortages (which are at a crisis stage in some localities), the need to provide appropriate wages and benefits for workers as incentives for recruitment and retention of staff, the fact that home care is without continuous on-site supervision, and the number of certifying or accrediting bodies with differing standards and procedures.

State licensure and Medicaid and Medicare certification are the fundamental systems for deterring poor quality care in the home care field. Voluntary accreditation standards have been developed by various professional organizations such as the National League of Nursing (NLN) through its Community Health Accreditation Program (CHAP), the National Home Caring Council, and the Joint Commission, but voluntary accreditation has not been widely sought because it is expensive and is not required by payers.

Medicare certification depends on replies to a survey that has relied heavily on structure and process measures to assess compliance with standards. New Conditions of Participation were published in August 1989, and Medicare is moving toward a deemed status program for home health agencies based on accreditation by, for instance, the Joint Commission and NLN's CHAP. State surveyors will be required to make home visits and to interview patients; however, they will continue to focus on structure and process measures such as training requirements, record-keeping, and practitioner credentials (Riley, 1988). The Omnibus Budget Reconciliation Act of 1987 (OBRA 1987) requires the distribution of a patient bill of rights and a complaint mechanism within state agencies.

Of 39 states that currently license home health agencies, only a minority impose requirements more stringent than the Medicare Conditions of Participation. For instance, 12 states mandate specific consumer rights, and 13 require specific training (Riley, 1988).

Several states (e.g., Oregon, Washington, Wisconsin, and Maine) have implemented "case management" models in which professionals work with consumers to "assess their needs, develop comprehensive plans of care, arrange for services, monitor service delivery, and reassess needs and revise plans regularly" (Riley, 1988). States view case-management (often administered through aging agencies) as an important quality assurance tool to develop client advocacy and provide services based on the needs of the client (Riley, 1988), but the success of these techniques for quality assurance remains unproven.

NLN CHAP accreditation standards require process measures of quality and client home visits. Similarly, Joint Commission accreditation standards stress critical elements of process such as patients' receiving care in a timely manner, the adequacy of instruction and supervision of staff on equipment use, patients' rights, care planning and provision, and internal quality assessment systems. The impact of these standards is also untested.

Detection

Medicare PROs currently review a small sample of postacute home care occurring between two related hospital admissions and are also required to investigate beneficiary complaints about quality. Both developments have heightened interest in how to review the quality of home health care.

In the home care field, the most fundamental problem for successful quality measurement is that care is both intermittent and rarely observed. Concern with patient abuse and theft are also raised as special issues for home health care. The process of care is typically evaluated according to whether it meets commonly accepted professional norms regarding the types of services a patient needs (Hawes and Kane, 1989). Common methods include chart review, peer review, worker skills checklists, and, to a lesser extent, patient interviews and supervisor visits.

Regulations pursuant to OBRA 1987 have called for emphasis on outcome-based measures and for the development of a patient needs assessment instrument for the use of hospital discharge planners and home health agencies. The Uniform Needs Assessment Instrument is briefly described in Chapter 6 and Volume II, Chapters 6 and 8.

Currently, review of records may provide information on whether services were provided as planned (number of visits), but patient outcomes are not regularly assessed (Hawes and Kane, 1989). LaLonde gives three reasons (cited in Riley, 1988): (1) the focus of accreditation and certification bodies on structure and process, (2) a scarcity of reliable and valid outcome scales to assess the quality of home care, and (3) limited resources within a home health care agency to modify existing scales or develop outcome scales and test them for reliability and validity.

Positive outcomes in home health might include improved physical or cognitive function, or both, at the time of discharge and satisfaction with care. The Home Care Association of Washington has recently developed a reliable and valid set of measures that include scales relating to patient outcomes (LaLonde, 1988). For much of the population in home care situations, improvement or full recovery may be unlikely. Thus, comparative statistics may be particularly important. Negative outcomes might be death, lack of improved functioning, bedsores, or urinary tract infection. Assessment of outcomes must depend on documentation in the medical record, a visiting nurse assessment, patient or family report, or a home visit by someone other than the provider of care.

The medical record is not, however, a highly developed instrument in the home care setting. Home health providers are not reimbursed for time spent documenting their care, and many home health aides are barely literate. Records generally have not supported elaborate record review to compare a plan of care with care received, progress in medical recovery or rehabilitation, recovery from cognitive and functional disability, or recovery of the capacity for self-care. As in any assessment based on medical record review, lack of documentation does not necessarily mean that a service was not provided.

Correction

Seventy-five percent of states report terminating contracts with home health agencies as their most common enforcement mechanism in the provision of home health services. Many withhold funds or recoup money already paid out. Some states impose intermediate sanctions for noncompliance, such as cutting off the intake of new clients or reassigning caseloads to other providers (Riley, 1988).

A more appealing method of improving quality (in home care as in other settings) would be the feedback of timely information to providers on their patterns of care with enough specificity and precision to generate improved performance. Such feedback, although it may occur as informal evaluation by supervisors, has not been as fully developed in home health care agencies as in hospital care.

PAYMENT SYSTEMS

The organizational, financial, and philosophical differences between traditional fee-for-service (FFS) practice and prepaid group practice in this country have been the subject of very intense examination over the past two decades—yielding a literature far too extensive to recount here (Luft, 1981, 1988; Brown, 1983). As the prepaid capitated approach has matured, it has spawned several variants and hybrids, complicating the task of specifying what systems factors are likely to encourage or impede successful quality assurance. This section attempts to highlight some key variables that should be taken into consideration in designing a quality assurance strategy for Medicare.

Today, three-quarters of nonfederal, nonresident physicians have a practice (including those who belong to preferred provider organizations, or PPOs[9]); that is, approximately 300,000 physicians practice through FFS rather than salaried or capitated arrangements. The percentage of FFS physicians is falling, however, and differences by age of physician are impressive. For example, excluding residents, 47 percent of physicians under age 36 are now (at least partly) salaried, compared to only 19 percent over age 55 (cited in Feinglass and Salmon, forthcoming).

Still, 97 percent of Medicare beneficiaries remain in FFS arrangements, despite substantial growth in capitated and salaried payments systems and strong promotion by the Health Care Financing Administration (HCFA) of beneficiary enrollment in Medicare HMOs and competitive medical plans. Thus, for the purposes of this study, the factors that must be considered in designing a strategy for quality assurance for Medicare are overwhelmingly those of the FFS sector.

Fee-for-Service Practice

Fee-for-service office practice has not generally been a focus of quality assurance programs.[10] A strategy for quality review for FFS practitioners would require a system to choose review methods and topics, to establish review criteria, to gather data, to disseminate results, to monitor change, and to intervene when necessary to correct problems. No such systems are currently in place. Hence, we have little past history or experience to guide the design of such a strategy.[11]

Data

In the FFS system (with billing to an insurance carrier), virtually all services paid by a health plan will be recorded and coded. In principle, this makes case-finding for quality assessment possible. In practice, many obstacles to the use of claims data must be overcome. They include incomplete or inaccurate recording or coding of diagnoses and services; noncovered (but key) services that are not recorded at all (e.g., prescription drugs for Medicare); covered services for which no claims are made; and noncovered services that are miscoded as covered ones (e.g., preventive services, such as screening mammography coded as diagnostic mammography). Most important, because billing systems are not created to provide any clinical data (e.g., results of laboratory tests, measures of severity of illness, or even accurate diagnoses), quality review that uses claims data as a screen must eventually look to other sources of information to assess the actual care rendered.

As mentioned earlier with respect to ambulatory care generally, medical records are scattered in individual physician offices and use nonstandardized recording systems. Practitioners may develop their own terminology, check-off lists, and flow sheets to record progress. They may use the briefest of notations knowing that no other practitioner (other than, perhaps, a practice partner) is likely to need or read them (the main exceptions to this statement are when a patient transfers to another physician or an attorney requests the record pursuant to malpractice action). Thus, the office medical record may be a very poor or uneven source of information nationally about either the process or the outcome of patient care, especially if that care involves a considerable amount of listening and counseling (as contrasted with provision of diagnostic tests and procedures or prescriptions).

HCFA is now requiring diagnostic coding on ambulatory Part B claims. Both the reliability and validity of that information will have to be assessed before it can be considered a useful data source for quality assurance. For instance, because most of the elderly have multiple diagnoses and the diagnostic codes have no impact on payment or treatment, many physicians may merely note a legitimate diagnosis, such as hypertension, even though another condition was the primary reason for a visit. If reliability of diagnostic data is established, it may be possible to apply automated logic programs to assess the appropriateness of ambulatory services based on acute or recurring diagnoses. Also the possibility exists that services can be linked across settings (such as hospital to outpatient), but, again, this deserves careful investigation.

Types of Problems

Because of the fundamental financial incentives for overuse of services, FFS quality assurance systems need to look carefully for overuse. When the FFS coverage has large deductibles and copayments or major coverage exclusions, however, then underuse also becomes a concern. The underuse problem may especially manifest itself among people never "entering the system," whereas overuse may occur through additional services even within a single visit. Procedure-oriented practices may make overuse more likely because of a reimbursement structure that rewards procedures at the expense of counseling, cognitive services, or lengthy personal interaction between patient and physician; in this sense, the payment scheme may underwrite the cost of other services such as patient education and preventive care. In all cases, however, attention must be given to finding poor technical quality (PPRC, 1989).

Prepaid Capitated Systems

In some ways the prepaid group practice sector, although small, has advanced on the quality assurance front more than the FFS sector has. Prepaid plans were developing quality assurance programs long before the HMO Act of 1973 (P.L. 93-222) required federally qualified HMOs to have ongoing programs that "stress health outcomes" (see Weiner and Densen, 1958; Shapiro et al., 1960, 1967, 1976; Morehead et al., 1964). Federally qualified HMOs have to meet certain financial and structural requirements, to have ongoing quality assessment programs, and to be able to demonstrate this to outside reviewers. Even nonfederally qualified HMOs and HMOs serving Medicaid patients are often called on by state departments of health to demonstrate their quality assurance programs. For instance, in California the Knox-Keene Health Care Service Plan Act of 1975 stipulated that California HMOs assess the acceptability and accessibility of care and the adequacy with which the HMO met the health needs of the served population. In Kansas, a new law requires independent, on-site quality-of-care inspections at least once every three years. Despite these regulatory requirements, in practice HMO quality assurance programs have ranged from "paper plans" with little substance to extensive and well-supported internal programs with research components.

More recently, Medicare PROs have begun to review the ambulatory care for the one million Medicare beneficiaries belonging to HMOs and competitive medical plans (CMPs) with Medicare risk contracts (see Chapter 6 and Volume II, Chapter 8). PRO review, which is fairly complex and exceeds what is required for the FFS sector, includes review of ambulatory care in addition to inpatient and other settings and calls for an emphasis on "episodes of care." For instance, the records of outpatient care for patients admitted for any of 13 specified diagnoses that might indicate substandard ambulatory management can be subjected to review. Moreover, some HMOs and CMPs that opt for so-called limited review are subject to evaluation of both their existing quality assurance program and a periodic sample of the cases that their program itself is investigating.

Data

Data systems in the prepaid practice sector can be both better and worse than those in the FFS sector. The major difference, of course, is that there are generally no claims forms—a source of appreciable problems in implementing Medicare PRO review of HMO and CMP care.

In principle, an advantage of prepaid over FFS systems is that the former can describe and document their enrolled populations (and can correlate use of services to this base). In practice, problems arise because people are enrolled in multiple systems, for example when each employed spouse covers all family members under his or her employer's health plan. When this occurs, an apparent "nonuser" may actually be receiving services in another system.

Management information systems (MIS) in HMOs typically have minimal clinical information. They may, for instance, use CPT-4[12] codes for classifying procedures or ICD-9-CM codes for hospital diagnoses, but the quality of these data might be suspect because they are for information management use, not for payment per se. MIS data are typically recorded in modules, such as membership-information files, specialty referrals, and encounter (usually a patient visit) information. A hospitalization module may include dates of admission and discharge, summary charges and diagnoses, but no more detailed information. Encounter forms may record aspects of the clinical encounter (e.g., date, practitioner, type of visit, disposition, and primary diagnoses), but there are no strong incentives or disincentives (other than the time required of the practitioner to complete the form) to record services or aspects of the visit accurately. Other information may be retrievable from the MIS (e.g., registration and demographic data on members and authorized specialty referrals), but integration of the data may be cumbersome, not especially timely, and expensive. The MIS may be developed internally or be commercial with major modification by software vendors. As a result, the definitions of basic terms, coding, and recording systems are idiosyncratic and vary widely from one HMO to another.

Clinical data for review of care are typically available only in the medical record and supplemented by other sources such as laboratory or pharmacy logs. The medical record system within any one HMO may have a standard format, and a unit record may be designed so that information about care in many settings (e.g., emergency room visits, hospital discharge summary, and specialty referrals) are recorded in the primary care chart. As in the FFS system, however, medical records may differ dramatically across different HMOs.

Group and staff models have the benefit of one or several practice locations in which records are gathered. Independent practice association (IPA) and network models, on the other hand, can resemble FFS practice. An IPA would find it very difficult to require participating physicians to use common data systems because physicians often participate in many different IPAs with only a small proportion of their practice enrolled in any given IPA.

Types of Problems

Because of the financial incentives for restricting access to expensive services such as specialty care or elective hospitalization, HMOs need to look carefully for underuse. The structure of financial incentives in HMOs may lead fewer people to be nonusers, but it may also reduce services among users. HMOs are also especially prone to "procedural" barriers to access (e.g., lengthy queues for appointments) and to barriers to physician-initiated or authorized services where "gatekeeper" physicians are at financial risk for patient use of these services. HMOs tend not to have incentives that favor overuse in general or procedures over cognitive services, but they can nevertheless be subject to problems of overuse of services. Problems of poor technical care must be sought as vigorously as in FFS system.

OTHER SETTING AND SYSTEM FACTORS

We emphasized in Chapter 1 that our definition of quality of care—and by extension, the quality assurance system that should be designed to reflect that definition—was intended to include both individuals and populations. Thus, a feature of singular importance to a quality assurance system that crosses both setting and payment systems is its ability to define the population *intended* to be served and the population *actually* served.

For the HMO and the Medicare program, the populations of users as well as nonusers can be defined (subject to the caveats noted above). In the hospital setting, in ambulatory FFS practice, and in home care, however, only the population served is defined. For these settings and payment systems, quality assessment systems can develop such measures as rates of compliance with standards, rates of adverse occurrences, and rates of patient satisfaction for those who receive services, but they cannot evaluate the status of those who do *not* obtain care.

Furthermore, we also emphasized "desired patient outcomes" as the central focus of our definition. Leaving aside the appreciable (but not insurmountable) difficulties with defining and measuring outcomes, it is important to note that outcome measures that are applied only to those who receive care may be misleading. They may point to ostensible differences in outcome that are in fact caused by differences in access. A quality assurance program must be able to correct for this problem in one of two ways (or both). It must be able to adjust for case mix before comparing care rendered in different institutions, settings, and payment systems. It should also be able to assess population-wide outcomes through mechanisms that will reach both users and nonusers.

SUMMARY

This chapter has introduced issues for quality assurance that are related to the setting of care (hospital, physician office-based care, and home health care) and to the payment mechanism (FFS and prepaid capitated systems). The more highly organized and integrated the provider setting, the more likely it is to have in place the informal and formal mechanisms (for example, specifications for granting practice privileges; good data systems; and formal peer review activities) that help to assure the quality of care delivered. Thus, the barriers to successful internal quality assurance are lower for hospitals than for ambulatory and home care. With respect to payment systems, FFS and HMO provider groups probably have offsetting advantages and disadvantages relating to availability of data, types of problems, and focus on individuals versus populations. In general, the design of a quality assurance strategy for Medicare faces more difficulties for the ambulatory and home health settings than for hospitals, regardless of payment systems. For that reason and because of the overwhelming preference of Medicare beneficiaries for the FFS system, the challenge to designing such a strategy for that system is greater than for the HMO sector.

NOTES

1. Conditions of Participation for hospitals to be reimbursed by the Medicare program, and the role of Joint Commission accreditation by which accredited hospitals are "deemed" to meet those conditions, are discussed more fully in Chapter 5 and in Volume II, Chapter 7.

2. This aspect of quality assurance is emphasized by the Joint Commission and is receiving increasing attention as a result of passage of the Health Care Quality Improvement Act (1986). For more discussion, see Chapter 9 and Volume II, Chapter 6.

3. International Classification of Diseases, 9th Revision, Clinical Modification.

4. Cox and Zeelenberg, 1987; DeTore, 1988; Kaplan, 1988.

5. At the National Institutes of Health Clinical Center, for example, orders for antibiotics entered on the clinical management information system are screened for appropriateness.

6. The need for defining an episode of illness is sometimes voiced. Defining an episode of illness is even more difficult than defining an episode of care because of the complexities of establishing either a beginning or an ending to the illness, both of which occur outside the physician's office and are unlikely to be recorded systematically, if at all, in the office records.

7. Mammography guidelines, for instance, are the subject of considerable controversy among various medical groups (McIlrath, 1989).

8. Much of this section is based on a paper prepared for this study by Catherine Hawes and Robert Kane on measuring outcomes in noninstitutional long-term care, hereafter referred to as Hawes and Kane, 1989.

9. PPOs are organizations or insurers that contract with practitioners to provide services to enrollees on a discounted FFS basis. The attraction to physicians is mainly a more stable, "guaranteed" patient population without the constraints or requirements of belonging to a traditional group or staff model HMO.

10. The most prominent exception may have been the efforts of the Experimental Medical Care Review Organizations (EMCROs) and Professional Standards Review Organizations (PSROs) to carry out ambulatory care review efforts in the 1970s. Efforts of earlier foundations of medical care were also carried out by physicians in "traditional" practices. The Association for Accreditation of Ambulatory Health Care also promotes ambulatory care review. One major research effort concerned the California Medicaid program, in particular, the Prepaid Health Research and Evaluation Demonstration (PHRED) project in which reviewers took microcomputers to physicians' offices to evaluate process of care. None of these efforts, however, has been translated into a widely accepted, national consensus or activity for review of care rendered in physicians' offices.

11. The Medical Outcomes Study (Tarlov et al., 1989) is measuring the process and outcomes of care in both capitated and fee-for-service settings. See Volume II, Chapter 6.

12. Current Procedural Terminology, fourth edition.

REFERENCES

Brown, L.D. *Politics and Health Care Organization: HMOs as Federal Policy.* Washington, D.C.: The Brookings Institution, 1983.

Buehler, J.W., Smith, L.F., Wallace, E.M., et al. Unexplained Deaths in a Children's Hospital: An Epidemiologic Assessment. *New England Journal of Medicine* 313:211-216, 1986.

Burnum, J.F. The Misinformation Era: The Fall of the Medical Record. *Annals of Internal Medicine* 110:482-484, 1989.

Chassin, M.R., Kosecoff, J., Park, R.E., et al. Does Inappropriate Use Explain Geographic Variations in the Use of Health Care Services? A Study of Three Procedures. *Journal of the American Medical Association* 258:2533-2537, 1987.

Cox, J.R. and Zeelenberg, C. Computer Technology: State of the Art and Future Trends. *JAAC* 9:204-214, 1987.

Craddick, J.W. and Bader, B.S. *Medical Management Analysis: A Systematic Approach to Quality Assurance and Risk Management.* Volume I. Auburn, Calif.: J.W. Craddick, 1983.

Darling v. Charleston Community Memorial Hospital, 33 ILL. 2D 326, 211 N.E.2d 253 (1965), *cert denied,* 383 U.S. 946 (1966).

DHHS (Department of Health and Human Services). *Uniform Ambulatory Medical Care. Minimum Data Set.* A Report of the United States National Committee on Vital and Health Statistics. DHHS Publ. No. (PHS) 81-1161. Washington, D.C.: U.S. Government Printing Office, 1981.

Dubois, R.W., Rogers, W.H., Moxley, J.H., et al. Hospital Inpatient Mortality: Is it a Predictor of Quality? *New England Journal of Medicine* 317:1674-1680, 1987.

DeTore, A.W. Medical Informatics: An Introduction to Computer Technology in Medicine. *American Journal of Medicine* 85:399-403, 1988.

Eddy, D.M. and Billings, J. The Quality of Medical Evidence. *Health Affairs* 7:19-32, Spring 1988.

Feinglass, J. and Salmon, J.W. Corporatization and the Use of Medical Management Information Systems: Increasing The Clinical Productivity of Physicians. *International Journal of Health Services,* forthcoming.

Felts, W.R. Need for Standardized Ambulatory Care Data: National Provider Perspective. Paper presented at the American Public Health Association annual meeting, Chicago, Ill., October, 1989.

Flood, A.B. and Scott, W.R. Professional Power and Professional Effectiveness: The Power of the Surgical Staff and the Quality of Surgical Care in Hospitals. *Journal of Health and Social Behavior* 19:240-254, 1978.

GAO (General Accounting Office). *VA Health Care: VA's Patient Injury Control Program Not Effective.* HRD-87-49, Washington, D.C.: General Accounting Office, May 1987.

GAO. *Improving Quality of Care Assessment and Assurance.* PEMD-88-10, Washington, D.C.: General Accounting Office, May 1988.

Hawes, C. and Kane, R.L. Issues Related to Quality Review and Assurance in Home Health Care. Paper prepared for Institute of Medicine Study to Design a Strategy for Quality Review and Assurance in Medicare, 1989.

Hetherington, R.W. Quality Assurance and Organizational Effectiveness in Hospitals. *Health Services Research* 17:185-201, 1982.

Hsia, D.C., Krushat, W.M., Fagan, A.B., et al. Accuracy of Diagnostic Coding for Medicare Patients Under the Prospective-Payment System. *New England Journal of Medicine* 318:325-355, 1988.

Istre, G.R., Gustafson, T.L., Baron, R.C., et al. A Mysterious Cluster of Deaths and Cardiopulmonary Arrests in a Pediatric Intensive Care Unit. *New England Journal of Medicine* 313:205-211, 1985.

Joint Commission (Joint Commission on Accreditation of Healthcare Organizations). Agenda for Change *Update* 1:1, 1987.

Joint Commission. Agenda for Change *Update* 2:1,5, 1988.

Kaplan, B. Development and Acceptance of Medical Information Systems: An Historical Overview. *Journal of Health and Human Resources Administration* Summer:9-29, 1988.

Komaroff, A.L. The Doctor, the Hospital, and the Definition of Proper Medical Practice. Appendix E. in President's Commission. *Summing Up. The Ethical and Legal Problems in Medicine and Biomedical and Behavioral Research.* Washington, D.C.: President's Commission for the Study of Ethical and Legal Problems in Medicine and Biomedical and Behavioral Research, 1983.

LaLonde, B. *Quality Assurance Manual of the Home Care Association of Washington,* 2nd Edition. Edmonds, Wash.: The Home Care Association of Washington, 1988.

Lohr, K.N. Outcome Measurement: Concepts and Questions. *Inquiry* 25:37-50, 1988.

Luft, H.S. *Health Maintenance Organizations: Dimensions of Performance.* New York, N.Y.: Wiley, 1981.

Luft, H.S. HMOs and the Quality of Care. *Inquiry* 25:147-156, 1988.

Luke, R.D. and Modrow, R.E. Professionalism, Accountability, and Peer Review. *Health Services Research* 19:113-123, 1982.

Lynch, P. and Jackson, M.M. Monitoring: Surveillance for Nosocomial Infections and Uses for Assessing Quality of Care. *American Journal of Infection Control* 13:161-173, 1985.

McDonald, C.J., Hui, S.L., Smith, D.M., et al. Reminders to Physicians from an Introspective Computer Medical Record. *Annals of Internal Medicine* 100:130-138, 1984.

McIlrath, S. 11 Medical Groups Endorse Mammogram Guidelines. *AMA News,* July 14, 1989, pp. 3,48.

Meyer, H. Peer Review's Limits Visible Once Again. *AMA News,* May 5, 1989, p. 1, 9-12.

Morehead, M.A., Donaldson, R.S., Sanderson S., et al. *A Study of the Quality of Hospital Care Secured by a Sample of Teamster Family Members in New York City.* New York, N.Y.: Columbia University School of Public Health and Administrative Medicine, 1964.

O'Leary, D.S. The Need for Clinical Standards of Care. Editorial. *Quality Review Bulletin* 14:31-32, 1988.

Palmer, R.H. and Reilly, M.C. Individual and Institutional Variables Which May Serve As Indicators of Quality of Medical Care. *Medical Care* 17:693-714, 1979.

Palmer, R.H. *Ambulatory Health Care: Evaluation Principles and Practice.* Chicago, Ill.: American Hospital Association, 1983.

Palmer, R.H. Beyond Hospital Inpatient Care: The Challenges and Prospects for Quality Assessment and Assurance in Ambulatory Care. *Inquiry* :119-131, 1988.

Palmer, R.H. and Adams, M.E. Considerations in Defining Quality of Health Care. Paper prepared for Institute of Medicine Study to Design a Strategy for Quality Review and Assurance in Medicare, 1988.

PPRC (Physician Payment Review Commission). *Annual Report to Congress. 1989.* Washington, D.C.: Physician Payment Review Commission, 1989.

Rhee, S.O. Organizational Determinants of Medical Care Quality: A Review of the Literature. Pp. 127-146 in *Organization and Change in Health Care Quality Assurance,* Luke, R.D., Krueger, J.C. and Modrow, R.E., eds. Rockville, Md.: Aspen Systems Corporation, 1983.

Riley, P.A. *Quality Assurance in Home Care.* Report prepared for the National Academy for State Health Policy, an affiliate of the Center for Health Policy Development. Washington, D.C., December 1988.

Sacks, J.F., Stroup, D.F., Will, M.L., et al. A Nurse-Associated Epidemic of Cardiac Arrests in an Intensive Care Unit. *Journal of the American Medical Association* 259:689-695, 1988.

Scott, W.R. Managing Professional Work: Three Models of Control for Health Organizations. *Health Services Research* 17:213-240, 1982.

Shapiro, S., Jacobziner, H., Densen, P., et al. Further Observations on Prematurity and Perinatal Mortality in a General Population and in the Population of a Prepaid Group Practice Medical Care Plan. *American Journal of Public Health* 50:1304-1317, 1960.

Shapiro, S., Steinwachs, D.M., Skinner, E.A., et al. *Survey of Quality Assurance and Utilization Review Mechanisms in Prepaid Group Practice Plans and Medical Care Foundations.* Baltimore, Md.: Johns Hopkins Health Services Research and Development Center, 1976. (HEW contract HSM 110-73-435).

Shapiro, S., Williams, J., Yerby, A., et al. Patterns of Medical Use by the Indigent Aged under Two Systems of Medical Care. *American Journal of Public Health* 57:784-790, 1967.

Shortell, S.M. and LoGerfo, J.P. Hospital Medical Staff Organization and Quality of Care: Results for Myocardial Infarction and Appendectomy. *Medical Care* 19:1041-1055, 1981.

Steinwachs, D.M., Weiner, J.P., and Shapiro, S. Management Information Systems and Quality. Pp. 160-182 in *Providing Quality Care: The Challenge to Clinicians.* Goldfield, N. and Nash, D.B., eds. Philadelphia, Pa.: American College of Physicians, 1989.

Tarlov, A.R., Ware, J.E., Greenfield, S., et al. The Medical Outcomes Study. *Journal of the American Medical Association* 262:925-930, 1989.

Tierney, W.M., Hui, S.L., and McDonald, C.J. Delayed Feedback of Physician Performance Versus Immediate Reminders To Perform Preventive Care. *Medical Care* 24:659-666, 1986.

Tierney, W.M., McDonald, C.J., Hui, S.L., et al. Computer Predictions of Abnormal Test Results: Effects On Outpatient Testing. *Journal of the American Medical Association* 259:1194-1198, 1988.

Weiner, L. and Densen, P. Comparison of Prematurity and Perinatal Mortality in a General Population and in the Population of a Prepaid Group Practice Medical Care Plan. *American Journal of Public Health* 48:170-185, 1958.

Wennberg, J.E., Freeman, J.L., and Culp, W.J. Are Hospital Services Rationed in New Haven or Over-Utilised in Boston? *The Lancet* i:1185-1188, May 23, 1987.

9

Methods of Quality
Assessment and Assurance

A quality assurance program can have several purposes, each of which may be emphasized to varying degrees. In working toward its goals, a quality assurance program can try to prevent problems from occurring, detect and correct those problems that do occur, and encourage higher standards of care. It can attempt to remove or rehabilitate poor practitioners and providers, improve the average level of practice, reward excellence, or use some combination of those goals. The methods used in a quality assurance program may be as sharply focused as finding and reacting to isolated events involving a single patient and practitioner, such as a surgical mishap. They may be as broad as conducting continuing education, disseminating practice guidelines, initiating institution-wide "continuous improvement," designing management information systems with uniform clinical data elements, and conducting research on effectiveness at a national level. Ideally, the choice of methods for a strategy for Medicare quality review and assurance should be based on an assessment of the burdens of harm from different quality problems (Chapter 7), an understanding of important features of health delivery systems that affect our current ability to measure care and effect change (Chapter 8), and the strengths and limitations of major methods of quality assessment.

INTRODUCTION

In this chapter we describe selected methods of quality assessment and assurance and discuss how well they meet the criteria for successful quality assurance efforts outlined in Chapter 2. (Chapter 6 in Volume II goes into more detail and differentiates methods by purpose, agent, and setting. It includes methods in use, methods derived from research studies, and methods described during site visits.) We have here focused on methods for preventing, detecting, and correcting quality problems for three settings of care: hospital-based care, office-based care, and home health care. Some approaches are directed at individuals; others are directed at institutions. Some are used primarily by health care organizations; others principally by external regulatory groups. Some have been developed for research projects; others have evolved in clinical and administrative departments in health care facilities.

Methods of preventing problems described in this chapter include accreditation and licensure for health care organizations and licensure and board certification for individual practitioners. Other methods include patient management guidelines and clinical reminders.

Approaches in detecting problems include analysis of administrative data bases, retrospective chart review, nonintrusive outcome measures, generic screening for adverse events using medical records, clinical indicators, and assessments of patient outcomes (such as health status and satisfaction). Detection methods based on aggregate data include the use of administrative data bases for analyzing outcomes such as mortality and complication rates. Individual-case sources of information about quality include autopsy, case conferences, and patient complaints.

Our discussion of methods of correcting problems emphasizes factors that are thought to impede or enhance the effectiveness of interventions intended to change behavior. Some interventions may be quite informal, for example telephone conversations with individual practitioners. Others, such as financial sanctions, are more formal. Interventions based on poor practice patterns include remedial education, restrictions on practice, and penalties.

The final section of this chapter reviews current thinking about the advantages and disadvantages of educational approaches, incentives (including rewards), and disincentives (including penalties) for individual physicians both for improving average and outlier practitioners. Because there has been little evaluation of methods of intervention, this section does not lend itself well to discussions of known strengths and limitations. Therefore, we confine our discussion to a description of factors and variables that are thought to influence ways of changing behavior in health care organizations.

Important Attributes of Methods

When considering the strengths and limitations of quality assurance methods, one should consider several features. Among these are reliability and validity. Reliability refers to consistency in results, that is the degree to which measures of quality agree either when repeated over time or when applied by different people or in different settings. To assess the reliability of a credentialing system, for instance, one might evaluate the consistency of information obtained about applicants for hospital privileges or how often review committees agree in their recommendations. To determine the reliability of a method to detect quality problems, one might calculate how often chart reviewers identify the same adverse events. Reliability in correcting problems is more theoretical, but one might envision measuring whether comparable corrective action plans (e.g., continuing education courses or reading designated literature) consistently improve tested knowledge.

Validity in this context refers to whether a method acts as intended. For one to consider board specialization a valid method of ensuring high quality, for instance, one would look for proof that those who are board certified provide a demonstrably higher quality of care than those who are not. Likewise, the validity of an outcome measure of quality could be assessed by determining whether patients with poor outcomes received deficient care and whether the deficiency produced the poor outcome. To demonstrate the validity of a method of correcting problems one would look for evidence that a specific intervention brought about the desired change. For instance, required consultation with a colleague before treating certain cases should result in fewer problem cases.

Assessment methods may be valid in that they detect real problems in quality, but even valid tools may be inefficient (if they detect a great many events that are not quality problems) or ineffective (if they fail to detect many important quality problems).

For virtually no method of assessment do we know the effect on provider behavior or the effect of practitioner change in behavior on patient outcomes. These are the ultimate tests of validity. Although methods may be accurate at identifying problems, they are valuable for quality assurance only if, or to the extent that, identification leads to changed behavior and to improved patient outcomes. Measures of these two demanding but critical factors are almost nonexistent, and this shortfall must temper any recommendations for specific approaches.

Assessment methods have important attributes other than reliability and validity. These include their practicality, ease of application, lack of unintended negative effects, inclusion of patient views and preferences, and ability to detect poor technical quality, overuse, and underuse. It is also useful to consider whether various methods of assessment provide timely information to improve performance and whether they yield information that accords with ideas about how professionals learn.

PREVENTION OF PROBLEMS

Accreditation and Licensure for Organizations

Hospitals, ambulatory care facilities, managed care organizations, and home health agencies can be accredited on a voluntary basis by the Joint Commission on Accreditation of Healthcare Organizations (Joint Commission). Approximately 77 percent of the approximately 7,000 Medicare participating hospitals have received Joint Commission accreditation. The remaining 1,600 hospitals that are not accredited are, for the most part, small rural institutions with 50 or fewer beds (see Chapter 5 in this volume and Chapter 7, Volume II for an extensive discussion of the evolution of the Joint Commission's accreditation process).

The accreditation manuals for each type of facility are designed for hospital use in self-assessment and for the Joint Commission to use for on-site surveys. For hospitals in "substantial compliance" such a survey occurs every three years. Scheduled at least four weeks in advance, the survey is conducted by a physician, nurse, and administrative surveyor over a three-day period using explicit scoring guidelines. After a concluding educational exit interview, the facility may receive full accreditation or may be notified that accreditation is contingent on its carrying out a plan of correction. A hospital with contingencies may submit written evidence or may undergo a return site visit. It may then may be fully accredited or, in due course, nonaccredited.

In 1981, the Joint Commission replaced their prescriptive, structure-oriented standards and numerical audit requirements with a standard requiring ongoing, facility-wide monitoring of care. Monitoring was intended to permit the identification of problems and ways to improve the delivery of care and to promote solutions to any problems identified. Nevertheless, structural standards designed to prevent problems and to ensure the capacity of the hospital to operate safely are still in effect. Three such areas of emphasis include (1) a standard specifying that the governing body is to hold the medical staff responsible for establishing quality assurance mechanisms, (2) medical staff standards requiring regular review, evaluation and monitoring of the quality and appropriateness of services provided by the medical staff, and (3) a standard calling for the establishment of coordinated hospital-wide quality assurance activities.

In addition to the Joint Commission, accreditation for ambulatory facilities can also be sought on a voluntary basis from the Accreditation Association for Ambulatory Health Care (AAAHC), for HMOs from the National Committee on Quality Assurance (NCQA), and for home health agencies from the National League for Nursing (NLN) through its Community Health Accreditation Program. To date nonhospital providers have sought accreditation infrequently. These accrediting organizations, however, have become increasingly active, and some states, such as Pennsylvania and Kansas, have determined that these accrediting groups are acceptable to provide external review for HMOs.

Strengths

Standards for accreditation are publicly available. If the standards are unambiguous, and if reviewers are consistent in applying them, then information on accreditation status provides comparable information on health facilities. If accreditation standards were more widely accepted by external regulators (e.g., eligibility for third-party payers or state licensure boards), this might reduce overlapping requirements.

Because accreditation is conferred voluntarily by a body representing the kind of facilities being reviewed, it represents a quasi-internal process that is, at least in theory, responsive to member organizations, yet accountable to the industry as a whole and to the public. Depending on the perceived value of accreditation and the stringency of the review process, the organization may make substantial efforts to comply with standards. A variable rating system in accreditation could recognize outstanding performance.

Limitations

Accreditation is evidence that certain quality assurance efforts such as requiring specific credentials, staffing policies, or grievance procedures are being pursued. However, unless the accreditation process is itself evaluated and found to be based on reliable and valid methods, it cannot be relied on as a method of ensuring quality, and it may divert resources from more effective approaches. Accreditation can be very expensive and cumbersome, and this may discourage its voluntary use.

Credentials, Licensure, and Specialty Certfication[1]

The examination of credentials is regularly used as a method of assuring high quality. The process is used (1) by state boards in granting licenses to practice, (2) by specialty and subspecialty boards in granting certification, (3) by hospital committees in reviewing applications to the medical staff, and (4) by payers in determining eligibility to be paid for services (Chassin et al., 1989a). The decisions of these groups may themselves constitute credentials. Licensure and board certification are particularly important.

Physician Licensure

Each state has statutes regulating the practice of medicine through physician licensure. Most of these laws define the practice of medicine and prohibit those who are unlicensed from engaging in it.

State medical practice acts are administered by state boards of medical examiners. Those who apply for licensure are judged on the basis of their education, postgraduate training, experience, results on licensing examinations, and moral character. Applicants for licensure must be graduates of schools of medicine or osteopathy that are accredited by the Liaison Committee on Medical Education, with special provisions being made for graduates of foreign medical schools. A postgraduate internship of one year is required by approximately three-quarters of the states, and applicants must successfully pass a licensing examination. All states currently use the Federation Licensing Examination (FLEX), prepared by the National Board of Medical Examiners (NBME) for the Federation of State Medical Boards. Most states will also accept the so-called National Boards, prepared by NBME or by the National Board of Examiners for Osteopathic Physicians and Surgeons. These examinations are administered in three stages as the student progresses through his or her education (Havighurst, 1988).

Some states have reciprocity agreements, whereby licenses granted by one state are recognized in another state. Some states require that applicants go through the procedures specified in their medical practice acts regardless of whether they are already licensed elsewhere (Havighurst, 1988).

Strengths. Licensure provides a minimum standard of quality for the individual health care practitioner. It does not meet any of the other goals of quality assurance listed in Chapter 2.

Limitations. The authority to practice medicine, once licensure has been obtained, is legally constrained only by criminal and medical malpractice law. Physician licensure is generally for life, and where licenses must be renewed, no new demonstration of competence is required. Many states have instituted certain continuing medical education (CME) requirements as a condition of license renewal. Attendance at approved CME is sufficient to meet the statutory mandate; those attending need not take and pass any examinations or show any other sign of accomplishment (Davis et al., 1984; Havighurst, 1988).

The physician's license is also unlimited in scope, permitting the physician to engage in areas of practice for which he or she may have little training (Havighurst, 1988). This lack of limits stands in sharp contrast to the strict limitations placed on other health professionals subject to licensure. Licensure in no way guarantees competence across the wide range of medical practice or over time.

Specialty Certification and Recertification

The American Board of Medical Specialties (ABMS) recognizes 23 specialty boards that certify physicians as medical specialists in carefully delineated areas of practice. Several other entities also certify physicians, but because the ABMS system is so dominant, "board certification" is generally understood to mean certification in a medical specialty by a board recognized by ABMS (Havighurst and King, 1983).

For a board to achieve accreditation status, it must be sponsored both by a professional group, such as a specialty society, and the appropriate scientific section of the American Medical Association (AMA). All the boards are evaluated for recognition according to the ABMS "Essentials for Approval of Examining Boards in Medical Specialties." Each board thus requires similar levels of training and experience.

The residency program must be approved by the Accreditation Council for Graduate Medical Education (ACGME), an organization composed of members of the ABMS, the AMA, and other concerned organizations. Together with appropriate specialty boards, the ACGME develops accreditation standards for each specialty residency program. These are regularly modified in conjunction with changing specialty board requirements and must be approved by the AMA's Council on Medical Education (Havighurst and King, 1983). Ultimately, candidates must also pass comprehensive examinations administered by the specialty board.

Candidates for certification must receive and complete specialty training in an approved graduate medical program, the length and extent of which vary somewhat among the specialties. A majority of physicians in the United States identify themselves as specialists, but only about one-half are actually certified by an ABMS board. The number seeking certification has grown and continues to grow rapidly. Almost all physicians newly entering practice now seek some sort of certification. Of those who designate themselves as specialists, an increasing number are actually board certified.

Strengths. Certification in a medical specialty is widely accepted as an indication that certified physicians possess a superior level of training and skill in their area of specialization. Information on certification is readily available from such sources as county medical societies, the ABMS, AMA, American Medical Directory, and the AMA Physician Masterfile. Certification has been endorsed by the Joint Commission as an "excellent benchmark for the delineation of clinical privileges" (Joint Commission, 1989, p. 106).

Limitations. Ramsey and his co-workers (1989) compared the performance of board-certified and noncertified practitioners in internal medicine using measures of knowledge, judgment, communications skills, and humanistic qualities. Scores of board-certified internists on a written examination were significantly higher than those of noncertified internists, but ratings by professional associates, patient satisfaction scores, and performance in the care of common illnesses (as measured by medical record review) showed few differences. There were modest differences in preventive care and patient outcomes that favored the certified physicians.

The Office of Technology Assessment (OTA, 1988) reviewed 13 studies on the adequacy of physician specialization as a measure of quality and found little evidence that board certification accurately predicts high-quality care. Studies that use process criteria tend to show that specialists trained in their area of practice (the modal specialist) provide higher quality than those who have not been so trained, but this higher quality of process has not been linked to superior patient outcomes. Nor has a relationship been established between specialist care and patient satisfaction (Chassin et al., 1989a). Even if superior performance is associated with specialty training or board certification in one area, such evidence would not necessarily be generalizable to other specialties, diagnoses, or procedures (OTA, 1988).

In the past, boards granted certification for unlimited periods. There has been a move over the past 10 years toward recertification requirements, so that 15 of the 23 specialty boards have now adopted or decided to adopt time-limited certification with intervals between reevaluations ranging from six to 10 years. One board offers voluntary recertification, and seven specialty boards have no recertification procedures (Havighurst and King, 1983).

Some experts have recommended that the certification and recertification processes should shift from one that is knowledge-based to a more "performance-based" assessment that reflects actual practice such as a review of a sample of records or observation. This, it is believed, will reflect more accurately the physician's practice and thereby increase the validity of board certification (Havighurst and King, 1983).

Appropriateness and Patient Management Guidelines[2]

In medicine, and particularly in organized ambulatory care practices, guidelines serve many purposes, but they are intended primarily for education. They may specify appropriate and inappropriate uses of medical interventions, act as reminders for relatively simple tasks (e.g., provision of vaccinations), or serve as shorthand reminders for complex clinical decision making. For this last use they are sometimes called patient care algorithms. In all these applications, practice guidelines can help to forestall the occurrence of problems in patient care. In modified formats, they can also be used for retrospective quality review. Numerous groups, including medical specialty groups, have formulated such appropriateness and patient management guidelines. They are also frequently developed by interested clinicians within health care facilities and by health services researchers. They take on a variety of formats, depending on their highly individualized purpose.

Strengths

Patient management guidelines can be viewed as the translation of a medical text into a focused, often graphic, and sometimes computerized format. The use of branched reasoning and flow diagrams allows for great complexity and logically complete presentations. Well-constructed guidelines can allow patient preferences to be elicited and taken into account.

Limitations

Few (perhaps no) algorithms in use today are based entirely on scientific evidence of effectiveness. Generally, some or all of the available evidence is augmented by the clinical experience of the formulators. Many guidelines are nothing more than lists of ambiguous or vague statements about appropriate care that lack any guidance on their implementation.

Guidelines are frequently put into practice with no or only haphazard pretesting or evaluation. Often they lack provisions for updating or modification based on new knowledge, on their usefulness to clinicians, or on their impact on care. Guidelines may be of limited use for patients with multiple chronic conditions because the formats rapidly become too complex for easy reference.

Clinical Reminder Systems

Clinical reminder systems are computerized methods used in some managed care plans, clinics, and office practices to remind clinicians of preventive tests that should be performed, of laboratory monitoring that is due for patients with chronic disease, and of potential drug interactions (McDonald, 1976; Barnett et al., 1978, 1983; McDonald et al., 1984; Tierney et al., 1986). For instance, when printing out a list of scheduled patients a reminder system may use an age, sex, and risk-adjusted algorithm to specify screening tests or laboratory monitoring for individual patients. Other reminders may be used interactively to warn of possible drug interactions or to query the physician and advise on appropriate antibiotic prescriptions.

Strengths

A computerized reminder system can alert a practitioner to patient needs and potential problems at the time patient care is provided, making it a truly concurrent quality assurance system. Such systems can be tailored to individual risk factors and previous medical history. Clinical reminder systems can incorporate probabilities of various outcomes and references to journal citations for further information and can be updated frequently. Their value in improving clinical process has been well demonstrated.

Limitations

These systems require readily available computer equipment, a rapid response time, and enough practitioner familiarity with the software to be feasible for use during practice hours. Their relationship to improved patient outcomes remains unevaluated.

DETECTION OF PROBLEMS

Use of Large Administrative Data Sets[3]

Large data sets refer to claims-based administrative data bases such as those for Medicare Part A and Part B claims. Roos et al. (1989) distinguish three types of data bases and the kinds of studies that are feasible with each. A Level 1 data base contains only hospital discharge abstracts and will permit aggregate studies of, for instance, in-hospital mortality rates and lengths of stay, by geographic region or over time. A Level 2 data base contains, in addition, unique patient-identifying numbers. It can be used to study, for instance, short-term readmissions and volume and outcome relationships at a hospital-specific level. A Level 3 data base (the most comprehensive) will also have information from health program enrollment files, including when eligibility begins and ends. This data base permits the highest quality longitudinal studies, short- and long-term outcomes studies, and population-based (system-wide coverage) studies. Studies can include outcomes for intervention-free individuals and for poor outcomes or other complications that are not recorded as part of the hospital stay.

Weiner et al. (1989) have provided examples of quality-of-care indicators that might be developed from ambulatory care data bases. These include system measures such as the rate of hospitalizations, of readmissions, and "avoidable disease" or disease first diagnosed at an advanced stage. Other examples include (1) preventive-care indicators, such as the percentage of eligible persons receiving a recommended number of periodic screening tests or exams within a given time period and the documented incidence of newly diagnosed disease versus the expected incidence; (2) diagnostic indicators, such as the number or proportion of patients who receive unnecessary diagnostic tests or procedures; and (3) treatment indicators, such as the percentage of patients with a given diagnosis who receive the appropriate medication, the percentage of patients undergoing ambulatory surgical procedures who experience complications including hospitalizations, and the percentage of all visits to the patient's primary provider.

Strengths

All large administrative data bases have several theoretical advantages for quality assessment. First, the accuracy of various types of data (e.g., medications, previous hospitalizations, and numbers of physician visits and medical conditions treated) is unaffected by errors in patient or practitioner recall. Second, the use of these data bases is unobtrusive; patient consent for individual studies is not required, and no bias is introduced from individuals' knowing that they are being studied. Unobtrusiveness may also contribute to their acceptability to practitioners and health care facilities. Third, assessors can create and test different statistical models or approaches to risk adjustment. They can also alter study designs or use several different study designs to test findings; for instance, they can use both cohort and case-control designs to examine the effect of different intervention periods.

Fourth, the same files can be applied in different ways, for instance, tracking outcomes of surgery, computer modeling of readmission, examining changes in complication rates over time, or studying outcomes of care for patients in different geographic areas. Fifth, investigators can accurately assess risks as well as benefits associated with treatment, especially for areas of medical uncertainty. The data bases can provide inputs for clinical decision making by allowing calculation of the probability of complications of treatment or of mortality at varying lengths of time after treatment. Sixth, the use of administrative data bases is relatively inexpensive in comparison to methods that require large-scale primary data collection.

An important strength of Level 3 data bases is that they contain population data, and thus they permit some assessment of population access and outcomes. Comparative studies should be able to identify possible areas of underuse.

Limitations

Administrative data bases have considerable drawbacks for quality assessment. First, data bases may exclude important information such as certain events, information on location of service and provider, or costs, and may assemble the elements in ways that complicate linkage to other files.

Second, the precision of the coding schemes (primarily the ICD-9-CM[4] and CPT systems) is of great concern, particularly for medical conditions that encompass a broad range of clinical severity and contain important clinical subgroups, such as congestive heart failure and diabetes mellitus. The ICD-9-CM coding system does not distinguish procedures performed on the right side of the body from those performed on the left. For this reason, a data base with ICD-9-CM codes will not allow a reviewer to determine whether a second hip replacement, for instance, is a reoperation or a new operation. Of equal concern is the poor ability of data bases to distinguish the order of events during a single episode of care (e.g., a pulmonary embolus that was present at the time of admission versus one that developed after surgery). Although administrative data bases record the occurrence of events such as x-rays and diagnostic tests, the results of these tests (whether positive or negative, or specific findings) are typically not recorded. New technologies or established technologies used in totally new ways may not be given codes for several years (PPRC, 1989).

Third, errors in recording and coding events can threaten the validity of the data. Some errors in recording are random, but some are systematic, especially if there are financial incentives for "upcoding" (systematic coding for services that are more intense or extensive and thus better reimbursed than the one actually provided) and "unbundling" (billing every component of a procedure separately) (PPRC, 1989). Depending on who is completing a form, and his or her incentives and training, the data will vary in accuracy. Diagnoses on hospital records are more likely to be accurate than diagnoses on outpatient-visit claims, although sometimes outpatient diagnoses can be grouped around a type of problem (e.g., gynecologic problems) to minimize this weakness.

Fourth, the data bases include only contacts with the health care system and of these, only contacts that generate a claim. A person who is ill but has no encounter with the health care system produces no record. Copayments and other barriers to access may accentuate this bias and lead to underestimates of poor outcomes.

Fifth, measuring the benefits of treatment is very difficult because positive outcome measures are not part of administrative data bases. Approximations may sometimes be attempted based on a decreased frequency of hospitalization or the length of intervention-free periods.

Sixth, analysis of large administrative data bases is a slow process. Even with major improvements in electronic data transfer and processing that are envisioned, it is not well-suited to rapid feedback of practice patterns.

Small Area Variations Analysis (SAVA)

SAVA is a way of using administrative data bases that has become a major area of research in its own right (Paul-Shaheen et al., 1987). Small area variations analysis can identify areas of high, average, and low rates of hospital services usage, but the methodology cannot discriminate appropriate from inappropriate care. As a problem-detection method, SAVA should be regarded as a screening methodology for alerting analysts about areas where quality problems may be occurring and for which more focused review may be needed. A strength of SAVA is that it can direct attention to potential areas of underuse as well as overuse.

Volume of Services (Individual or Organization)

After reviewing the literature on the possible relationship between volume of procedures done by institutions and the outcomes of those procedures, OTA (1988) concluded that good evidence exists that higher volume is associated with higher rates of good outcomes for a number of diagnoses and procedures. They cautioned, however, that the causal relationship is by no means clear, with controversy about whether higher volume permits the development of proficiency (e.g., in the surgeon or surgical team) or whether better practitioners attract a higher volume of patients. It is also not yet clear over what range of volume and under what circumstances the volume-outcome relationship holds.

Future Steps

Research using aggregate data has demonstrated their value for studying small area variations, length of stay, and variations in practice patterns and complications over time. Although work is underway to develop methods of risk adjustment, to improve linkages among data bases, and to validate and improve the accuracy of diagnosis and procedure codes, administrative data bases lack specificity in identifying quality problems for a given patient or for a particular episode of care. As a near-term strategy, these data bases are best suited to directing quality assessment efforts toward topics, populations, or providers requiring further study. Currently Medicare data bases do not include clinical data, measures of patient need, or outcome assessments. Efforts to devise a Uniform Needs Assessment instrument, to develop a Uniform Clinical Data Set, and to include patient functional status could greatly augment the value of administrative data bases for internal and external quality assurance programs (see also Chapter 6).

Retrospective Evaluation of Process of Care

Process studies review the provision of preventive, acute, and chronic care. Retrospective review of records using explicit criteria is the classic approach to assessing quality. Criteria and standards may be developed by a consensus of experts using their knowledge of the scientific literature and their clinical experience as guidance. Chapter 10 discusses issues in the development, validation, and evaluation of criteria for evaluating patient care.

Using an abstracting form developed for review, quality assessors cull information from the medical record and judge the quality of that care, usually against explicit process-of-care criteria. Sometimes the level of compliance with criteria is given a score; in other formats, care is simply rated as acceptable or unacceptable. Although some criteria sets are poorly constructed, others, such as patient management guidelines, may use branched criteria and an inclusive range of options in an attempt closely to approximate the clinical decision making process.

Palmer et al. (1984) and Greenfield (1989) have described the development of what are generally considered to be well-constructed algorithms for ambulatory patient care evaluation. They have been used to evaluate a range of medical situations such as compliance with preventive and well-child care, relatively simple interventions such as management following an abnormal Papanicolaou (Pap) smear, treatment of streptococcal sore throat or middle ear infection, and complex evaluation of patients presenting to the emergency room with chest pain (Greenfield et al., 1981).

The Committee on Practice Assessment of the Ontario Chapter, College of Family Physicians of Canada (CFPC) (Borgiel et al., 1985; Borgiel, 1988) conducted a pilot research effort during 1987 to develop a practical, economical, and acceptable method of practice assessment appropriate for use in office practice of family physicians. Its conceptual base was the notion of tracers (Kessner et al., 1973), in which general conclusions about care provided by the practitioner or facility are drawn on the basis of tracer (indicator, or representative) conditions and problems that are intensively studied. The CFPC computerized process evaluation focused on chart review for a set of tracer conditions to evaluate routine care for common ailments.

Although the study is still in a pilot phase, it provides a promising method of ambulatory office-based assessment. It also has potential for selecting doctors for participation in managed care organizations and for physician recertification (Chassin et al., 1989a). Moreover, the computerized algorithms developed for this study have continued to be adapted and extended. Some 280 screens cover about 85 percent of all primary care diagnoses, including condition-specific history and physical examinations, laboratory tests, therapies, and patient education (Michael McCoy, personal communication).

Strengths

Retrospective review of care using criteria developed by practitioners is likely to have face validity for professionals and for the public. Process criteria can address poor technical quality, overuse, and underuse because of undertreatment. Individual criteria can be evaluated for validity and reliability. Retrospective review can be used to identify outliers and to evaluate and provide specific information to improve the practices of outlier practitioners and raise the average level of performance. Information can document improvement in quality and can be used for comparisons over time and across sites of care.

Limitations

The development of criteria and standards requires evidence of efficacy or at least effectiveness. This evidence is often unavailable or contradictory. Even if available for certain patient populations, it is not available for every combination of patient risk factors (e.g., age, family history, or health habits) and other coexisting patient conditions, nor for all possible interventions and their combinations.

Retrospective review, which is commonly based on medical record review for reasons of cost, feasibility, and unobtrusiveness, is subject to well-known limitations of medical record review. The validity of recorded information such as patient history and physical exam findings must be assumed, but this may not be a legitimate assumption. Care provided may not be recorded; Gerbert et al. (1988) agreed with earlier researchers that the concordance among methods such as record review, videotaped observation, physician interview, and patient interview was not high. Interpersonal aspects of care, such as patient inability to follow a given medical regime or refusal of care, may also not be recorded. When care involves multiple practitioners with multiple medical charts, only a portion of that care may be retrieved for review. Even when data are recorded by practitioners or others they must be accurately retrieved from the medical record and accurately coded. This is a special challenge in ambulatory care, given the lack of uniformity in describing many ill-defined conditions.[5] Chart review using explicit criteria followed by implicit review raises additional problems in reliability.

Outcome Data

General Points

Outcome data are attractive for quality assessment because they address the primary goals of health care. These include cure, repair of injured or dysfunctional organs, relief of pain or anxiety, rehabilitation of function, and prevention of or delay in the progression of chronic disease. Sources of outcome data include administrative data bases (e.g., deaths, complications of treatment, and readmissions), medical records (e.g., infections and return to the operating room), questionnaires and interviews about health status, and surveys of patient satisfaction.

To be valid as methods of quality assessment, approaches based on outcomes must direct users to areas of likely deficiency so that further study and appropriate interventions may occur at the institutional or subinstitutional level. At an institutional level, medical staff and administrators must be able to identify problem practitioners and decide what actions are needed to change a pattern of unsatisfactory outcomes.

Linking process and outcome depends to some degree on the timing of measurement. The closer an outcome measurement is to the time of medical intervention, the more likely it is that the outcome may be at least partly attributable to medical care rather than to some intervening event. For instance, reduction in blood pressure for patients with hypertension is a short-term outcome that might be helpful in assessing care of an individual patient or practitioner. Morbidity or mortality 10 or 20 years after diagnosis is a long-term outcome that would be more useful for comparing different populations or modes of therapy.

Validity is also affected by the quality of data recorded and retrieved and by the accuracy of patient (and "proxy") reports on functional outcome status or satisfaction. Data must be adequately adjusted for factors other than medical or nursing care, for example other chronic conditions, severity of illness, and patient age. To assess the care provided by an individual practitioner, there must be a sufficient number of cases of any one diagnosis to provide statistically reliable data—a condition not often met except over a long time period, in specialty care, and for some conditions frequently treated by primary care physicians, such as hypertension and diabetes.

Hospital Mortality Rates

Strengths. Hospital-specific mortality rates are potentially useful nonintrusive screens for poor quality care. Death is obviously an important outcome of health care, and a substantial portion of hospital deaths is believed to be avoidable (OTA, 1988). Data are relatively easy to obtain; most hospital discharge abstracts and many claims systems have information on death.

The first public release by the Health Care Financing Administration (HCFA) of hospital-specific mortality elicited bitter accusations of inaccuracy and the potential for misunderstanding of data that were not adjusted for severity. Since then, considerable work has gone into the development of methods of adjustment; the model now includes such variables as hospital admission during the previous year and comorbid conditions.

Limitations. For hospital-specific mortality rates to be a valid screen for poor quality, hospitals with high mortality would have to be shown to provide poorer quality of care than hospitals with low death rates, as measured by an analysis of the process of care. Such a determination is limited by (1) unreliable diagnosis and procedure coding and (2) a lack of sufficient clinical detail to adjust adequately for the patients' severity of illness at the time of admission (Chassin et al., 1989a, 1989b).

Hospital-specific mortality rates are further limited in their usefulness unless they use large numbers of hospitals, large numbers of patients from each hospital, comparisons over time to minimize the effect of chance variation, and adjustments for key hospital characteristics (Dubois, 1989). Only if all such information is complete and accurate can mortality data be adequately adjusted for severity and used as a screen for further review.

Medical Complications

Strengths. As with mortality rates, the use of complication rates as a measure of quality is attractive as a nonintrusive measure because it is believed that at least a portion of complications is preventable.

Limitations. The use of administrative data bases to identify complications that are the consequence of poor-quality care is hampered by the lack of accuracy of diagnostic and procedure coding, by the need for accurate and complete data, and by further variability and inconsistency in the recording of major complications (usually recorded as a secondary diagnosis). Methods have not yet been developed to distinguish complications ensuing from poor care from those occurring because of the degree of illness. For instance, cardiac arrest (a serious complication of heart attack) may occur because the heart is already severely damaged or because irregularities in the heart rhythm are not monitored and recognized (Chassin et al., 1989a). Another limitation, as with the use of mortality data, is the lack of sufficient clinical detail to adjust adequately for the patients' severity of illness at the time of admission.

Generic Screening

Rutstein et al. (1976) first used the term "sentinel event" to describe adverse outcomes that can be closely linked with poor process of care. Each sentinel event is chosen because it is thought to have a high probability of indicating poor quality and therefore to warrant further review and possible intervention.

Generic screening is a method of identifying adverse, or sentinel, events by medical record review. Screens are "generic" in the sense that they apply broadly to the institution rather than to specific departments or diagnoses. Examples of generic screens are "unplanned repair or removal of organ," "severe adverse drug reaction," and "inpatient admission after outpatient surgery." Events subject to screening include those in which patient harm occurs (such as ocular injury during anesthesia care) and events with the potential for harm (such as equipment malfunctions or patient falls).

Generic screening, now widespread in hospitals, is a two-stage system of medical chart screening by nurse reviewers, followed by implicit physician review. Data may be recorded on worksheets that are also used for admission, continued stay, and discharge review. Data are collected within a designated period after admission (e.g., 48 hours), at periodic intervals (e.g., every three days), and after discharge when all services provided have become part of the medical record. Individual events that meet certain explicit criteria (sometimes called screen failures or variations) are further reviewed by a physician advisor. Direct action is taken if a quality problem is confirmed and action directed toward an individual practitioner is appropriate. Data are later aggregated (e.g., by time, service, shift) to determine trends. PROs use generic screening as their primary method of chart review.

Strengths

Many adverse events (for instance, many nosocomial infections, especially surgical wound infection) are preventable (OTA, 1988). Characteristics of patients at high risk of such events have been identified (Larson et al., 1988). By focusing on an adverse event rather than a disease-specific process, generic screening can help to focus attention on interdisciplinary problems. The generic screening process is an appealing method for directing quality resources to serious problems of poor technical quality, overuse, and underuse (although underuse can only be detected for those already receiving care). All these features lend credibility to the general approach, although not necessarily to individual screening criteria.

Screening for adverse events is easy to implement. If it is done at frequent intervals and data are reviewed and collated promptly, screening for adverse events can result in immediate action. When potentially dangerous conditions exist, response can be timely enough to prevent further harm to an individual patient and to other patients exposed to similar risks. If data are retrieved by well-trained reviewers and combined with other tasks such as utilization review and discharge planning, screening supports coordination of care and efficient use of resources. Well-developed screening criteria sets could be generalizable to many sites and could provide benchmark data for comparison across sites and over time.

Limitations

Generic screening is inefficient in identifying quality problems. Reports of the percentage of cases that fail initial screens and must be further reviewed range from 14 to 30 percent (Craddick and Bader, 1983; Meyer et al., 1988; Hiatt et al., 1989). Only a fraction of those cases will be shown to have true quality problems.[6]

Some screen items are much less efficient than others. Inefficiency occurs because the criteria for determining a screen failure are often ambiguous. For instance, one criterion for the PRO generic screen that assesses medical stability at discharge is "abnormal results of diagnostic services which are not addressed or explained in the medical record." Yet determination of what is properly considered abnormal and what is adequate attention to the abnormality varies with a patient's condition, other medical problems, and severity of illness; this is difficult for a reviewer to determine without more specific guidance. Such inefficiency is costly in terms of resources and reviewer patience. Ambiguity of screening criteria is also likely to make them unreliable, which is another limitation.

Generic screens have not been well evaluated. The value of screening for adverse events depends on how well adverse events are recognized by medical practitioners, documented in the medical record, and then identified by reviewers. Screens may miss as many problems as they find (see Chapter 6). Some screen items are much less efficient than others. It is not known how often generic screens miss serious problems in quality that are also missed by risk-management programs because the screening instrument is insensitive to them, because they are not recognized by the reviewer, or because they do not become evident until after discharge. For instance, Hiatt et al. (1989) found a 7.9 percent false-negative rate attributable to reviewers not recognizing events that were recorded; only 3.4 percent of very severe adverse events identified by a risk management program were missed because they were not recorded at all in the medical chart. On the other hand, a GAO study of occurrence screening in the Department of Defense found that about 65 percent of occurrences were missed by hospital reviewers (GAO, 1989). The findings were attributed to (1) lack of sufficient guidance for reviewers, especially when more than one event was found in a patient's medical record, (2) insufficient medical expertise by corpsmen reviewers, and (3) physicians screening their own records.

Because documentation is more extensive and adverse events more easily observed in the hospital during the longer period of observation, generic screening seems more suited to the hospital setting than to most ambulatory care where visits are brief and outcomes are unseen and unrecorded. The method might, however, also be suitable for long-term-care screening.

Generic screen data applied by internal quality assurance programs are most frequently reviewed long after the patient has been discharged; generic screening by PROs occurs six months or more after discharge. Thus, as most commonly used, they are not helpful for concurrent intervention. Instead, their value for patient care thus depends on dissemination of data on patterns of problems. The study committee was unable to assemble evidence, however, that this dissemination occurs routinely in hospitals.

Clinical Indicators

Clinical indicators of care can refer to several quite different things. They can refer to adverse events or to measures of process recorded routinely by clinical care and ancillary departments. They can also be written screens of acceptable practice that are objective, measurable, and applied consistently to the review of care by nonphysician reviewers (see O'Leary, 1988; Lehmann, 1989). Finally, they can be appropriateness protocols (based on adherence to condition- or procedure-specific standards) or be positive or negative health status outcomes.

The Joint Commission distinguishes sentinel events and comparative indicators. Sentinel events are serious complications or outcomes that should always trigger a more intensified review, such as maternal death or craniotomy more than 24 hours after emergency room admission. Comparative indicators establish rates over time or rates in comparison to other institutions. A particularly high or low rate may trigger further review, for example, the rate of death after coronary artery bypass graft surgery, the rate of wound infections, and the rate of vaginal births after cesarean delivery.

Strengths and Limitations

By and large, the same advantages and drawbacks to generic screening and retrospective review of the process of care apply to clinical indicators. A possible advantage of clinical indicators over standard generic screens is a presumed higher face validity for physicians and other practitioners. A possible drawback is their relative newness.

Patient Reports and Ratings

Patient reports refer broadly to interviews and surveys of patients that are conducted either at the time care is provided or later, by telephone or by mail. Surveys can include potential patients, for example Medicare beneficiaries or HMO members who have not used care. Interviews and surveys may ask patients to report on the process of care (both technical and interpersonal) and its outcome and to rate the quality of the care they received and their satisfaction with it.

Strengths

Surveys can investigate such aspects of patient experience as access to care, amenities of care, interpersonal and technical aspects of care, health status, understanding of instructions, experience in comparison to expectations (including a judgment of outstanding as well as poor care), and unmet needs. Detailed satisfaction surveys are fielded by many HMOs and, increasingly, by hospitals. In addition to compiling assessments of care received in primary care facilities, some surveys also include questions about care provided by specialists and affiliated hospitals.

Patient assessments are commonly sought internally by organizations (although they are not necessarily fielded by or used by the quality assurance program), and only rarely by external groups. Patient reports can provide information about (1) underuse (such as perceived lack of access, underdiagnosis, or undertreatment), (2) interpersonal aspects of care, and (3) expectations and preferences. Most problem detection methods do not tap these aspects of quality. Patient surveys that provide for free responses (for example, asking if the respondent has comments to make) can identify unexpected problems and elicit useful suggestions. Satisfaction questionnaires that are sensitive to specific elements of care and to change over time can be a valuable way of documenting improvement and excellence. Survey results can be used to compare sites if data are properly adjusted for differences in populations and expectations.

Recently a great deal of work has gone into the development of valid and reliable patient assessment instruments (Davies and Ware, 1988). The increasing availability of such instruments may bring a degree of standardization of methods and instruments to the health care field for use by the Medicare program as well as by internal quality assurance programs.

Limitations

Patient reports are prone to the usual sources of error in survey methodology, such as bias due to nonresponse by certain population subgroups and errors in recall. General questions inquiring about satisfaction typically result in overstated patient assessments in comparison to specific questions. The ability or inability of patients to judge technical quality of care is also a problem as is accounting for the effect of illness and the effect of the health care environment on patients' assessments. Surveys have the potential, as well, to disrupt the doctor-patient relationship. Like other assessment methods, patient assessments must be able to adjust for differences in access, patient characteristics, and expectations if assessments are to be used for comparisons.

Survey data have not in the past generally been accorded high priority as sources of information about quality or as forces for change within health care organizations. Often they were poorly constructed and implemented without pretesting. In many settings, patient surveys are fielded by marketing departments and have little or no linkage to quality assurance efforts; typically there is no feedback of data on patient satisfaction to practitioners, administrators, policymaking groups, or governing boards. More recently, however, proponents of continuous improvement have placed increased emphasis on knowing the needs of those served, whether patients or other "customers."

If such information were to be collected and used by purchasers of health care, incentives to change processes in areas of dissatisfaction would probably be reinforced. The effect on quality of care and on health, however, would depend on whether areas that are changed are "amenities" of care or important elements of effective health care.

Health Status Assessment

Outcomes of care are the ultimate criteria for judging the quality of care and thus have great face validity for both patients and caregivers. Outcome measures include disease-specific clinical endpoints of care such as physiologic outcomes, a broad set of generic measures of functional and emotional status, and measures of well-being (see Chapter 2).

Strengths

Outcomes, such as patient health status measured at some transitional point in care, can help to evaluate preceding care in another setting such as at the time of admission to the hospital or admission to home health care. Similarly, periodic health status measurement can provide information about changes in status compared with expected status.

Limitations

Comparing observed health with expected health requires empirical data on the natural history of illness and on the effects of treatment. Such information is still lacking for many conditions. More important, linking lower-than-expected health status to a deficient and identifiable element of care is often difficult and limits the value of outcome-based methods for quality assessment. This variant of the "process-outcomes" link problem lies at the heart of difficulties with outcome measurement as a quality assurance tool.

Health outcome measures appropriate for office practices, such as physical and emotional functioning, are not in wide supply, although they are available (Nelson and Berwick, 1989). The Medical Outcomes Study (MOS) (Tarlov et al., 1989; Stewart et al., 1989) has shown promising interim results using the MOS Short Form (Stewart et al., 1988), a generic measure of functional status. The MOS Short Form has been used to demonstrate distinct functional profiles for patients with nine different chronic diseases (e.g., hypertension, coronary heart disease, diabetes, and depression) and might prove useful as benchmarks for evaluating care. An innovative set of visual charts, called COOP charts, tap areas of physical, mental, role, and social functioning and is also being tested for use in ambulatory practice (Nelson et al., 1987).

Individual-Case Methods

Several methods of case-by-case problem detection, such as autopsy and case conferences, have been developed and implemented in health care settings. Other approaches have administrative or even legal purposes, such as patient complaint and incident-reporting systems. Still others might be considered monitoring devices to identify poor practitioners after lengthy external processes. These include PRO sanctions, disciplinary actions by state medical boards, and malpractice settlements.

Two general problems limit the value of case-by-case systems as problem-detection methods. First, these systems have generally not been aggregated nor findings classified consistently so that patterns could be identified. Second, these systems are usually not linked to quality assurance efforts directly or indirectly through a common reporting pathway (for example, a hospital governing board). As a result, they do not contribute to the analysis of patient problems or integrated feedback of information to practitioners (see Nelson, 1976). The specific strengths and weaknesses of three methods, autopsy, case conferences, and patient complaints, are discussed below.

Autopsy

Strengths. Unexpected findings at autopsy are considered to be an excellent way to refine clinical judgment and identify possible misdiagnosis. Landefeld and Goldman (1989) summarized the value of autopsies. In 5 to 10 percent of cases "treatable, major unexpected findings have been discovered that, if known premortem, would probably have improved the patient's chance of survival. Other major unexpected findings were revealed in another 10 percent of cases" (Landefeld and Goldman, 1989, p. 42). Autopsies can provide information on the rates of and reasons for discrepancies between clinical diagnoses and postmortem findings.

Limitations. Several aspects of autopsy have limited its usefulness for quality assessment. There are no standard methods for classifying unexpected autopsy findings nor any formal system of feedback from pathologists to quality assurance programs. Autopsy reports may lag death by one to three months. Moreover, the proportion of hospital deaths that are accompanied by autopsy has declined greatly in recent years (from 50 percent in the 1940s to 14 percent in 1985) (Geller, 1983; MMWR, 1988). The decline in autopsy rates has been attributed to lack of insurance reimbursement and to practitioner reluctance to request permission for autopsy from the patient's family. Landefeld and Goldman (1989) have suggested several strategies for increasing the rate of autopsies, including requesting permission for possible autopsy at the time of admission and reimbursement by HCFA and other third-party payers; they believe reimbursement is justified on the basis of its value for quality assurance.

Case Conferences

Case conferences are primarily educational meetings in which physicians review the care of difficult cases. The case may be presented because it was unusual or complex, required difficult clinical management choices, or had an adverse outcome. The discussion may cover a great many topics such as the value of new technologies, approaches to care that might have been more conservative, clinical findings that were overlooked, or an ethical dilemma presented by the case.

The Morbidity and Mortality (M&M) conference is a department-based conference that occurs after an adverse event such as a death or complication, typically after a surgical procedure. The course of illness and diagnostic, autopsy, and pathology findings are presented and discussed by the attending physician and pathologist.

Strengths. Case conferences are highly valued by clinicians as an effective method of learning. They are conducted in a nonjudgmental atmosphere and are considered clinically pertinent. They accord with medical training in that they focus on individual cases.

Limitations. Case conferences are believed to be very effective in monitoring and assuring high quality of care in hospitals. They do not, however, result from or lead to systematic information about practice patterns and outcomes that might advance the institutions' understanding of patterns of care in unanticipated ways.

Patient Complaints

Reviewing complaints can be a method of detecting problems in care. Responding to complaints may have two valuable functions. It indicates to patients that the organization takes problems seriously, and it may prompt intraorganizational reforms that would never be suggested by formal quality assurance mechanisms. Complaint reporting programs are also used by external regulators, such as state and local departments of health and insurance commissioners. At least one PRO visited in this study believed that patient (or other) complaints were useful in identifying problem practitioners and that PRO review of patient complaints helped foster better relations with the patient community.

Strengths. Review of complaints, like patient assessments, includes patients in the quality review process and permits the identification of unexpected problems. A systematic classification and review of complaints has the potential to identify underservice, including lack of access to services. It can also identify interpersonal issues; like malpractice allegations, complaints about health practitioners are probably less likely when the interpersonal process has been good.

Limitations. The value of using rates of complaints for detecting quality problems depends on the relationship between the rate of complaints and the rate of quality problems, about which virtually nothing is known. Nor is it known whether serious problems in care are more likely than trivial problems to result in complaints. According to the New York State Department of Health (personal communication), only a small percentage of complaints received are confirmed as quality problems. In short, patient complaints may be highly idiosyncratic, so that patterns of complaints may be very difficult to detect or interpret.

The degree of patient vulnerability probably affects the likelihood of lodging a complaint. For instance, healthy HMO patients may not hesitate to register complaints about overlong waits. By contrast, elderly, frail, and isolated patients receiving home health care may be more reluctant to complain about home health aides on whom they are dependent, yet the danger to the patient's health in the latter situation may be far more grave.

FACTORS THAT IMPEDE OR ENHANCE THE EFFECTIVENESS OF QUALITY INTERVENTIONS TO CORRECT PROBLEMS

It is difficult to overstate, although not difficult to understand, our lack of knowledge about useful strategies for changing professional and organizational behavior. If the science of quality assessment is considered to be in its infancy, then we must regard our knowledge of strategies for quality assurance to be embryonic. Arguably, we know more about how to change patient behavior (e.g., see Haynes et al., 1979) than how to change the behavior of health professionals and organizations.

The study committee asked Avedis Donabedian, an eminent observer and writer in the field of quality assurance, to reflect on barriers to effective quality assurance. In preparing this discussion, we have drawn heavily on the paper he prepared in response to that request (Donabedian, 1989). The remainder of this section considers the key attributes of the medical profession that should be taken into account in designing a quality assurance effort. It also considers important aspects of changing practice behaviors of both individuals and organizations in response to quality assurance findings.

Special Characteristics of the Medical Profession

Donabedian (1989) argues that to appreciate the factors that promote or hinder quality assurance and to evaluate methods commonly used to change individual behavior, one must understand several special characteristics of the medical profession. These include professional autonomy and accountability, training and socialization of physicians, traditions of informal peer review, and unfamiliarity with quality assurance as a formal process.

Autonomy and Accountability

The tension between autonomy in the practice of medicine and accountability for its quality is a hallmark of this profession. In granting the medical profession primary responsibility for quality, society has recognized the special expertise required to determine what constitutes goodness in technical care and has insulated physicians from interference by outside interests that might subvert clinical judgment. At the same time, it has expected a reasonable degree of public accountability. These are principles that the medical profession has espoused and to which society has largely adhered.

The desires of the medical profession to define quality and to control the means for assuring it have been recognized by delegating the monitoring function outside hospitals to organizations controlled by or responsive to physicians (such as the Medicare PROs). Within hospitals, the organized medical staff is entrusted with that responsibility. The medical profession also controls the criteria and standards by which quality of care is to be judged.

Opinions differ as to which societal requirements constitute interference with professional prerogatives and which are legitimate demands for accountability. In this tension between accountability and professional autonomy, one finds the origin of much that troubles quality assurance efforts today.

Socialization and Peer Relations

Two related characteristics of medicine are (1) the emphasis placed on recruitment, training, and socialization and (2) the significance accorded to informal rather than formal quality assurance interventions carried out by fellow clinicians. Both mechanisms are intended to produce professionals who are both technically competent and morally equipped to be self-critical and self-correcting. In professional training and in later practice, monitoring individual performance has been informal rather than formal. Individual conduct has been regulated indirectly through inclusion in or exclusion from the network of professional referrals and by other, more or less subtle indicators of professional approval.

Medical professionals depend economically and to some extent emotionally on one another. The careers of physicians depend on the approval of colleagues who vouch for their competence by sending them patients. Colleagues also offer encouragement and support for what may be regarded as an intrinsically uncertain and hazardous profession, not only because of the substantial likelihood of mistakes, but also because of the perceived litigiousness of the public and the unsympathetic scrutiny of external monitors. Quality monitoring, when it progresses to the point of identifying individual practitioners directly or by implication, requires that some physicians sit in judgment over others. Even though the participants in this monitoring may be legally protected from reprisal, they are subject to other powerful modifying motivations.

Distrust of Externally Imposed Efforts

The medical profession would like to see the traditions of professionalism and informal peer review preserved and incorporated into quality assurance efforts. This stance is very different from recent developments often feared and opposed by physicians. Although quality monitoring in hospitals and PRO review are under physician control, physicians are warned that if they will not do the job, others can be found who will. Moreover, what physician-directed review agencies do is more and more externally prescribed, often in painful detail. What physicians do and accomplish is subject to external verification.

To many physicians, the objectives of the monitoring enterprise are often suspect. They have reason to believe that much of what is done in the name of quality is, in fact, cost control.

Also alien (and alienating) is the insistence by external controllers that monitoring extend to the identification of individual malfeasance, leading to disciplinary action. Some physicians claim that the "body count" (meaning the number of physicians censured) has become the measure of success in federal performance monitoring. In some ways, federal agencies have bypassed the medical profession altogether, for instance, by releasing to the public information such as hospital-specific mortality rates that could create mistrust and discord between physicians and patients. In such circumstances, one can expect monitoring to be resisted and, when possible, weakened, perhaps to the point of nullification.

Unfamiliarity with Quality Assurance Purposes and Methods

Physicians are not generally familiar with methods of quality assessment and have only recently moved into clinical management in any numbers. They are trained to be concerned with the care of individual patients, not with patterns of care. Epidemiological and statistical skills are recent additions to medical training. Further, few trainees have participated in quality assessment.

This lack of familiarity makes leadership in quality assurance efforts both scarce and crucial, and it points to the need for educational reform in building the capability of professionals to act with confidence. We return to this point in Chapter 11.

Changing Practitioner Behavior

Changing professional behavior in the long run requires persuading the professional of the need to change. The most persuasive data are those that are credible, complete, timely, and pertinent to an individual's practice.

Educational Approaches

Good education and training are regarded by the health care professions to be the foundation for good practice. Beyond a lengthy and rigorous initial experience, a lifetime characterized by continuous learning is the ideal. Professionals hold educational interventions to be the preferred method for obtaining behavior change, especially if the method does not single out individuals.

Although education may be the most useful first approach to changing professionals' behavior, the kinds of problems or practitioners that are most amenable to educational interventions are not clear. Respected clinicians providing feedback in relatively informal settings may be the most effective agents for change. Lohr et al. (1981, p. vii), in referring to technology diffusion, state that "in general, professional colleagues are considered more potent legitimizing agents than any other single influence, and the most effective force for physicians' adoption of medical innovations is professional, face-to-face contact with recognized peers." The same can also be said for adoption of new practice behaviors (Eisenberg, 1986; Schroeder, 1987; Davidoff et al., 1989).

After reviewing the literature, Eisenberg (1986) reported that some studies show continuing education to be effective, others show it to be ineffective, and many other studies are inconclusive because of deficiencies in their methods or ambiguities in their findings. Guided by this picture and principles of adult education, he surmised that successful approaches to modifying physician behavior should have the following features. First, a practitioner should have accepted (presumably on the basis of valid evidence) that he or she has a need to learn. Second, the educational content should be specific to the need already identified. Third, education should be conducted face-to-face. Fourth, if possible, it should be conducted one-to-one. Fifth, it should be conducted by an "influential" person—a person the practitioner trusts and respects. Presumably, many educational efforts fail because one or more of these conditions are not met.

Education is called for when insufficient knowledge or skill are at least in part the reason for deficient care. How often ignorance and ineptitude are a cause of poor care, and to what degree, is not known, but their contribution can be expected to vary considerably from setting to setting. McDonald and his co-workers (McDonald, 1976; McDonald et al., 1984; Tierney et al., 1986) concluded after a controlled study that errors in ambulatory care occurred more often because of overload of tasks and information than because of lack of knowledge. To the extent that mistakes are caused by lack of access to current knowledge, online computer-aided management, warning, and reminder systems may hold promise for affecting physician behavior. We do not, however, know a great deal about the circumstances in which these systems are used or are useful, and we recognize that available tools and attitudes may be changing dramatically as the professionally trained population becomes increasingly computer literate.

The conditions detailed above underscore the importance of establishing a clearly defined link between quality monitoring and continuing education, as typified by the "bi-cycle" model proposed many years ago by Brown and Uhl (1970) and repeatedly advanced since.[7] Donabedian (1989) believes that the relative effectiveness of alternative ways of linking monitoring to education, and of conducting the educational effort itself, should be high on the agenda of research on the effectiveness of quality assurance through monitoring.

Incentives and Disincentives

Professional behavior can also be changed by directive. The net effect of such an approach on the health of patients and the morale of professionals has not been explored. Likewise, little is known about the effects of positive versus negative incentives or ways to link informal professional incentives to quality assurance activities.

Feedback and education are meant to appeal to internalized values and to mobilize the personal resources of practitioners. Various factors in the environment may well enhance or diminish these efforts. Much depends on the implicit expectations and informal understandings of medical colleagues, but a great deal may also depend on the structure of a more formalized system of rewards and penalties. The relative impotence of quality assurance efforts in directly modifying practitioner behavior may be attributable to the absence of a clearly defined, consistently operative link between the results of monitoring and the career prospects of practitioners. Thus, the formal system of incentives and disincentives deserves particular attention in any analysis of effectiveness.

Incentives are commonly regarded as rewards and disincentives as penalties, but not receiving a reward when a system of rewards has been instituted can be a disincentive, and not being penalized when a system of penalties has been established can be an incentive. A system based on recognizing and rewarding, rather than ferreting out and punishing error, would very likely differ in its acceptability to professionals and perhaps also in its effectiveness. One might also hypothesize that a system having features of both approaches could be the most effective.

Rewards and penalties might also be distinguishable by whether they are professional, financial, or both, and by whether they are generalized or particularized. For example, a promotion connotes both professional and financial rewards that are not necessarily related to any particular meritorious action; rather, a general pattern of laudable behavior is being recognized. By contrast, withholding payment for an unapproved procedure is a particularized penalty. A proposal that physicians be awarded part of the savings that accrue from their maintaining a lower-than-average length of hospital stay is an positive financial reward related to a pattern of behavior. The traditional incentives of the professional culture such as career advancement, salary, risk-sharing and bonus arrangements, and esteem of colleagues are more individualized.

The magnitude of the rewards or penalties might affect their impact. This may be especially true if penalties are matched to the seriousness of the offense (Vladeck, 1988), to the credibility and legitimacy of the judgments that lead to them, to the presence of procedural and legal safeguards against arbitrary action, and to evidence that penalties are used fairly and consistently.

Eisenberg (1986) reached two conclusions about the use of penalties. First, penalties do modify physician behaviors. Second, they are deeply resented and may have unexpected or unwanted consequences—a "backlash," as he calls it. Such backlash undoubtedly would create political and administrative problems, but its effect on the quality of care is not clear.

Changing Systems and Organizations

Berwick (1989) has stated that "flaws come more often from impaired systems than from impaired people." Many quality assurance professionals concurred with this view during our site visits, and this viewpoint has led many to focus not only on average practice rather than outliers but on organizational factors that affect quality and on ways of changing them.

Despite a voluminous literature on planned organizational change (Johnson, 1989), its principles have not been extensively applied to the health care organization. In particular, the implementation of continuous improvement models (discussed in Chapter 2) has not yet progressed far enough to demonstrate their effectiveness in modifying clinical and organizational behavior.

In a discussion of barriers limiting implementation of quality assurance programs, Luke and Boss (1981, p. 148) stated that the ineffectiveness of educational strategies results from a "failure to conceptualize quality assurance primarily as a problem of organizational and behavioral change." They further asserted that ". . . the real barriers to quality assurance are not the impediments to data acquisition and analysis but the points of resistance to change within health institutions." They identified 10 barriers to change that must be recognized and addressed if interventions are to be effective. These barriers are: (1) autonomy expectations of health professionals; (2) collective benefits of stability; (3) calculated opposition to change; (4) programmed behavior; (5) tunnel vision; (6) resource limitations; (7) sunk costs; (8) accumulations of official constraints on behavior; (9) unofficial and unplanned constraints on behavior; and (10) interorganizational agreements.

Many organizational factors may influence the effectiveness of quality assurance efforts. Particularly important may be the collaborative nature of medical practice and its dependence on institutional (mainly hospital) support (Knaus et al., 1986). Physicians, as a group, may be able to control only a part of what is done for patients; any one physician can control even less. Palmer et al. (1985) found that physicians in ambulatory practices were more likely to improve their care in response to failures revealed by monitoring when the change to be made was more directly under their own control.

Organizational Factors Influencing the Form and Effectiveness of Quality Assurance

Quality monitoring is most likely to occur when care is provided in or through institutions or organized programs. Thus, the forms it takes as well as its effectiveness can be expected to reflect the characteristics of these organizations.

Variations in quality among institutions are probably at least partly attributable to the fact some institutions have better developed and functioning quality monitoring systems than others. When care is made more "visible" to colleagues (for example, through sharing responsibility for care, consultation, teaching rounds, clinical conferences, and the like), then the quality of that care is likely to be higher (Neuhauser, 1971; Shortell et al., 1976). Other advantages in quality have been attributed to controls over recruitment and staffing, to equipment and material resources, to direct supervision of professional work, and to more subtle attributes such as coordination, communication, and tightness of organizational control (Georgopoulos and Mann, 1962; Scott et al., 1976; Flood and Scott, 1978). The role of formal monitoring mechanisms, as a separable organizational feature, in influencing the quality of care provided is as yet unexplored.

Several features of the organizational environment might influence the implementation and effectiveness of quality monitoring. These include ideology, leadership, and baseline performance.

Ideology

The importance accorded to quality, both in absolute terms and relative to competing objectives (particularly cost containment), may be an important determinant of the effectiveness of quality monitoring. The sources of concern for quality may derive from the perception of a social responsibility, a professional imperative, a prudent yielding to coercion, or the prospect of a profitable response to market forces. All these factors may also bear on the effectiveness of quality assurance, particularly if all motivations impel in the same direction (Donabedian, 1989).

The relative importance given to technical care as compared to the interpersonal process may also influence the form and success of quality assurance. To some extent this choice is ideological; it reflects or is influenced by the views of the organization's leadership, the values and traditions of the major constituencies to which the organization is answerable, and the functions an organization serves. For instance, the quality of technical care is likely to be the dominant concern of a major teaching center. In contrast, a long-term care facility under religious auspices is impelled, in part, by the values of its sponsors to emphasize the amenities and the interpersonal aspects of care. In the first instance, the interpersonal process may be at risk, whereas in the second situation technical care may be in jeopardy.

Leadership

Leadership as a component of the organizational environment is least amenable to control and often dependent on serendipity. Donabedian (1989) points out that whether leadership is provided by a member of the governing board or a senior administrator, he or she must be a trusted and respected colleague who is directly involved in the program. Although the evidence is weak, it seems to suggest that quality monitoring is more effective in altering physician behavior when clinical leaders participate in it and alter their own behavior in response to its findings (Palmer et al., 1988).

Baseline Performance

The baseline level of clinical performance that characterizes an organization may be an important determinant of the perceived need for quality monitoring and may affect both the design of the monitoring enterprise and its effectiveness. In this regard, the shared perceptions of the level of performance may be as important as the actual level, more objectively assessed.

When the actual or perceived level of performance is exceedingly high, formal monitoring may seem redundant. When such review is externally imposed, it may be resented and at best perfunctorily performed. Major teaching institutions may be particularly prone to these behaviors.

When actual performance is at an uncommonly low level, quality monitoring may be regarded as a threat. Where monitoring is introduced, it may be ineffective because poor practice is usually the consequence of deep-seated organizational pathology. Disbelief, defensiveness, and low expectations may lead to weak internal criteria and standards that fail to challenge. Even when external criteria and standards are held out as an example, they are likely to be countered by a host of arguments seeking to show why the criteria do not apply to the peculiarities of the local situation.

SUMMARY

The variety of techniques for quality review and assurance used in the United States is enormous and rich. Some activities are intended to prevent quality problems; some are designed to detect them; and still others are efforts to correct problems once they are identified.

This chapter has provided a highly selective sampler of methods for quality review and assurance. It illustrates the considerable range of efforts beyond those of the federal PRO program and shows there is much to learn from the professional and provider communities' own efforts. All these methods have strengths and limitations, which we have cited here. We have, however, taken no position on the quality of those efforts. The techniques and approaches described are not necessarily the best, although some may well be state-of-the-art.

Our review here of quality assessment methods currently in use (and the descriptions of methods in various settings in Volume II) reveals inadequacies, in particular, the weak focus on the continuum of care across multiple providers for patients, especially those with chronic illness, who move from one setting of care to another. Review tends to focus on single events and single settings rather than episodes of care.

By and large, review techniques look at the technical quality of care and specifically at the physician component of decision making. For those receiving care, undertreatment, and to a lesser degree, overuse may be identified. The quality of interpersonal care and the use of patient outcomes in evaluating care are only now beginning to be incorporated into quality review efforts.

This chapter highlights the need for a much better understanding of how effectively to bring about change in provider performance and practice patterns. Available intervention methods include information feedback on performance, financial incentives and disincentives and penalties, and organizational development and change techniques. The emphasis is often on overcoming deficiencies in knowledge or skills, indifference, or impairment. The limited repertoire of practitioner-oriented interventions (e.g., education, exhortation, surveillance, and sanctions) is insufficient to address what may be far more complex reasons for inappropriate or poor technical care. These include the nature of medical work, its collaborative nature, the lack of physician control over many aspects of health services, and the organizational environment of practice.

Most quality assurance professionals have at one time or another become discouraged at the results of providing information on practice and hoping that a change in behavior would result. The likelihood of change may be linked to the seriousness of the deficiency, the relevance of the practitioner's behavior to that deficiency, and the ease of changing behavior. The most promising strategies for changing individual behavior are likely to be those that act in concert with the training and practice characteristics of doctors in conforming to the medical culture, that help the already good practitioners as well as the outliers, and that recognize the limited ability of any given practitioner to change the delivery system.

Leadership and commitment in concert with other organizational goals may be the most important factors in organizational change. Organization and funding of quality assurance programs likely influence their effectiveness. The baseline level of performance and the external regulatory environment are also likely to influence an organization's response to purported deficiencies.

NOTES

1. Some of the discussion of licensure and board certification has been drawn from a paper, "Medicare Quality Assurance Mechanisms and the Law," by A.H. Smith and M.J. Mehlman prepared for this study and referred to hereafter as Smith and Mehlman, 1989.
2. See Chapter 10 for a more extended discussion of appropriateness (practice) guidelines, patient management criteria sets, and algorithms.
3. Much of this discussion has been drawn from a paper by L.L. Roos, N.P. Roos, E.S. Fisher, and T.A. Bubolz prepared for this study and hereafter referred to as Roos et al., 1989. Some of the material will appear in Roos et al. (forthcoming) and Roos, 1989.
4. International Classification of Diseases, ninth revision, clinical modification. The Medicare hospital (Part A) files for instance, use ICD-9-CM codes, and diagnosis-related groups (DRGs) are based on them as well.
5. The development and testing of coding dictionaries that manage multiple medical terms such as those in use with the Computer Stored Ambulatory Record (COSTAR) have demonstrated promise in improving coding accuracy in ambulatory care.
6. Calculations done from data supplied by HCFA for the Second Scope of Work through February 1989 of review of more than 6.1 million records show the

following: Of all records reviewed, nearly 24 percent failed at least one screen. Of those that failed at least one screen, physician advisors confirmed quality problems in 30 percent, or about 7 percent of all records reviewed (HCFA, 1989).

7. The bi-cycle model is one in which problems are identified, analyzed, attacked, and then reevaluated. In the case of problems caused by lack of practitioner knowledge or skills the methods of correction should involve highly targeted, pertinent continuing education.

REFERENCES

Barnett, G.O., Winickoff, R.N., Dorsey, J.L., et al. Quality Assurance Through Automated Monitoring and Concurrent Feedback Using a Computer-Based Medical Information System. *Medical Care* 16:962-970, 1978.

Barnett, G.O., Winickoff, R.N., Morgan, M.M., et al. A Computer-Based Monitoring System for Follow-up of Elevated Blood Pressure. *Medical Care* 21:400-409, 1983.

Berwick, D.M. The Ideal of Continuous Improvement. Reply to Letters to the Editor. *New England Journal of Medicine* 320:1425, 1989.

Brown, C.R. Jr. and Uhl, H.S. Mandatory Medical Education: Sense or Nonsense? *Journal of the American Medical Association* 213:1660-1668, 1970.

Borgiel, A.E. Assessing the Quality of Care in Family Physicians' Practices by the College of Family Physicians of Canada. Pp. 63-72 in *Quality of Care and Technology Assessment*. Lohr, K.N. and Rettig, R.A. eds. Washington, D.C.: National Academy Press, 1988.

Borgiel, A.E., Williams, J.I., Anderson, G.M., et al. Assessing the Quality of Care in Family Physicians' practices. *Canadian Family Physician* 31:853-862, 1985.

Chassin, M.R., Kosecoff, J., and Dubois, R. *Value-Managed Health Care Purchasing. An Employer's Guidebook Series. Volume II: Health Care Quality Assessment*. Chicago, Ill.: Midwest Business Group on Health, 1989a.

Chassin, M.R., Park, R.W., Lohr, K.N., et al. Differences Among Hospitals in Medicare Patient Mortality. *Health Service Research* 24:1-31, 1989b.

Craddick, J.W. and Bader, B.S. *Medical Management Analysis: A Systematic Approach to Quality Assurance and Risk Management*. Vol. I. Auburn, Calif.: J.W. Craddick, 1983.

Davidoff, F., Goodspeed, R., and Clive, J. Changing Test Ordering Behavior: A Randomized Controlled Trial Comparing Probabilistic Reasoning With Cost-Containment Education. *Medical Care* 27:45-58, 1989.

Davis, D., Haynes, R.B., Chambers, L., et al. The Impact of CME: A Methodologic Review of the Continuing Medical Education Literature. *Evaluation and the Health Professions* 7:251-284, 1984.

Davies, A.R. and Ware, J.E. Involving Consumers in Quality of Care Assessment. *Health Affairs* 7:33-48, Spring 1988.

Donabedian, A. Reflections on the Effectiveness of Quality Assurance. Paper prepared for the Institute of Medicine Study to Design a Strategy for Quality Review and Assurance in Medicare, 1989.

Dubois, R.W. Hospital Mortality as an Indicator of Quality. Pp. 107-131 in *Providing Quality Care: The Challenge to Clinicians*. Goldfield, N. and Nash, D.B., eds. Philadelphia, Pa.: American College of Physicians, 1989.

Eisenberg, J.M. *Doctor's Decision and the Cost of Medical Care*. Ann Arbor, Mich.: Health Administration Press, 1986.

Flood, A.B. and Scott, W.R. Professional Power and Professional Effectiveness: The Power of the Surgical Staff and the Quality of Surgical Care in Hospitals. *Journal of Health and Social Behavior* 19:240-254, 1978.

GAO (General Accounting Office). *DOD HEALTH CARE. Occurrence Screen Program Undergoing Changes, but Weaknesses Still Exist*. GAO/HRD-89-36. Washington, D.C.: General Accounting Office, January 1989.

Geller, S. Autopsy. *Scientific American* 248:124-135, 1983.

Georgopoulos, B.S. and Mann, F.C. *The Community General Hospital*. New York, N.Y.: MacMillan, 1962.

Gerbert, B., Stone, G., Stulbarg, M., et al. Agreement Among Physician Assessment Methods: Searching for the Truth Among Fallible Methods. *Medical Care* 26:519-535, 1988.

Greenfield, S., Cretin, S., Worthman, L.G., et al. Comparison of a Criteria Map to a Criteria List in Quality-of-Care Assessment for Patients with Chest Pain: The Relation of Each to Outcome. *Medical Care* 19:255-272, 1981.

Greenfield, S. Measuring the Quality of Office Practice. Pp. 183-198 in *Providing Quality Care: The Challenge to Clinicians*. Goldfield, N. and Nash, D., eds. Philadelphia, Pa.: American College of Physicians, 1989.

Havighurst, C.C. and King, N.M. Private Credentialing of Health Care Personnel: An Antitrust Perspective. *American Journal of Law & Medicine* 9:131-201, 1983.

Havighurst, C.C. *Health Care Law and Policy: Readings, Notes, and Questions*. Westbury, N.Y.: Foundation Press, 1988.

Haynes, R.B., Taylor, D.W., and Sackett, D.L., eds. *Compliance in Health Care*. Baltimore, Md.: Johns Hopkins University Press, 1979.

Hiatt, H.H., Barnes, B.A., Brennan, T.A., et al. Special Report: A Study of Medical Injury and Medical Malpractice. *New England Journal of Medicine* 320:480-483, 1989.

Johnson, K.W. Knowledge Utilization and Planned Change: An Empirical Assessment of the A VICTORY Model. *Knowledge in Society* 2:57-79, 1989.

Joint Commission. *1990 AMH. Accreditation Manual for Hospitals*. Chicago, Ill.: Joint Commission, 1989.

Kessner, D.M., Kalk, C.E., and Singer, J. Assessing Health Quality: The Case for Tracers. *New England Journal of Medicine* 288:189-194, 1973.

Knaus, W.A., Draper, E.A., Wagner, D.P., et al. An Evaluation of Outcome from Intensive Care in Major Medical Centers. *Annals of Internal Medicine* 104:410-418, 1986.

Landefeld, C.S. and Goldman, L. The Autopsy in Quality Assurance: History, Current Status, and Future Directions. *Quality Review Bulletin* 15:42-48, 1989.

Larson, E., Oram, L.F., and Hedrick, E. Nosocomial Infection Rates as an Indicator of Quality. *Medical Care* 26:676-684, 1988.

Lehmann, R. Forum on Clinical Indicator Development: A Discussion of the Use and Development of Indicators. *Quality Review Bulletin* 15:223-227, 1989.

Lohr, K.N., Winkler, J.D., and Brook, R.H. *Peer Review and Technology Assessment in Medicine.* R-2820-OTA. Santa Monica, Calif.: The RAND Corporation, 1981.

Luke, R.D. and Boss, R.W. Barriers Limiting the Implementation of Quality Assurance Programs. *Health Services Research* 16:305-314, 1981.

McDonald, C.J. Protocol-Based Computer Reminders, the Quality of Care and the Non-Perfectibility of Man. *New England Journal of Medicine* 295:1351-1355, 1976.

McDonald, C.J., Hui, S.L., Smith, D.M., et al. Reminders to Physicians From an Introspective Computer Medical Record: A Two-Year Randomized Trial. *Annals of Internal Medicine* 100:130-138, 1984.

Meyer, W., Clinton, J.J., and Newhall, D. A First Report of the Department of Defense External Civilian Peer Review of Medical Care. *Journal of the American Medical Association* 260:2690-2693, 1988.

MMWR. Morbidity and Mortality Weekly Report. Autopsy frequency—United States (1980-1985). 37:191-194, 1988.

Nelson, A.R. Orphan Data and the Unclosed Loop: A Dilemma in PSRO and Medical Audit. *New England Journal of Medicine* 295:617-619, 1976.

Nelson, E.C. and Berwick, D.M. The Measurement of Health Status in Clinical Practice. *Medical Care* 27: S77-S90, (March Supplement) 1989.

Nelson, E.C., Wasson, J.H., Kirk, J.W., et al. Assessment of Function in Routine Clinical Practice: Description of the COOP Chart Method and Preliminary Findings. *Journal of Chronic Diseases* 40:55S-63S, (Supplement) 1987.

Neuhauser, D. *The Relationship Between Administration Activities and Hospital Performance.* Chicago, Ill.: The University of Chicago Center for Health Administrative Studies, Research Series 29, 1971.

O'Leary, D. *Future Trends in Evaluating Quality Care.* Lecture delivered at the McCormick Center Hotel, Chicago, Ill., May 13, 1988.

OTA (Office of Technology Assessment). *The Quality of Medical Care. Information for Consumers.* OTA-H-386. Washington, D.C.: U.S. Government Printing Office, June 1988.

Palmer, R.H., Strain, R., Maurer, J.V., et al. Quality Assurance in Eight Adult Medicine Group Practices. *Medical Care* 22:632-643, 1984.

Palmer, R.H., Louis, T.A., Hsu, L.N., et al. A Randomized Control Trial of Quality Assurance in Sixteen Ambulatory Care Practices. *Medical Care* 23:751-768, 1985.

Palmer, R.H., Hall, J.A., Hargraves, L., et al. Internal Leadership versus External Review for Ambulatory Care Quality. *Outline of Talk* (Draft) September 28, 1988.

Paul-Shaheen, P., Clark, J.D., and Williams, D. Small Area Analysis: A Review and Analysis of the North American Literature. *Journal of Health Politics, Policy and Law* 12:741-809, 1987.

PPRC (Physician Payment Review Commission). *Annual Report to Congress. 1989.* Washington, D.C.: Physician Payment Review Commission, 1989.

Roos, L.L. Nonexperimental Data Systems in Surgery. *International Journal of Technology Assessment in Health Care* 5:341-386, 1989.

Roos, L.L., Roos, N.P., Fisher, E.S., et al. Strengths and Weaknesses of Health Insurance Data Systems for Assessing Outcomes. Paper prepared for the Institute of Medicine Study to Design a Strategy for Quality Review and Assurance in Medicare, 1989.

Roos, L.L., Sharp, S.M., Cohen, M.M., et al. Risk Adjustment in Claims-based Research: The Search for Efficient Approaches. *Journal of Clinical Epidemiology,* 42:1193-1206, 1989.

Ramsey, P.G., Carline, J.D., Inui, T.S., et al. Predictive Validity of Certification by the American Board of Internal Medicine. *Annals of Internal Medicine* 110:719-726, 1989.

Rutstein, D.D., Berenberg, W. B., Chalmers, T.C., et al. Measuring the Quality of Medical Care (Tables Revised, 9/1/77) A Clinical Method. *New England Journal of Medicine* 294:582-588, 1976.

Scott, W.R., Forrest, W.H. Jr., and Brown, B.V. Hospital Structure and Postoperative Mortality and Morbidity. Pp. 72-89 in *Organizational Research in Hospitals.* Shortell, S.M. and Brown, M., eds. Chicago, Ill.: Blue Cross Association, 1976.

Schroeder, S.A. Strategies for Reducing Medical Costs by Changing Physicians' Behavior. *International Journal of Technology Assessment in Health Care* 3:39-50, 1987.

Shortell, S.M., Becker, S.W., and Neuhauser, D. The Effects of Managerial Practices on Hospital Efficiency and Quality of Care. Pp. 90-107 in *Organizational Research in Hospitals.* Shortell, S. M. and Brown, M. eds. Chicago, Ill.: Blue Cross Association, 1976.

Smith, A.H. and Mehlman, M.J. Medicare Quality Assurance Mechanisms and the Law. Paper prepared for the Institute of Medicine Study to Design a Strategy for Quality Review and Assurance in Medicare, 1989.

Stewart, A.L., Hays, R.D., and Ware, J.E. The MOS Short-form General Health Survey: Reliability and Validity in a Patient Population. *Medical Care* 26:724-732, 1988.

Stewart, A.L., Greenfield, S., Hays, R.D., et al. Functional Status and Well-being of Patients with Chronic Conditions: Results from the Medical Outcomes Study. *Journal of American Medical Association* 262:907-943, 1989.

Tarlov, A.R., Ware, J.E., Greenfield, S., et al. The Medical Outcomes Study. An Application of Methods for Monitoring the Results of Medical Care. *Journal of the American Medical Association* 262:925-930, 1989.

Tierney, W.M., Hui, S.L., and McDonald, C.J. Delayed Feedback of Physician Performance Versus Immediate Reminders to Perform Preventive Care: Effects on Physician Compliance. *Medical Care* 24:659-666, 1986.

Vladeck, B.C. Quality Assurance through External Control. *Inquiry* 25:100-107, 1988.

Weiner, J., Powe, N., Steinwachs, D., et al. Quality of Care Indicators for Potential Application to Insurance Claims/Encounter Data. Report to the Cigna Foundation. Johns Hopkins University Research and Development Center, 1989.

10

Critical Attributes of Quality-of-Care Criteria and Standards

The rapid growth in health care expenditures has prompted third-party payers, both governmental and private, to institute programs that try to control costs by restraining the use of health care services. These programs range from direct efforts to identify and discourage specific unnecessary services (e.g., prior review of proposed care) to financial incentives for providers and consumers to reduce services (e.g., capitated payments to health care providers and cost-sharing by patients). These steps, if successful, can not only control costs but also improve the quality of care by reducing exposure to iatrogenic illness and injury. However, these programs could also over-reach to discourage the provision or use of needed services.

Good criteria for assessing quality of care and for distinguishing appropriate from inappropriate care can operate at the intersection between cost and quality concerns in two major ways. On the one hand, they can strengthen the clinical basis for prior review activities aimed at detecting and avoiding unnecessary care. On the other hand, they can help to identify or to prevent the underuse of care that might be an undesirable side effect of review programs, financial incentives, and other methods of controlling costs. It was against this background that Congress mandated the Medicare quality assurance study and specified as one task the "development of prototype criteria and standards" for defining and measuring quality of care.

Developing quality-of-care criteria is not a simple task, and the results are not uniformly helpful. Criteria sets vary considerably in their method of development and their substance, depending on the objectives, focus, skills, and experience of their creators. Even when criteria sets have a basic approach and specific application in common (as described in the next sections of this chapter), their formulations may differ substantially in scope, explicitness, flexibility, and scientific support. Not surprisingly, criteria sets vary in their utility and acceptability.

A prerequisite for developing useful and acceptable quality-of-care criteria is a consensus on the characteristics of sound criteria sets and acceptable methods for constructing them. The immediate goal in this chapter is to propose a basis for such a consensus. The actual development and implementation of sound guidelines will require a commitment of considerable time, resources, and expertise over a period of years.

The Institute of Medicine (IOM) study committee believed that the best way for it to move toward a framework for developing sound criteria was to convene a panel of respected experts in guideline formulation from various organizations active in this field. The main purpose of the panel was to reach agreement on the desirable attributes of quality-of-care criteria. These attributes would be standards against which old or newly developed criteria could be compared and evaluated. The panel's focus was thus on the formulation of "criteria for judging criteria" rather than on the endorsement of specific sets of criteria. Appendix A describes the composition and activities of the panel.

The remainder of this chapter discusses the conceptual issues presented to the panel. These included: three types of quality-of-care criteria sets, the range of attributes and characteristics that might be considered desirable or necessary for such criteria sets to have, the uses to which such criteria sets can be put in a quality assurance context (such as education or quality review), and key attributes for such criteria sets.

Producing criteria sets that meet the standards proposed by the panel calls for a complex and sophisticated development strategy, or perhaps several strategies depending on the type of criteria set in question. Later sections of this chapter briefly discuss methods for developing criteria with particular emphasis on stages in the development process, priority-setting, and affordability.

TYPES OF CRITERIA SETS

Different kinds of criteria sets have evolved to meet different needs. The expert panel identified three broad types: appropriateness guidelines, patient care evaluation and management criteria, and case-finding screens. Each of these is discussed below.

Appropriateness Guidelines

Appropriateness guidelines describe accepted indications for using particular medical interventions and technologies, ranging from surgical procedures to diagnostic studies. Some guidelines specify under what circumstances a particular service is appropriate (indicated). For instance, one indication for colonoscopy might be lower gastrointestinal tract bleeding. Guidelines may also describe when an intervention is not indicated. One example might be performing a carotid endarterectomy on an asymptomatic patient when the carotid angiography shows stenosis of less than 50 percent (Merrick et al., 1986). Finally, guidelines may identify equivocal indications or areas of uncertainty where consideration might be given to complex or hard-to-enumerate patient factors or where different clinicians simply disagree. For example, the indications for an exercise test to detect coronary artery disease may be "equivocal" for asymptomatic male patients over age 40 in special occupations involving public transportation or safety, including pilots, railroad engineers, and police officers (American College of Cardiology, 1986a).

Appropriateness is an integral part of quality health care (Brook, 1988b; Greenfield, 1988). In this context appropriateness generally means that the service in question has demonstrated clinical benefit for a particular indication and that the likelihood of benefits outweighs the likelihood of harm. Good quality care does not include surgery or other services that are technically flawless but not indicated or necessary. Thus, some experts have begun to explore whether economic costs ought to be factored into definitions of appropriateness, but there is no clear agreement on this point (Paterson, 1988; see also the discussion in Chapter 1 of this report).

Many organizations formulate appropriateness guidelines. The National Institutes of Health (NIH) consensus conference represents one forum for guideline development (Kanouse et al., 1987; Kosecoff et al., 1987; PPRC, 1988a). Particularly active in recent years have been technology assessment committees of several medical specialty societies. The best known effort may be that of the Clinical Efficacy Assessment Project (CEAP) of the American College of Physicians (ACP) (Sox, 1987; Steinberg, 1988). In addition, endoscopy guidelines have been developed by the American Society for Gastrointestinal Endoscopy (ASGE, 1986) and guidelines for various cardiovascular procedures by the American College of Cardiology (ACC) and American Heart Association (AHA) Task Force (ACC, 1986a, 1986b).[1]

Third-party payers such as Blue Cross and Blue Shield Association (BCBSA) and Medicare also develop standards identifying appropriate indications for various medical procedures and technologies. Their primary purpose is to serve as bases for making coverage or utilization review decisions that are intended to control costs by reducing payments for inappropriate or unnecessary services. Examples of such criteria include the preadmission review criteria developed or adopted by the Medicare Peer Review Organizations (PROs) for specified procedures and the guidelines for appropriate use of selected medical technologies developed by the BCBSA

Medical Necessity Program (IOM, 1988; Schaffarzick, 1988). The BCBSA has also supported the CEAP work and has worked with different specialty and research groups to develop guidelines that are disseminated to hospitals and physicians for educational and quality assurance purposes (not payment decisions).

Independent research organizations also have been involved in developing guidelines for the appropriate use of various medical technologies. One example is represented by The RAND Corporation's appropriateness criteria for coronary angiography, coronary artery bypass surgery, carotid endarterectomy, cholecystectomy, and diagnostic upper gastrointestinal endoscopy and colonoscopy[2] (Chassin et al., 1986a, 1986b; Kahn et al., 1986a, 1986b; Merrick, 1986; Park et al., 1986; Solomon et al., 1986; Chassin et al., 1987; Chassin, 1988; Winslow et al., 1988a, 1988b).

Patient Care Evaluation and Patient Management Criteria Sets

A second type of criteria set has evolved to help assess or guide the management of particular outpatient or inpatient medical problems rather than use of a specific service or technology.[3] These criteria sets often involve medical conditions that are characterized by ill-defined symptom complexes or that require multiple discrete clinical decisions over time. For example, they may define the range of appropriate services and care for problems such as hypertension, right lower quadrant pain, or post-operative fever, or they may specify various screening and preventive services.

A major challenge for evaluation and management criteria is variability in patients' clinical status, sociodemographic characteristics, and treatment preferences. For example, the appropriate diagnostic work-up of right lower quadrant pain may differ for a young male with fever, a young woman with an intrauterine device, or a middle-aged woman with a history of irritable bowel syndrome. Similarly, the appropriate management strategy for an elderly person with Type II (adult onset) diabetes who has difficulty checking fingersticks (home tests for blood sugar levels) may differ from that for a more adept, medically sophisticated younger diabetic.

Traditionally, quality assurance criteria developed for evaluating patient care have dealt with this complexity and variability by identifying the minimum process elements for managing a particular condition.[4] Beyond this minimum, the criteria allow for substantial clinical judgment about patient management activities. This strategy reflects, in part, a dearth of clinical research that would permit greater specificity and, in part, a lack of resources that would allow the developers of the criteria to be more precise.

Recently, computerized software systems have helped extend the use of patient management criteria by making it faster and simpler to match specific diagnostic or treatment steps to a variety of medical conditions. For example, the management of hypertension for a particular patient might be evaluated through on-line scoring of the patient's medical record for compliance with criteria calling for documentation of a funduscopic examination of the eye, urinalysis, potassium measurement, dietary instruction, and medication for patients with diastolic blood pressure consistently over 100 mm Hg.

A related approach is represented by detailed algorithms, decision trees, or criteria maps that more comprehensively specify the steps for managing a problem (Greenfield et al., 1975, 1977, 1981; Stulbarg et al., 1985). Patient variability is addressed by constructing a "network," diagram, or flow chart that helps the practitioner choose which of several alternate pathways provides the best fit between treatment options and patient characteristics. These algorithms represent optimal rather than minimal standards. Compared to the latter, they tend to be more difficult to develop and validate, and consensus may be harder to achieve. Complex algorithms may be difficult for practicing physicians to understand or accept. Even when physicians do understand the algorithms, they may not find them practical in normal clinical or (especially) crisis situations or for routine quality-of-care evaluations.

Case-Finding Screens

Case-finding screens identify potential quality-of-care problems that warrant further evaluation. These screens are objective, easily used, and often related to outcomes such as surgical complications. They trigger more in-depth analysis and peer review to confirm the presence of the problem and to detect remediable defects in processes of care at a particular institution or by a particular provider. Their relative ease of application makes them appealing for monitoring the effects of changes in provider organizational features, process of care, or payment methods.

One variety of case-finding screen is represented by hospital generic screens, sometimes called "occurrence screens." These screens have traditionally focused on single, adverse, "sentinel" events, such as an unplanned return to an operating room (OTA, 1988). The PROs have used generic screens for several years (see Chapter 6). Their set includes occurrences or specific "flags" such as nosocomial infections, unexpected death, or a return to the intensive care unit (ICU) within 24 hours of discharge from the ICU. Hospital-wide process or outcome criteria are intended to be broadly applicable across clinical departments and specialties rather than specific to, say, a clinical department, the emergency room, or pediatric care. They have been adopted by the AHA as part of its "Integrated Quality Assurance" (IQA) program (Longo et al., 1989), which in turn is based on a complex IQA model developed by the Hospital Association of New York State.

Another variety of case-finding screen is represented by specialty-specific clinical indicators such as those being developed by the Joint Commission on Accreditation of Healthcare Organizations (Joint Commission) (Lehmann, 1989; Marder, 1989; Winchester, 1989). Like generic screens, these indicators can consist of sentinel events that trigger more in-depth review. Unlike generic screens, however, they are specific to a particular specialty, type of procedure, or clinical system for delivering care. One such sentinel event in obstetrics, for instance, is the delivery by planned cesarean section of an infant weighing less than 2500 grams or one with hyaline membrane disease. The indicator may be either an adverse outcome that is linked to a process under the practitioner's or institution's control or a process than has been clearly associated with an adverse outcome (Lehmann, 1989).

More complicated, less easily applied versions of screens also exist. With "threshold" criteria, the trigger is not a specific event, but a rate of events above or below a defined level; for example, more than a 10-percent rate of appendectomies where the appendix is normal. Other screens involve failure to follow up abnormal results of laboratory tests or diagnostic studies (for example, positive blood cultures, suspicious shadows on radiographic films, or abnormal Papanicolaou [Pap] smears). Hospital admissions for conditions that could indicate poor ambulatory care are a newer focus. The 13 sentinel conditions discussed in Chapter 6 (for example, diabetic complications and malignant neoplasm of the genitourinary organ) in the Third Scope of Work for PROs constitute another example.

Since the release of hospital mortality rates by the Health Care Financing Administration (HCFA) beginning in 1986, researchers and others have focused on using aggregate mortality rates or aggregate rates of other adverse occurrences to screen institutions or patient populations (with adjustments for severity of case mix) and flag possible institutional quality-of-care problems. This approach has generated a considerable literature in a comparatively short time (Dubois et al., 1987a, 1987b; Dubois, 1989; Daley et al., 1988; Jencks et al., 1988; Kahn et al., 1988; OTA, 1988; Chassin et al., 1989; Ente and Lloyd, 1989; Fink et al., 1989; Hannan et al., 1989) and is reviewed more thoroughly in Chapter 6, Volume II.

Relationships Among Criteria Sets

The above classifications do not imply that these groupings are mutually exclusive or in conflict. Criteria sets can be difficult to categorize, and it is probably not productive to draw distinctions too finely. The labels are less important than the purposes for which criteria sets are used, individually or together.

Case-finding screens, for instance, can be used in conjunction with either appropriateness guidelines or patient evaluation and management criteria. Screens are an initial, easily applied mechanism to locate cases for more detailed review. Items included in such screens could be selected from the more easily identified or discrete elements of a set of appropriateness or patient management guidelines. Cases failing the screen would then receive in-depth review against the more detailed guidelines, thus linking these different types of criteria sets in a review continuum.

For example, one element of an evaluation-management criteria set for hypertension, such as documentation in the medical record of a funduscopic examination of the eye, might serve as a case-finding screen that nonphysician reviewers could apply. Regardless of the element or elements used as screens, the in-depth review might draw on the complete set of evaluation criteria. Traditionally, in-depth assessment has consisted of subjective "implicit" review by peer physician reviewers, but evaluation guidelines might well serve as an objective aid to their efforts.

Traditional screens, whether based on sentinel adverse occurrences or elements of the process of care, have focused more on misuse of medical technology in the sense of poor technical quality than on problems of overuse or underuse of technology. Likewise, outcome data used to screen for statistical outliers are directed primarily at poor technical quality of services rather than at overuse or underuse of care. Screens adapted from appropriateness guidelines might complement existing screens by focusing on services performed for a clearly inappropriate indication.

EFFECT OF THE TYPE AND USE OF CRITERIA ON SPECIFICATION OF DESIRABLE ATTRIBUTES

All these criteria sets can be used in different contexts for different purposes. Three major purposes are to educate practitioners, to educate and empower consumers, and to establish minimum standards of care for use in quality-of-care review. Such reviews may be prospective, concurrent, or retrospective.

Third-party payers and others hope that certain types of criteria, especially appropriateness guidelines, can be used to reduce the costs of medical care. This study, however, differentiates quality of care from cost containment. To the extent that using such criteria reduces overuse of care, costs may be lower. The application of criteria also may identify underuse of services, and this could increase expenditures, at least in the short term. This chapter and this report focus on the quality-of-care applications of criteria sets, not their uses for cost control.

The desirable characteristics of a criteria set may vary somewhat according to its use. For example, guidelines used to educate health professionals almost surely need to be different from those used to review care. Complex, comprehensive algorithmic criteria useful for educational purposes might be difficult to apply in the emergency care of acutely ill patients (when speed and parsimony are important) or in retrospective review (where brevity is desirable).[5] Criteria for retrospective review may need to be different in some respects from those used for concurrent or prospective review. The same may be true for criteria for internal versus external review.

Greenfield (1989) discusses the differences between prospective and retrospective algorithms. Prospective algorithms are directive because care has not yet been rendered. They must be logically complete, include rare diagnoses and unlikely events, have a narrower range of options, and be independent of medical records. Retrospective algorithms, by contrast, review care already delivered. They tend to be used as screens for further review and thus do not need to be logically complete. They have a more extensive range of options to allow for variation in clinical practice, and they depend on information documented in the medical record.

The features of a criteria set may also differ by level of review, such as whether they are to be used for the initial screening by nonphysician reviewers or for in-depth physician review. If a criteria set is intended to support making judgments about individuals, individual cases, or individual episodes of care, then several attributes such as sensitivity, specificity, reliability, and validity are much more important than if the criteria are simply going to physicians or to patients for educational purposes.

The desirable attributes of a criteria set will also vary according to the type of criteria set. For example, whether they are manageable for nonphysician reviewers or whether they are easy to adapt for use by computer may be especially important for case-finding screens. By contrast, whether criteria sets have built-in flexibility or are demonstrably acceptable to professionals may be more important for technology-specific or patient management guidelines.

GENERAL ATTRIBUTES OF CRITERIA SETS

As a starting point for discussing desirable attributes of criteria sets, the IOM staff prepared an extensive list of possible attributes based on review of the limited literature on guideline development and technology assessment (Eddy, 1987, 1988, forthcoming; Brook, 1988a, 1988b; Greenfield, 1988; Lewin and Erickson, 1988; PPRC, 1988a, 1988b, 1989; Brook et al., 1989). The final list of general attributes as modified by the expert panel appears in Table 10.1. This section defines the basic concepts behind the short labels for attributes that are used to simplify discussion.

Attributes can usefully be divided into two basic categories: substantive (or structural) attributes and implementation (or process) attributes. Substantive attributes relate to inherent characteristics of a criteria set. Implementation attributes focus on the processes of developing and applying a criteria set.

Substantive Attributes

In the category of substantive attributes are concepts such as sensitivity, specificity, and predictive value. *Sensitivity* refers technically to the likelihood that a case will be identified as deficient given that it really is deficient, where deficient care is measured by some outside "gold" standard that reviews all care provided. *Specificity* refers to the likelihood that truly good care will be identified. The term predictive value is defined as the proportion of cases identified by screens or other criteria as presenting quality problems that subsequently prove to be true quality problems. It takes into account the prevalence of the quality problem being investigated as well as the screen's sensitivity.[6] The traditional computational definitions are shown Figure 10.1.

These terms have generally been used in the context of case-finding screens to measure how frequently the screen detects cases of deficient care for further review (sensitivity) while passing over cases of adequate care without triggering review (specificity). A screen or criterion has poor specificity if it flags a lot of cases for review when the care was satisfactory. This wastes time and money and leads to considerable frustration on the part of reviewers. Conversely, a screen or criterion has low sensitivity if it misses a lot of cases where care was poor. This means it is ineffective for its intended purpose. (Both these criticisms have been leveled at the case-finding generic screens used by the Medicare PROs; see Chapter 6.)

Sensitivity and specificity are also important attributes for technology-specific or evaluation-management guidelines. Indeed, with some modifications, these concepts can be applied to all three types of criteria sets. The sensitivity of technology-specific and patient management guidelines refers to their ability to detect and deal with all potential cases of inappropriate or deficient care. Their application should lead to the identification of most cases of inappropriate or poor quality care with high sensitivity. For instance, in retrospective review of care of patients with chest pain, sensitivity refers to the likelihood that the quality measure correctly identifies deficient care if the physician does not follow an indicated step in the guidelines, such as admitting a patient in cardiac shock.

Reliability requires that a criteria set be appropriate, and generate consistent results for all user groups for which it is intended and that it do so time and time again. Reliable criteria relating to, for instance, a cardiovascular procedure or problem must produce the same decisions or evaluation

TABLE 10.1 General Attributes of Criteria Sets: Final List

Attribute	Definition or Explanation
Substantive and Structural Attributes	
Sensitivity	High "true positive rate" in detecting deficient or inappropriate care
Specificity	High "true negative rate" in passing over cases of adequate care
Reliability	Known to produce same decisions or evaluations when applied by the user groups for which the criteria set is intended
Validity	Based on outcome studies or other scientific evidence of effectiveness
Documentation	A. Documents methods of development and cites literature (including estimates of outcomes) B. Documents how reliability was established
Patient Responsiveness	Allows for eliciting or taking account of patient preferences
Flexibility	Respects the role of clinical judgment, with "clinical judgment" explicable
Clinical Adaptability	Allows for or takes into consideration clinically relevant differences among different classes of patients; population to which criteria apply is specified
Inclusiveness	Covers all major foreseeable clinical situations and full range of clinical problems
Concordance	Reflects consensus of professionals with extensive experience in field, with input from academic and nonacademic practitioners, generalists and specialists
Acceptability	Acceptable to majority of professionals
Clarity	Written in unambiguous language; terms, populations, data elements, and collection approach clearly defined
Appropriateness	Specifies appropriate, inappropriate, and equivocal indications (procedure and technology appropriateness guidelines)
Implementation and Process Attributes	
Pretesting	Guidelines are tested before implementation
Dynamism	Mechanism and commitment exists for reviewing and updating criteria sets to incorporate new information and cover new situations
Evaluation	Mechanism exists to review and evaluate outcome or impact of guidelines
Comprehendability	A. Format understood by nonphysician reviewers B. Format understood by practitioners C. Format easily understood by patients/consumers

Attribute	Definition or Explanation
Manageability	A. Not unduly burdensome for nonphysician reviewers to apply
	B. Not unduly burdensome for physician reviewers to apply
	C. Not unduly burdensome for professional to follow
Nonintrusiveness	Minimizes inappropriate direct interaction with treating physicians
Appealability	Allows for appeals process by professionals and patients
Feasibility	Ease of obtaining information
Computerization	Has been or could easily be computerized
Executability	A. Includes instructions for implementation
	B. Includes instructions for scoring and quantification

	Standard	
Screen or Criterion	Poor Care	Good Care
Poor Care	a True Positive	b False Positive
Good Care	c False Negative	d True Negative

NOTE:

Sensitivity = True Positive/(True Positive + False Negative), or $a/(a + c)$

Specificity = True Negative/(False Positive + True Negative), or $d/(b + d)$

Predictive value (positive) = True Positive/(True Positive + False Positive), or $a/(a + b)$

Predictive value (negative) = True Negative/(False Negative + True Negative), or $d/(c + d)$

FIGURE 10.1   Computational Definitions of Sensitivity, Specificity, and Predictive Value

whether applied in the cardiology department of a university hospital or in a community setting. Similarly, case-finding criteria should identify the same kinds of cases regardless of who uses them.

For the purposes of this discussion, the attribute *validity* relates to outcomes and scientific evidence of effectiveness (if not efficacy). That is, a criteria set that contradicts clinical research data on effectiveness of health services, ignores them, or misuses them is not valid (and can be useless or even harmful). A valid criteria set should be based on or related to studies of patient outcomes or other scientific evidence of effectiveness to the extent such evidence is available.

This definition can be expanded to make more explicit the type of evidence used (e.g., randomized clinical trials or expert consensus) or to grade the quality of the supporting evidence. The type of evidence that is appropriate or available may vary considerably depending on the particular technology or problem in question. Some medical interventions have been heavily investigated, for instance, aspirin in the prevention of stroke in patients with transient ischemic attacks (TIAs) and coronary artery bypass grafting in patients with angina; others have not, for example, hysterectomy. Where the criteria begin with an outcome (as in many case-finding screens), there should be an effort to link the outcome to an identified process.

Whatever form the supporting evidence might take, the nature of that evidence should be made very explicit because users need to be able to assess the product. Thus, an important aspect of a criteria set's validity is clear *documentation*. Documentation should include (A) information about how the criteria were developed, including the literature on which it is based and what is known or not known about expected outcomes, and (B) how reliability of the criteria set was established.

Patient responsiveness refers to whether the guidelines have some mechanism for eliciting and taking into account patient preferences and values. In some chronic conditions, such as prostatic hypertrophy, it is not clinically obvious whether surgical intervention is the best course. For some patients, the probability of undesirable side effects of surgery might outweigh the symptoms. Patient values should be included, for instance, in decisions to forego potentially disabling or disfiguring interventions such as life-prolonging chemotherapy that may cause blindness as a side effect.

To make certain that guidelines are responsive to patient values and preferences, one might incorporate what some call patient decision nodes. For example, for an individual with chronic obstructive pulmonary disease, the node might be whether the use of a respirator had been discussed with the patient. For others, the patient-responsiveness elements might be reflected in a footnote listing reasons for making an exception to the guidelines. For instance, although a given medicine might prolong the life of a patient with acquired immunodeficiency syndrome, it may cause blindness and be refused by the patient. Eliciting patient preferences is not routine at present, but it is a worthwhile goal that is consistent with the overall strategy for quality assurance advanced in this report.

Flexibility reflects the extent to which a criteria set identifies and specifies exceptions to criteria. Quality review can be seen as a three-step process: (1) application of an initial screen, (2) in-depth or peer review, and (3) appeal. Flexibility may not be an important feature of an initial screen applied as a case-finding mechanism; the criteria at this initial stage should be clear (although exceptions may be stated). Flexibility is, however, an important aspect of the secondary, in-depth review process triggered by the screen, and substantial allowance should be made for clinical judgment at this stage. The less specific are guidelines used to aid secondary review, the greater the role of clinical judgment.

Particularly in areas of uncertainty in clinical medicine, greater leeway in decision making should be afforded to the practitioner. In the case of criteria sets for clinical management, psychosocial and interpersonal concerns justify preserving considerable discretion for clinical judgment. Too much leeway for clinical judgment, however, can undermine the criteria-setting effort. For this reason, guidelines should anticipate and make provision for the more common clinical exceptions and variations. When clinical judgment is invoked, the reasoning should be accurately described by the practitioner or reviewer. Such a situation might occur when an idiosyncratic patient factor or an extenuating circumstance that had not been taken into account in the criteria interacts with the characteristics of a specific patient to make that case an exception.

Whereas flexibility deals with the more idiosyncratic cases, *clinical adaptability* means that the criteria set takes into account the predictable clinically relevant differences among classes of patients. The criteria set should then specify the classes to which it is intended to apply. These classes may be based on age, sex, diagnosis, surgical risk, problem severity, or other factors.

Clinical adaptability is distinct from *inclusiveness,* which means that the criteria set applies to a large proportion of the patients to which it is addressed. For example, inclusive carotid endarterectomy guidelines would not be limited to assessing the need for that procedure in patients with transient ischemic attacks, but rather would address the full range of potential indications, from asymptomatic carotid bruits to strokes in evolution. Inclusiveness further implies that criteria sets collectively should cover the full range of surgical and medical problems encountered in the hospital or other setting being reviewed.

Several of the foregoing characteristics—in particular, patient responsiveness, flexibility, and clinical adaptability—underscore the point that criteria cannot be unremittingly rigid. If exceptions cannot be specified in the criteria set itself, then there must be an opportunity for recourse or appeal in special cases. The panel characterized this concept of appealability as an implementation or process attribute, rather than an inherent characteristic of a criteria set per se, and it is therefore discussed later.

Concordance can be considered an attribute either of substance or of implementation. It embodies the important concept that guideline development should reflect a consensus of professionals with extensive and appropriate clinical experience. The body that formulates guidelines should not be limited to "experts," but should have input from experienced generalists as well as specialists and from nonacademic as well as academic practitioners. This should be reflected in the documentation for the criteria set.

Acceptability refers to whether the guidelines are satisfactory and credible—that is, seem to have at least face validity—to the professionals who will be using them. It is differentiated from concordance in that it focuses on acceptance by the target user group as opposed to those formulating the guidelines.

Clarity requires that criteria sets can be easily understood and consistently interpreted and applied. This is the everyday version of reliability as discussed above. Clarity calls for unambiguous language and specific definitions of the terms, data elements, and the target population. Terms such as "persistent abdominal distress despite appropriate therapy" are too vague to be meaningful in a list of appropriate endoscopy guidelines. Similarly, vague language in some carotid endarterectomy guidelines include "transient speech dysfunction," "altered body sensation," or "angiography confirming an atherosclerotic lesion in the appropriate carotid artery." Table 10.2 includes more such examples of unclear language and some suggested alternatives that are less ambiguous.

Appropriateness refers to whether the criteria explicitly describe (1) what actions are clearly appropriate, (2) where there is divergence of or absence of evidence, and (3) what actions are clearly inappropriate. Guidelines should indicate whether these distinctions are based on scientific evidence or a preponderance of expert opinion. In addition, alternative approaches that may be appropriate for diagnosing or treating a problem should be listed. The terms indicated, equivocal, and not indicated are viewed by some practitioners as more neutral and therefore preferable terms.[7]

Implementation or Process Attributes

Before implementing criteria of all sorts, formulators should *pretest* them on a small scale to determine their effect on providers and patients. Pretesting also provides an opportunity to modify language and format and thus

TABLE 10.2 Examples of Vague and Clear Language for Criteria Sets

Vague	Clear
Unexplained weight loss	Weight loss of >15 percent of body weight during the preceding 4 months
Persistence of bleeding (or any sign or symptom)	Bleeding that continues for four or more months following initiation of therapy with oral contraceptives
Severe bleeding	Drop in hematocrit of >6 percent in less than eight hours
	Bleeding that has required transfusions on two or more occasions in the past six months
	Blood volume depletion greater than 2,000 ml
	Bleeding that requires the acute replacement of blood volume with two or more units of whole blood
Appropriate trial of therapy	At least one month of treatment with aspirin at a dose of 325 mg every other day or more
	Quadriceps strengthening exercises performed for at least 20 minutes per day, five days per week for at least six weeks
	Treatment for 10 to 14 days with penicillin or erythromycin at a dose of 250 mg four times a day
	Wearing a splint at least 12 hours a day for two months or more
Upper abdominal distress	Epigastric pain occurring one-half to two hours after eating
	Epigastric pain of more than one hour duration
	Discomfort consistently related to eating certain foods
Deteriorating (or unstable) vital signs	Blood pressure less than 90 mm Hg systolic, with a drop of at least 15 percent from average level of past 24 hours
	Temperature >101° F
	Pulse >120
Significant organ involvement	A process that causes loss of >20 percent of the function of an organ system (e.g., blood urea nitrogren, vital capacity, or left ventricular ejection fraction)
Evaluation should be efficient yet thorough	Evaluation should include history of exposure, physical examination of systems at risk, and laboratory testing capable of changing diagnostic logic
Positive stress test	A 1 mm or more horizontal or downsloping ST segment depression during exercise of patient who has normal electrocardiogram at rest

improve reliability. Pretesting can provide information about the extent to which a perceived problem even exists.

The attribute *dynamism* emphasizes a commitment to and a mechanism for ongoing review and updating of the criteria. Where controversy is high or change is rapid, reassessments and revisions will need to be more frequent. Dynamism means building feedback into the implementation system. That is, guidelines or interpretive material need to be modified to accommodate new scientific findings and lessons learned about practitioners' use of the criteria once they have been disseminated.

Closely related to dynamism is the need for periodic *evaluation*. A mechanism for evaluating the impact of criteria should be built into the implementation plan. Pretesting, dynamism, and evaluation all refer to the need for an iterative process for building and refining criteria sets.

Although the medical logic underlying guidelines may be very complex, their structure and elements should be comprehensible. For instance, complex algorithmic guidelines should probably read from top to bottom and from left to right.[8] If criteria cannot be understood by the intended users, whether they are trained reviewers, practitioners, or patients, they are likely to be improperly used or not used at all.

Along the same lines, criteria should be *manageable* for physician and nonphysician reviewers and for practitioners. Particularly with procedure and management guidelines, the practitioner should be able to internalize the practice standards rather than have to refer constantly to the written criteria.

The information-gathering process should be as *nonintrusive* as possible. Clinicians frequently complain that existing utilization and pre-procedure review programs require them to spend an inordinate amount of time interacting with reviewers. Although prior review necessarily entails some such interaction, well-designed and pretested criteria sets should keep interactions with treating physicians to the essential minimum.

Appealability is the extent to which exceptions to even the best criteria can be allowed. The point here is that each patient is unique, and thus even highly valid, sensitive, and specific criteria will not be appropriate for every case in every conceivable situation. A means by which this patient uniqueness can be taken into account is essential.

Another desirable attribute of criteria sets is the relative ease with which information for review can be obtained, that is, *feasibility*. There can be a delicate balance between avoiding unduly burdensome data collection and vitiating the pressure needed to raise the quality and availability of information in medical records and other sources. Only when the cost of acquiring the information is clearly out of balance with the value of the information should the criteria set be designed to exclude those elements.

Two last dimensions of guideline implementations are *computerization* and *executability*. Computerization refers to construction of criteria sets so that they can be translated into a computerized format for use by reviewers or practitioners as appropriate.[9] Guidelines are executable if they include specific instructions for implementation. This may require that a data collection format (abstracting form) be included. If a scoring system is used, the criteria set should include clear instructions for scoring and quantifying results. For instance, if several process-of-care evaluation criteria are to be combined into a single "index" score, the method of aggregation, whether simple addition or more complex arithmetic steps, should be described. If some variables are to be weighted more heavily than others, that must be clearly stated. Even if each variable in the index score is to be given equal weight (i.e., has a weight of 1), that should be specified.

DIFFERENCES AMONG KEY ATTRIBUTES FOR DIFFERENT CRITERIA SETS

Although each attribute defined in Table 10.1 is important, no criteria set is likely to conform equally well to all these requirements. Which, then, are the more critical?

As the expert panel considered this question, they arrived at somewhat different rankings for the three types of criteria sets, as reported in Table 10.3A. Each column in the table shows the attributes rated 4.5 or higher on a scale that rated 5 as most important and 1 as least important. (The data on which this table is based are found in Table A.4 of Appendix A. Because of possible interest in the "second tier" of desirable attributes, we have also included those attributes with ratings from 4.0 through 4.4 in Table 10.3B). The order of the attributes in the table reflects the frequency of their appearance across criteria sets, rather than how panelists rated them for each specific set.

Clarity was identified as a key attribute for all three types of criteria sets, and panelists repeatedly stressed the need for clarity during their discussions. The generality, vagueness, and convoluted nature of many existing criteria undoubtedly contributes to the emphasis, first, on clear and complete but also simple and parsimonious definitions of terms and, second, on straightforward descriptions of target populations, medical conditions, and patient variables.

Appropriateness Guidelines

Validity—scientific evidence of effectiveness—was identified as the most important attribute for technology- and procedure-specific appropriateness guidelines. This evidence, insofar as possible, should include assessments of patient outcomes and comparisons of principal alternatives, for example,

TABLE 10.3A Key Attributes of Criteria Sets, by Type of Criteria Set and Type of Attribute

Attributes	Type of Criteria Set		
	Appropriateness Guidelines	Evaluation and Management	Case-Finding Screens
Substantive			
	Clarity	Clarity	Clarity
	Validity	Validity	
	Sensitivity		Sensitivity
	Documentation-A[a]		
		Reliability	
		Flexibility	
		Clinical	
		Adaptability	
		Concordance	
Implementation			
	Appealability		Appealability
			Comprehendability[b]
			Evaluation
		Dynamism	
		Executability	

[a] Documents methods of development and cites literature.
[b] Comprehendability by nonphysician reviewers.

NOTE: See Table 10.1 for definitions of attributes. Criteria in this table are listed in order of frequency with which they appeared in the three tables of criteria sets (e.g., for all three criteria sets, for only two, or for only one). The decision cutoff for inclusion in this table was a mean score [on a scale of 1 (least important) to 5 (most important)] equal to or greater than 4.5 in the second round of ratings by the expert panel (see Appendix, Table A.4).

watchful waiting versus procedural intervention. When the evidence changes, the guidelines should be evaluated for continuing validity. The panelists indicated that many current criteria sets are not adequately validated and that validity must be emphasized as the field of criteria development progresses. In a related point, the panelists stressed that the evidence on which the guidelines are based must be clearly documented along with the processes by which criteria sets were created.

Another substantive attribute the panelists emphasized was sensitivity. This, to repeat, is the ability to identify cases appropriate for intervention and to avoid cases where the intervention would produce little or no net benefit or might harm the patient.

Among the process attributes, the panelists saw appealability as most important. Even if a set of guidelines includes detailed provisions for different classes of patients and clinical situations, there must be a means for "real time" responses to questions about how guidelines should apply to patients and situations that fall outside these classifications.

TABLE 10.3B Attributes of Criteria Sets, Rated Lower Than the Key Attributes, by Type of Criteria Set and Type of Attribute

Attributes	Type of Criteria Set		
	Appropriateness Guidelines	Evaluation and Management	Case-Finding Screens
Substantive			
	Clinical Adaptability Concordance Flexibility Reliability Appropriateness Documentation-B[a] Specificity	Appropriateness Sensitivity Documentation-A[d]	Clinical Adaptability Concordance Flexibility Reliability
Implementation			
	Comprehendability[b] Pretesting Dynamism Comprehendability[c] Evaluation	Comprehendability[b] Pretesting Comprehendability[c] Evaluation	Comprehendability[b] Pretesting Dynamism Manageability, MD Manageability, non-MD

[a]Documents how reliability was established.

[b]Comprehendability by physicians.

[c]Comprehendability by nonphysician reviewers.

[d]Documents methods of development and cites literature.

NOTE: See Table 10.1 for definitions of attributes. Criteria in this table are listed in order of frequency with which they appeared in the three types of criteria sets (e.g., for all three criteria sets, for only two, or for only one). The decision cutoff for inclusion in this table was a mean score [on a scale of 1 (least important) to 5 (most important)] equal to or greater than 4.0 but less than 4.5 in the second round of ratings by the expert panel (see Appendix, Table A.4).

Criteria for the Evaluation and Management of Patient Care

Clarity, flexibility, and clinical adaptability were rated as critical attributes for evaluation and management criteria, with reliability, validity, and concordance also rated as very important. For evaluation and management criteria sets, flexibility and clinical adaptability are central. The first attribute underscores the role of clinical judgment and expertise in making case-by-case evaluations of the care that individual practitioners render to individual patients. The second concept focuses on the need for the criteria sets to distinguish, when possible, the differences in classes of patients or clinical situations that warrant differences in the application of the criteria. Both attributes emphasize the continuing significance of peer review for the process of quality assurance.

The more advanced kinds of criteria sets can build in a considerable amount of flexibility and adaptability and thereby reduce the workload for peer reviewers. For instance, a simple and mechanically applied criteria set might flag the failure to do a funduscopic examination on a blind patient as a quality problem, and the peer review process would have to be activated to determine that no deficiency existed in fact. A more sophisticated criteria set would specify such foreseeable exceptions to basic evaluation criteria and allow reviewer judgment to be reserved for less straightforward cases.

The emphasis placed on flexibility and adaptability may vary depending on whether one is developing and applying prospective education protocols or algorithms or working with retrospective assessments of actual care, where the need for flexibility in peer review may be especially significant. Although the panelists did not mention it explicitly, responsiveness to patient preferences and sensitivity to the physician-patient relationship are also aspects of good clinical judgment and peer review.

More generally, criteria sets must recognize valid alternative approaches to patient evaluation and treatment. By analogy to the technology- and procedure-specific guidelines, developers of criteria sets could categorize different approaches to patient evaluation and management as being appropriate, equivocal, or inappropriate. A more-or-less equivalent tactic would be to assign grades of superior, acceptable, or unacceptable to different combinations of patient evaluation and management steps. Some patient management problems might be assessed as a series of discrete decisions, rather than as an overall process. Thus, an assessment would focus not on "how to treat a patient with a headache" but rather on "appropriate indications for use of Fiorinal" and other specific services that might be combined to treat a headache. In all these situations, however, the criteria must reflect concordance among practitioners with clinical experience.

Among implementation attributes, dynamism and executability stand out as important for patient evaluation and management criteria. In many areas of care for the elderly, standards of care of a decade ago might serve quite well today. Nevertheless, the advance of knowledge in medicine is swift, and process-of-care criteria risk obsolescence if they are not systematically reviewed and updated as appropriate. Outdated criteria sets may yield no better or even worse decisions about the adequacy of patient care than implicit peer review alone.

Finally, the developers of evaluation and management criteria must provide clear guidance about how the criteria sets are to be used, especially how elements in the criteria sets are to be quantified, scored, weighted, and aggregated. This is particularly true when criteria sets will be used for formal quality-of-care evaluation rather than simply education. Review decisions that label care as exemplary, acceptable, or substandard can have a considerable impact on practitioners' and institutions' reputations and financial well-being.

Case-Finding Screens

Many types of case-finding mechanisms exist, including the kinds of generic screens used by PROs and the specialty-specific clinical (outcome) indicators developed by the Joint Commission. In this study, the focus is on the former. Other than clarity, the only critical attribute the expert panel identified for generic screens was sensitivity, intended here to mean "a high true positive rate in detecting deficient care."

Because generic screens are meant to flag cases for in-depth review based on more rigorous criteria, it is not surprising that the panel emphasized the implementation aspects of case-finding screens more than their substance. Among the implementation attributes, appealability ranked high, reflecting the view that case-finding screens must be backed by a well-developed system of peer review that includes adequate avenues for appealing initial negative decisions. In addition, the case-finding screens must be comprehensible to nonphysician reviewers, and their usefulness must be periodically evaluated. The disappointing history of the generic screens in the Medicare program, as described in Chapters 6 and 9, probably accounts for the importance accorded these attributes.

METHODS AND STRATEGIES FOR DEVELOPING QUALITY-OF-CARE CRITERIA

General Stages of Criteria Development

Criteria development should follow several basic stages, which have been described in greater detail by Eddy (1988) and others (Chassin, 1988; PPRC,

1989).   First, a group of experienced clinicians should be convened (in person or by telecommunication) to review the relevant literature and the existing criteria sets in the area under consideration.   As previously indicated, this group should include generalists as well as specialists and nonacademic as well as academic practitioners.   The best of the existing criteria sets can be used as a starting point, with modifications and refinements based on the literature and the attributes discussed above.

Because evidence on which the experts' judgments are based should be clearly documented, a second requirement is a thorough literature review. Procedurally, this can and perhaps should precede the convocation of any expert group.   The literature review must specify both where data exist and where they are lacking.

Whether a specific approach to the literature review should be used is not a settled matter.   Opinions differ about the value of meta-analysis (a technique for quantitative synthesis of multiple studies with different methods and findings) over traditional literature reviews, and the merits of including unpublished information in the analysis are also debated.   Selection of particular approaches will depend on the issue under consideration and the quality and extent of the available literature.   It may not be productive to attempt to specify in advance rules as to the specific form and content of the literature review.   Some experts suggest that the criteria produced through such a literature review and deliberation by a group of experienced practitioners should be circulated to a second set of experts for further review before any attempt is made to implement them; this suggestion, too, occasions debate.

Third, the criteria should be pilot-tested before they are put into general use.   Fourth, a mechanism should be established to evaluate the impact of the criteria on patient care after general implementation.   This might involve a small number of systematic evaluation projects (which conceivably could use a randomized controlled trial approach) as well as ongoing monitoring.

Whether provision should be made for some form of consumer input into the process of criteria development remains an open question (as does provision for payer input).   If consumer representation is decided on, it might be most appropriate at the level of a steering or oversight committee that determined general strategy rather than at the technical level.   Consumer representatives must be made familiar with the issues.   As an alternative to direct consumer representation, provision might be made for seeking the assistance of public opinion specialists.

Priorities

With respect to strategies for criteria development, in general, priority should be given to high-risk, high-cost, high-volume, or problem-prone services. Examples include carotid endarterectomy (high risk), liver transplant (high cost), Pap smears (high volume), or nursing home care (problem prone). Emphasis might be placed on guidelines for technologies or management problems that may result in serious outcomes such as death or severe disability, although these may be areas where a clear consensus on standards does not exist. The absence of broad agreement may require greater flexibility in criteria, but it does not argue against the adoption of criteria. In fact, guidelines may be most useful where practices are most divergent, partly because they will make the divergence more obvious and partly because they will highlight where practice and data conflict.

Nonetheless, a headlong rush to formulate guidelines for the sake of having guidelines is not desirable. Criteria development is a vital component of quality assurance, but the necessary time and resources must be committed to this process if criteria that truly enhance quality of care are to emerge.

Affordability

The expert panel mentioned the need for cost-consciousness in developing and promulgating criteria. Resources to provide care, to do research, and to support quality assurance are scarce. The trade-offs can be difficult, and criteria development may have a lower priority. Thus, efficient mechanisms for building on existing criteria, disseminating and sharing criteria across organizations, and minimizing duplicate efforts are necessary. As with any endeavor in health care delivery, the value of the product—that is, the quality of the work in the face of its cost—needs to be optimal.

One must avoid, however, too narrow a view of the utility of good criteria and the contributions they can make to good patient care, research, and quality assurance. For instance, appropriateness guidelines can help curtail use of unnecessary services, potentially freeing resources for provision of additional care where it is needed. Patient management criteria can guide patient care more appropriately. Process and outcome criteria are the central issues of quality assurance. Finally, the process of developing criteria itself can highlight areas of medical practice in need of further research. Again, affordability is a legitimate concern, but excessive frugality in the resources devoted to criteria development may prove to be a false economy.

OTHER ISSUES

Larger Clusters

By the end of the expert panel discussion, it had become clear that the group was not entirely happy with the large number of atomistic attributes it had isolated and defined. Consequently, there was some sentiment for

TABLE 10.4 Possible "Larger Clusters" of Attributes for Quality-of-Care Criteria

Substantive Attributes	Implementation Attributes
Scientific Grounding	Implementation
Reliability	Feasibility
Validity	Computerization
Documentation	Executability
Latitude (clinical and patient	Ease of use
boundaries and judgment)	Comprehendability
Flexibility[a]	Manageability
Appealability[a]	Nonintrusiveness
Patient Responsiveness	Appealability
Clinical Adaptability	Flexibility[a]
Inclusiveness	Appealability[a]
Design	Dynamism
Clarity	Pretesting
Concordance	Dynamism
Acceptability	Evaluation
Appropriateness	
Efficiency	
Sensitivity	
Specificity	

[a]Both flexibility and appealability might be built into the criteria or their application and, depending on the type of criteria set, at various stages of review.

identifying larger groupings of attributes that would convey the basic ideas of scientific basis, ease of use, and so forth. One such grouping is proposed in Table 10.4.

The table groups the several substantive attributes into four major categories related to their scientific grounding, latitude, design, and efficiency. The implementation attributes fell into four categories as well: implementation, ease of use, appealability, and dynamism. The two attributes of flexibility and appealability were seen as important to both structure and process, and thus appear in both sets.

Concerns Raised But Not Addressed by the Panel

The panelists raised several issues that warrant considerable attention in the future but that they did not have time to pursue. First was the need for parsimony in articulating attributes, that is, for grouping attributes so that they are more easily understood and applied. The clusters in Table 10.4 offered earlier are one approach for doing this.

Second, the attributes for good criteria sets should be perceived as goals, not absolutes. Although most, if not all, criteria sets today would fail if evaluated against these attributes, they should be revised, not discarded. For instance, if the principal problem with guidelines today is that they are too vague or poorly written, then they can be more precisely and clearly stated. If the criticism is poor documentation, this fault, too, can be corrected.

The third point was that not all these attributes can be maximized simultaneously in any individual criteria set. The importance of an individual attribute may depend on the type of criteria set in question and its purpose. Furthermore, whether such criteria are used chiefly for cost containment or for quality assurance may change the weights given to different attributes. We tried to highlight the key attributes for criteria sets used in quality assurance programs (Table 10.3), but a good deal more work needs to be done in this area as the practice guidelines, effectiveness, and outcomes research efforts of the federal government and other parties expand.

Fourth, it is critical to ask about the impact of guidelines. Have they been shown to improve the quality of patient care? Do they misclassify cases of good or poor care? Have they prompted malpractice lawsuits? Do patients or clinicians get around them somehow? Do they save money? Again, with respect to the federal government's initiatives in this area, evaluation is essential.

Finally, some types of criteria, especially patient management algorithms, serve educational and decision-making needs of both practitioners and patients. Criteria sets can help practitioners educate themselves and can help patients and their families make better choices about when to seek care and how to assess diagnostic or therapeutic options. The concern for patient preferences is especially pertinent, given the emphasis on desired health outcomes in the committee's definition of quality of care.

Implications for Quality Assurance in Medicare Program

Development and use of guidelines for a geriatric population calls for great sensitivity to their special characteristics, such as multiple chronic problems and frailty. Moreover, in quality assurance, moving from single discrete procedures to episodes and longitudinal care is difficult. However, this broad approach is especially important for an elderly population.

The theme of education permeates the enterprise of quality assurance. The challenge is to define appropriate and effective ways to use medical care and to apply this knowledge whether one is teaching medical students, house staff, established clinicians, or oneself. This study accords considerable importance to fostering internal quality improvement programs for providers and practitioners, so that the external Medicare quality assurance program can be targeted more effectively and efficiently. Making good quality-of-care criteria a paramount concern for the federal quality assurance effort will strengthen both these processes.

SUMMARY

One congressional charge to the study committee was to develop prototype criteria and standards. Criteria sets vary considerably in their usefulness, depending on their objectives, their method of development, and the skills and experience of their creators. Three main kinds of criteria sets have evolved to meet different needs. Appropriateness guidelines describe indications for specific medical interventions and technologies, ranging from surgical procedures to diagnostic studies. Patient care evaluation and management criteria are intended to assess or guide the management of outpatient or inpatient medical problems. Case-finding screens identify potential quality-of-care problems that warrant further evaluation.

Because of the current interest in these types of criteria sets (particularly practice guidelines), the IOM study committee believed its best contribution was to provide preliminary guidance for their development, that is, to clarify the key "standards for standards." To this end, it convened a panel of experts in guideline formulation to elucidate the key attributes or characteristics of sound criteria sets and acceptable methods for constructing them. The expert panel reviewed the literature, completed ratings of proposed attributes of criteria sets, and attended a two-day meeting at which they examined examples of existing criteria sets and revised and re-rated attributes.

Attributes of good criteria sets can be divided into two categories: substantive (or structural) attributes related to the inherent characteristics of a criteria set and implementation attributes focused on the process of developing and applying a criteria set. Substantive attributes might be further categorized as those related to scientific grounding, latitude, design, and efficiency. Implementation attributes can be categorized as those concerning implementation, ease of use, appealability, and dynamism.

For each of the three types of criteria sets considered, the panel discussed the range of attributes and characteristics that might be considered desirable or necessary; ultimately, they arrived at somewhat different ratings of key attributes for each set. Among the substantive attributes, clarity (e.g., unambiguous language and clear definitions of terms) was a key attribute for all three types of criteria. Validity (criteria based on outcome studies or other scientific evidence of effectiveness) was considered very important for both appropriateness guidelines and patient evaluation and management criteria. Sensitivity (a high true positive rate in detecting deficient or inappropriate care) was rated very high for appropriateness guidelines and case-finding screens. Documentation (of methods of development and literature used) was voted very important for appropriateness guidelines. Several other characteristics were considered highly important for the patient evaluation and management criteria sets as well, including reliability (known to produce the same decisions when applied by user groups for the purposes for which the criteria set was intended), flexibility (respects the role of clinical judgment), clinical adaptability (allows for or takes into account clinically relevant differences among different classes of patients), and concordance (reflects consensus of professionals with extensive experience in the field). Among the implementation attributes, appealability (allows for appeals process by professionals and patients) was rated highly important for both appropriateness guidelines and case-finding screens. Two additional attributes were considered critical for patient evaluation and management criteria sets: dynamism (mechanism exists to review and update criteria sets to incorporate new information and to cover new situations), and executability (includes instructions for scoring, quantification, and implementation). Finally, two other additional characteristics were voted as highly important for case-finding screens: comprehendability (format understood by nonphysician reviewers) and evaluation (mechanism exists to review and evaluate the outcome or impact of the screens).

The panel emphasized that these attributes of criteria sets should be understood as goals, not absolutes. Most, if not all, criteria sets existing today would fail if evaluated against these attributes, and not all attributes can be maximized simultaneously in any individual criteria set. The panel also called for further work in this area, highlighting the need for better information about the impact of these types of criteria sets on patient care and about the best way to use criteria sets to help practitioners, patients, and family members make better decisions about health care.

NOTES

1. Summary descriptions of these and other criteria development activities can be found in IOM, 1988.
2. The RAND guidelines and methods were originally developed for and used in extensive research efforts supported by the Health Care Financing Administration and by several private foundations.
3. One might say that these patient management criteria start with a medical condition to which appropriate services are fit, whereas the criteria described in the section on appropriateness guidelines start with a procedure or service to which are fit medical conditions that warrant its use.
4. Typical process-of-care criteria are discussed or can be found in Lohr, 1980a, 1980b; Palmer et al., 1984; Borgiel, 1988; Palmer, 1988; and RTI, 1988.
5. For quality assurance efforts, the usefulness of algorithms, or protocols that follow algorithmic maps, remains somewhat controversial. At organizations such as Harvard Community Health Plan, for instance, algorithm-protocol for-

mulation is a collective process in which many clinicians participate. The process may be more valuable ultimately for those involved in developing these instruments than for those receiving them; it establishes a process of ongoing internal review under detailed, generally accepted guidelines. The more complex protocols, however, may amount to little more than "restatements of medical texts" and prove unwieldy to use; carried to the extreme they may limit the clinician to practicing "cookbook medicine."

6. Predictive value was suggested by some panel members as a separate attribute, distinct from sensitivity. The expert panel's discussion of this area indicated that correctly identifying problems of defective care (i.e, predictive value positive, as defined in Figure 10.1) is an integral part of sensitivity, and members of the panel in fact used the term sensitivity in this broader sense. Thus, defining sensitivity as high true positive rate in the list of attributes shown in Table 10.1 and omitting predictive value as a separate attribute from the final list of attributes reflect this approach.

7. Not indicated should be distinguished from contraindicated. Not indicated means that the acceptable (or even equivocal) indications are absent. Contraindicated means that there is some supervening medical condition or reason for not doing something that would otherwise be indicated (such as use of aspirin for persons suffering from blood-clotting disorders, use of virtually any drugs during pregnancy, or certain tranquilizers for persons on antihypertensive drugs).

8. One panelist shared the following "criteria for critiquing a clinical algorithm." Graphics should be (1) uncluttered, (2) read from top to bottom and from left to right, (3) use clear and consistent symbols, (4) provide clear and consistent referencing and numbering, and (5) include minimal redundant steps or boxes. For accuracy and logic, algorithms need (1) accurate definitions, (2) accurate and up-to-date information (e.g., on dosages, laboratory values, and diagnostic signs), (3) enumeration of all important steps in the medical care process, (4) annotation of all "essential" and "critical" actions or decision points, and (5) consistent and parsimonious logic (HCHP, 1986).

9. This is only recently being done in the quality and utilization review fields, especially for utilization management program. However, the translation of equivalent documents, such as survey questionnaires, into computerized forms (e.g., computer assisted personal interview or CAPI techniques) is much more highly developed. Clearly, this approach offers much for quality review methods.

REFERENCES

ACC (American College of Cardiology). Guidelines for Exercise Testing. (A Report of the American College of Cardiology and American Heart Association Task Force on Assessment of Cardiovascular Procedures (Subcommittee on Exercise Testing). *Journal of the American College of Cardiology* 8:725-738, 1986a.

ACC. Guidelines for Clinical Use of Cardiac Radionuclide Imaging. (A Report of the American College of Cardiology and American Heart Association Task Force on Assessment of Cardiovascular Procedures (Subcommittee on Nuclear Imaging). *Journal of the American College of Cardiology* 8:1471-1483, 1986b.

ASGE (American Society for Gastrointestinal Endoscopy). *Appropriate Use of Gastrointestinal Endoscopy,* Manchester, Mass.: American Society for Gastrointestinal Endoscopy, 1986.

Borgiel, A.E. Assessing the Quality of Care in Family Physicians' Practices by the College of Family Physicians of Canada. Pp. 63-72 in *Quality of Care and Technology Assessment.* Lohr, K.N. and Rettig, R.A., eds. Washington, D.C.: National Academy Press, 1988.

Brook, R.H. Practice Guidelines and Practicing Medicine: Are They Compatible? Paper prepared for the Physician Payment Review Commission. Santa Monica, Calif.: The RAND Corporation, 1988a.

Brook, R.H. Quality Assessment and Technology Assessment: Critical Linkages. Pp. 21-28 in *Quality of Care and Technology Assessment.* Lohr, K.N. and Rettig, R.A., eds. Washington, D.C.: National Academy Press, 1988b.

Brook, R.H., Kamberg, C.J., Mayer-Oakes, A., et al. Appropriateness of Acute Medical Care for the Elderly: Analysis of the Literature. R-3717-AARP/RWJ/RC. Santa Monica, Calif.: The RAND Corporation, 1989.

Chassin, M.R. Standards of Care in Medicine. *Inquiry* 25:437-453, Winter 1988.

Chassin, M.R., Kosecoff, J., Park, R.E., et al. *Indications for Selecting Medical and Surgical Procedures—A Literature Review and Ratings of Appropriateness: Coronary Angiography.* R-3204/1-CWF/HF/HCFA/PMT/RWJ. Santa Monica, Calif.: The RAND Corporation, 1986a.

Chassin, M.R., Kosecoff, J., Solomon, D.H., et al. How Coronary Angiography Is Used. *Journal of the American Medical Association* 258:2543-2547, 1987.

Chassin, M.R., Park, R.E., Fink, A., et al. *Indications for Selecting Medical and Surgical Procedures—A Literature Review and Ratings of Appropriateness: Coronary Artery Bypass Surgery.* R-3204/2-CWF/HF/HCFA/PMT/RWJ. Santa Monica, Calif.: The RAND Corporation, 1986b.

Chassin, M.R., Park, R.E., Lohr, K.N., et al. Differences among Hospitals in Medicare Patient Mortality. *Health Services Research* 24(1):1-31, 1989.

Daley, J., Jencks, S., Draper, D., et al. Predicting Hospital-Associated Mortality for Medicare Patients. *Journal of the American Medical Association* 260:3617-3624, 1988.

Dubois, R.W. Hospital Mortality as an Indicator of Quality. Pp. 107-131 in *Providing Quality Care: The Challenge to Clinicians.* Goldfield, N. and Nash, D.B., eds. Philadelphia, Pa.: American College of Physicians, 1989.

Dubois, R.W., Brook, R.H., and Rogers, W.H. Adjusted Hospital Death Rates: A Potential Screen for Quality of Medical Care. *American Journal of Public Health* 77:1162-1167, 1987a.

Dubois, R.W., Rogers, W.H., Moxley, J.H., et al. Hospital Inpatient Mortality. Is It a Predictor of Quality? *New England Journal of Medicine* 317:1674-1680, 1987b.

Eddy, D.H. Clinical Policies. Pp. 47-54 in *Proceedings. Standards of Quality in Patient Care: The Importance and Risks of Standard Setting.* Invitational Conference, Council of Medical Specialty Societies, Washington, D.C., September 1987.

Eddy, D.H. Methods for Designing Guidelines. Paper prepared for the Physician Payment Review Commission. Durham, N.C.: Duke University, 1988.

Eddy, D.H. *A Manual for Assessing Health Practices and Designing Practice Policies.* (In collaboration with the Council of Medical Specialty Societies Task Force on Practice Policies.) Forthcoming.

Ente, B.H. and Lloyd, J.S. *Taking Stock of Mortality Data. An Agenda for the Future.* Proceedings of a 1988 Conference. Chicago, Ill.: Joint Commission on Accreditation of Healthcare Organizations, 1989.

Fink, A., Yano, E.M., and Brook, R.M. The Condition of the Literature on Differences in Hospital Mortality. *Medical Care* 27:315-336, 1989.

Greenfield, S. The Challenges and Opportunities that Quality Assurance Raises for Technology Assessment. Pp. 134-141 in *Quality of Care and Technology Assessment.* Lohr, K.N. and Rettig, R.A., eds. Washington, D.C.: National Academy Press, 1988.

Greenfield, S. Measuring the Quality of Office Practice. Pp. *183-200* in *Providing Quality Care: The Challenge to Clinicians.* Goldfield, N. and Nash, D.B., eds. Philadelphia, Pa.: American College of Physicians, 1989.

Greenfield, S., Cretin, S., Worthman, L.G., et al. Comparison of a Criteria Map to a Criteria List in Quality-of-Care Assessment for Patients with Chest Pain: The Relation of Each to Outcome. *Medical Care* 19:255-272, 1981.

Greenfield, S., Lewis, C.E., Kaplan, S., et al. Peer Review by Criteria Mapping: Criteria for Diabetes Mellitus. *Annals of Internal Medicine* 83:761-770, 1975.

Greenfield, S., Nadler, M.A., Morgan, M.T., et al. The Clinical Investigation and Management of Chest Pain in an Emergency Department: Quality Assessment by Criteria Mapping. *Medical Care* 12:807-904, 1977.

Hannan, E.L., Bernard, H.R., O'Donnel, J.F., et al. A Methodology for Targeting Hospital Cases for Quality of Care Record Reviews. *American Journal of Public Health* 79:430-436, 1989.

HCHP (Harvard Community Health Plan). Criteria for Critiquing a Clinical Algorithm. Unpublished mimeo. Boston, Mass.: HCHP, 1986.

IOM (Institute of Medicine). *Medical Technology Assessment Directory.* Washington, D.C.: National Academy Press, 1988.

Jencks, S.F., Daley, J., Draper, D., et al. Interpreting Hospital Mortality Data. The Role of Clinical Risk Adjustment. *Journal of the American Medical Association* 260:3611-3616, 1988.

Kahn, K.L., Brook, R.H., and Draper, D. Interpreting Hospital Mortality Data. How Can We Proceed? *Journal of the American Medical Association* 260:3625-3628, 1988.

Kahn, K.L., Roth, C.P., Kosecoff, J., et al. *Indications for Selecting Medical and Surgical Procedures—A Literature Review and Ratings of Appropriateness: Diagnostic Upper Gastrointestinal Endoscopy.* R-3204/4-CWF/HF/HCFA/PMT/RWJ. Santa Monica, Calif.: The RAND Corporation, 1986a.

Kahn, K.L., Roth, C.P., Fink, A., et al. *Indications for Selecting Medical and Surgical Procedures—A Literature Review and Ratings of Appropriateness: Colonoscopy.* R-3204/5-CWF/HF/HCFA/PMT/RWJ. Santa Monica, Calif.: The RAND Corporation, 1986b.

Kanouse, D.E., Brook, R.H., Winkler, J.D., et al. *Changing Medical Practice Through Technology Assessment: An Evaluation of the NIH Consensus Development Program.* R-3452-NIH. Santa Monica, Calif.: The RAND Corporation, 1987.

Kosecoff, J., Kanouse, D.E., Rogers, W.H., et al. Effects of the National Institutes of Health Consensus Development Program on Physician Practice. *Journal of the American Medical Association* 258:2708-2713, 1987.

Lehmann, R. Joint Commission Forum: Forum on Clinical Indicator Development: A Discussion of the Use and Development of Indicators. *Quality Review Bulletin* 15:223-227, 1989.

Lewin, L.S. and Erickson, J.E. Leadership in the Development of Practice Guidelines: The Role of the Federal Government and Others. Paper prepared for the Physician Payment Review Commission. Washington, D.C.: LEWIN/ICF, October 1988.

Lohr, K.N. *Quality of Care for Respiratory Illness in Disadvantaged Populations.* P-6570. Santa Monica, Calif.: The RAND Corporation, 1980a.

Lohr, K.N. Quality of Care in the New Mexico Medicaid Program (1971-1975). *Medical Care* 18:1-129 (January Supplement), 1980b.

Longo, D.R., Ciccone, K.R., and Lord, J.T. *Integrated Quality Assessment. A Model for Concurrent Review.* Chicago, Ill.: American Hospital Association, 1989.

Marder, R.J. Joint Commission Plans for Clinical Indicator Development for Oncology. *Cancer* 64:310-313, 1989 (Supplement).

Merrick, N.J., Fink, A., Brook, R.H., et al. *Indications for Selecting Medical and Surgical Procedures—A Literature Review and Ratings of Appropriateness: Carotid Endarterectomy.* R-3204/6-CWF/HF/HCFA/PMT/RWJ. Santa Monica, Calif.: The RAND Corporation, 1986.

OTA (Office of Technology Assessment). *The Quality of Medical Care: Information for Consumers.* Chapter 5: Adverse Events. Washington, D.C.: U.S. Government Printing Office, 1988.

Palmer, R.H., Louis, T.A., Thompson, M.A., et al. Final Report of the Ambulatory Care Medical Audit Demonstration Project (ACMAD). Boston, Mass.: Harvard Community Health Plan and Harvard University, March 1984.

Palmer, R.H. The Challenges and Prospects for Quality Assessment and Assurance in Ambulatory Care. *Inquiry* 25:119-131, 1988.

Park, R.E., Fink, A., Brook, R.H., et al. *Physician Ratings of Appropriate Indications for Six Medical and Surgical Procedures.* R-3280-CWF/HF/PMT/RWJ. Santa Monica, Calif.: The RAND Corporation, 1986.

Paterson, M.L. The Challenge to Technology Assessment: An Industry Viewpoint. Pp. 106-125 in *Quality of Care and Technology Assessment.* Lohr, K.N. and Rettig, R.A., eds. Washington, D.C.: National Academy Press, 1988.

PPRC (Physician Payment Review Commission). Improving the Quality of Care: Clinical Research and Practice Guidelines. Draft Background Paper for Conference. Washington, D.C.: Physician Payment Review Commission, September 28, 1988a.

PPRC. Chapter 13. Increasing Appropriate Use of Services: Practice Guidelines and Feedback of Practice Patterns. *Annual Report to Congress.* Washington, D.C.: Physician Payment Review Commission, March 1988b.

PPRC. Chapter 12. Effectiveness Research and Practice Guidelines. *Annual Report to Congress.* Washington, D.C.: Physician Payment Review Commission, April 1989.

RTI (Research Triangle Institute). *Nationwide Evaluation of Medicaid Competition Demonstrations.* Final Report. Research Triangle Park, N.C.: RTI, 1988.

Schaffarzick, R.W. Technology Assessment: Perspective of a Third-Party Payer. Pp. 98-105 in *Quality of Care and Technology Assessment.* Lohr, K.N. and Rettig, R.A., eds. Washington, D.C.: National Academy Press, 1988.

Solomon, D.H., Brook, R.H., Fink, A., et al. *Indications for Selecting Medical and Surgical Procedures—A Literature Review and Ratings of Appropriateness: Cholecystectomy.* R-3204/3-CWF/HF/HCFA/PMT/RWJ. Santa Monica, Calif.: The RAND Corporation, 1986.

Sox, H.C., Jr., ed. *Common Diagnostic Tests. Use and Interpretation.* Philadelphia, Pa.: American College of Physicians, 1987.

Steinberg, E.P. Technology Assessment: A Physician Perspective. Pp. 79-88 in *Quality of Care and Technology Assessment.* Lohr, K.N. and Rettig, R.A., eds. Washington, D.C.: National Academy Press, 1988.

Stulbarg, M.S., Gerbert, B., Kemeny, M.E., et al. Outpatient Treatment of Chronic Obstructive Pulmonary Disease—A Practitioner's Guide. *Western Journal of Medicine* 142:842-846, 1985.

Winchester, D.P. Assuring Quality Cancer Care in an Evolving Health Care Delivery System. *CA—A Cancer Journal for Clinicians* 39:201-205, 1989.

Winslow, C.M., Kosecoff, J.B., Chassin, M., et al. The Appropriateness of Performing Coronary Artery Bypass Surgery. *Journal of the American Medical Association* 260:505-509, 1988a.

Winslow, C.M., Solomon, D.H., Chassin, M.R., et al. The Appropriateness of Carotid Endarterectomy. *New England Journal of Medicine* 318:721-727, 1988b.

APPENDIX A
CRITERIA-SETTING EXPERT PANEL ACTIVITY

The Institute of Medicine (IOM) study committee and staff determined that conducting an expert panel activity could be the best way to discharge the study's congressional request to develop prototype criteria and standards. The panel members are listed in Table A.1. The remainder of this Appendix describes this activity, which included a literature review, a homework exercise for the panelists, a two-day meeting in June 1989, and staff analysis of all products of these steps; it also provides more details about the results of the homework task and meeting discussions.

Homework Exercise

As a starting point for discussion of desirable attributes of different types of criteria sets, the IOM staff reviewed the existing literature on guideline development (see Chapter 10 reference list); on the basis of that review, the staff prepared an extensive list of possible general attributes. Three catego-

TABLE A.1 Criteria-Setting Expert Panel for Study to Design a Strategy for Quality Review and Assurance in Medicare

William A. Causey, M.D., F.A.C.P.
Jackson Medical Association
Jackson, Mississippi
(Representing American College of Physicians)

Mark R. Chassin, M.D.
Value Health Sciences, Inc.
Santa Monica, California

Arthur J. Donovan, M.D., F.A.C.S.
University of Southern California
Los Angeles, California
(Representing American College of Surgeons)

Leonard S. Dreifus, M.D., F.A.C.C.
Lankenau Hospital
Philadelphia, Pennsylvania
(Representing American College of Cardiology)

David M. Eddy, M.D., Ph.D.[a]
Duke University
Durham, North Carolina and Jackson, Wyoming

Lesley Fishelman, M.D.
Harvard Community Health Plan
Boston, Massachusetts

Sheldon Greenfield, M.D.
New England Medical Center and Tufts University School of Medicine
Boston, Massachusetts

Robert J. Marder, M.D.
Joint Commission on Accreditation of Healthcare Organizations
Chicago, Illinois

Jane L. Neumann, M.D.
Wisconsin Peer Review Organization and Waukesha Hospital
Waukesha, Wisconsin

Bruce Perry, M.D., M.P.H.
Group Health Cooperative of Puget Sound
Seattle, Washington

Ralph W. Schaffarzick, M.D.
Center for Quality Health Care of the
Blue Cross and Blue Shield Association
Auburn, California

[a]Was unable to attend meeting

ries of criteria were identified for special attention: (1) procedure- and technology-specific appropriateness guidelines, (2) criteria for evaluation of patient care and patient management, and (3) case-finding screens.

This list was incorporated into a homework exercise questionnaire, Possible General Attributes of Criteria Sets, which was mailed to panel members for response before the panel meeting. Panel members were requested to rate the listed attributes on a scale of 1 to 5, with 1 signifying not important attributes and 5 as very important attributes. Space was provided at the end of the questionnaires for respondents to suggest additional attributes or modification of listed attributes and to make any other comments. To help determine in what ways the attributes and their ratings might differ for the three types of criteria sets, the staff provided the questionnaire in triplicate.

The results of the first round of the homework exercise (done at home) are given in Table A.2. As reflected in the large number of 4 or 5 ratings and absence of very low ratings, the panel considered all of the listed attributes important in varying degrees. To obtain more spread in subsequent ratings, we revised the 1 to 5 scale for the second round of balloting (at the meeting) to read least important (1) and most important (5).

Several attributes were rated of less importance for all types of criteria sets; these included simplicity from the patient standpoint and generalizability-compatibility with existing quality assurance approaches (with suggestions that the latter attribute be deleted from the list). Several attributes were rated as more important for some types of criteria sets than others. For example, ease of computerization, feasibility (ease of obtaining data), and reviewer manageability were rated as more important for case-finding screens than for appropriateness guidelines and evaluation-management criteria.

The homework exercise suggested that various modifications in the list of proposed attributes and their definitions warranted further consideration at the expert panel meeting. It also identified several important underlying issues, such as the impact of differences in use on the definition and ratings of attributes of criteria sets. These issues were introduced at the meeting (and were discussed in Chapter 10).

Meeting

The expert panel meeting opened with a general discussion of attributes of criteria sets (Table A.3). The panel first discussed some fundamental issues raised by the homework exercise regarding standards for judging criteria sets, in particular the impact of use or purpose when considering desirable attributes of criteria sets. It then returned to the original list and proposed many modifications and clarifications for the items on it. These are embodied in the final list of general attributes of criteria sets in Table 10.1 of Chapter 10.

In subsequent sessions, the panel considered the proposed general attributes in the context of each of the three major types of criteria sets. Specific examples of each type of criteria set were used as a mechanism for examining the proposed attributes more closely; the advantages and limitations identified for these illustrative criteria sets helped the process of defining important attributes. In each session, the attributes for the particular type of criteria set under consideration were reformulated and re-rated (Table A.4). The highest-rated attributes (separately, for substantive and for implementation attributes) for each type of criteria set were extracted from these data and summarized in Table 10.4A of Chapter 10; the selection criterion was a mean score on the second round of voting of 4.5 or greater. Table 10.4B shows those attributes that were given an average rating of at least 4.0 but less than 4.5. In the final session, methods and strategies for guideline formulation were discussed.

TABLE A.2 Expert Panel Homework Exercise: First Round Ratings of Attributes

Attributes	Appropriateness			Evaluation/Management			Case-Finding		
	n[a]	Mean[b]	SD[c]	n	Mean	SD	n	Mean	SD
Sensitivity	9	4.9	.33	8	4.5	.53	10	4.7	.67
Specificity	9	4.7	.71	8	4.6	.52	10	3.9	1.10
Reliability	10	4.4	.84	10	4.5	.71	10	4.6	.52
Validity	10	4.7	.48	10	4.8	.42	10	4.4	.70
Dynamism	10	4.5	.53	10	4.3	.48	10	4.0	.67
Flexibility	10	4.4	.70	10	4.3	.82	10	3.8	1.14
Clinical Adaptability	10	4.4	.70	10	4.5	.71	10	4.0	1.05
Responsiveness	10	3.4	1.17	10	3.6	1.17	9	2.9	1.27
Inclusiveness	9	3.3	1.10	9	2.9	1.17	10	2.7	.95
Concordance	10	4.0	.94	10	4.1	1.10	10	3.9	.88
Acceptability	10	4.0	1.05	10	4.1	.99	10	4.0	1.05
Clarity	10	4.6	.52	10	4.6	.52	10	4.5	.71
Simplicity (non-MDs)	10	4.4	.70	10	4.1	.99	10	4.3	.82
Simplicity (MDs)	10	4.5	.71	10	4.6	.52	10	3.9	.99
Simplicity (patients, consumers)	10	3.5	1.27	10	2.9	.88	10	2.7	1.25

Attribute	n	Mean	SD	n	Mean	SD	n	Mean	SD
Manageability (reviewers)	10	4.4	.70	9	3.7	1.22	10	4.2	1.03
Manageability (professionals)	10	4.6	.52	9	4.6	.53	10	4.3	.82
Feasibility	9	4.2	.67	8	4.1	.64	10	4.3	.67
Computerization	10	4.0	1.05	9	3.7	1.00	10	4.4	.84
Priority (hi-risk,hi-cost)	10	4.8	.42	9	4.6	.73	10	4.4	.70
Priority (consensus exists)	10	3.8	.63	10	4.1	.88	10	4.1	.74
Generalizability	10	3.6	1.07	10	3.1	1.20	10	3.4	1.17
Affordability	10	4.2	.63	10	4.1	.99	10	4.2	.63
Appealability	10	4.5	.53	10	4.0	1.33	10	4.0	1.63
Documentation (outcome estimates)	10	4.0	.94	9	3.8	.83	9	3.8	.83
Documentation (methods)	10	4.1	.88	10	4.2	.92	9	3.9	.93
Executability	10	4.2	.63	9	4.4	.88	10	4.4	.70

[a] n is the number of respondents. There were 10 respondents to the homework exercises. Where $n < 10$, the attribute was rated not applicable by one or more respondents. One non-response (to inclusiveness on the evaluation/management criteria homework) was also coded as not applicable.

[b] Mean is the mean rating or score among those rating the attributes.

[c] SD is the standard deviation of the mean.

TABLE A.3 Activities and Discussion Topics for Criteria-Setting Expert Panel

General Discussion of Proposed Attributes for Criteria Sets
    Presentation: Results of homework exercise
    Discussion:
        Extent to which attributes of criteria sets might differ according to their use or purpose
        Definitions of listed attributes and of any additional attributes
Application of Attributes to Three Types of Criteria Sets
    Discussion:
        Proposed attributes for each type of criteria set
    Examine illustrative criteria sets:
    Technology- or procedure-specific appropriateness guidelines
        (a) American Society of Gastroenterology's upper endoscopy guidelines
        (b) Pre-procedure criteria for carotid endarterectomy from Delmarva PRO,[a] New York PRO, and St. Luke's Hospital, Houston
    Criteria for evaluation and management of problems and conditions
        (a) UCLA/McCoy versus Medicaid hypertension management review criteria
        (b) Stulberg chronic obstructive pulmonary disease management algorithm
    Case-finding screens
        (a) Ear, nose and throat screening criteria from Medical Management Analysis
        (b) Hospital Association of New York State hospital-wide indicators
    Reformulate attributes for each type of criteria set
General attributes: revisited
Discussion of Methods for Criteria Development
    Literature review, expert panel, and other approaches
    Stages of guideline development process and the appropriate forum for each stage
    Differences in methodology for formulation according to type and purpose of criteria set

[a]Utilization and Quality Control Peer Review Organization (PRO).

TABLE A.4 Expert Panel Homework Exercise: Second Round Ratings of Attributes

Attributes	Appropriateness			Evaluation/Management			Case-Finding		
	n^a	Mean^b	SD^c	n	Mean	SD	n	Mean	SD
Sensitivity	10	4.5	.53	9	4.4	.73	10	4.9	.32
Specificity	10	4.0	.67	9	3.7	.83	10	3.0	.94
Predictive Value	10	3.7	.82	9	3.8	1.17	10	3.9	.88
Reliability	10	4.2	.79	10	4.5	.71	9	4.1	.78
Validity	10	4.6	.84	10	4.5	.71	9	4.0	.87
Documentation-A^d	10	4.6	.70	10	4.3	.67	8	3.9	.83
Documentation-B^e	10	4.2	.92	10	3.9	.99	9	3.9	.78
Flexibility	9	4.3	1.12	10	4.8	.42	7	4.1	.90
Clinical Adaptability	10	4.4	.84	10	4.8	.42	7	4.3	.95
Responsiveness	10	2.7	.95	10	2.9	.88	6	2.7	1.03
Inclusiveness	10	2.8	1.55	10	3.4	1.17	9	4.2	.97
Acceptability	10	2.8	1.40	10	3.6	.97	8	2.9	.99
Clarity	10	4.5	.71	10	4.8	.42	9	4.8	.44
Appropriateness	10	4.2	.63	9	4.0	1.12	4	2.6	1.71
Pretesting	10	4.2	.92	10	4.0	1.15	9	4.2	1.09
Dynamism	10	4.4	.70	10	4.6	.70	10	4.4	.70
Evaluation	10	4.1	.74	9	4.3	.5	10	4.5	.53
Comprehendability (non-MD)	10	4.3	1.25	10	4.2	.63	10	4.6	.52
Comprehendability (MD)	10	4.3	.82	10	4.3	.48	10	4.2	.63

Table A.4 continues

TABLE A.4 Continued

	Appropriateness			Evaluation/Management			Case-Finding		
Attributes	n^a	Mean[b]	SD[c]	n	Mean	SD	n	Mean	SD
Comprehendability-Patient	10	3.2	1.48	10	2.9	1.20	9	3.0	1.41
Manageability (non-MD)	10	3.7	1.06	10	3.6	.84	10	4.0	.67
Manageability (MD)	10	3.8	1.03	10	3.3	.95	10	4.2	.79
Manageability (Professional)	10	3.7	.82	10	3.6	.84	10	3.8	1.23
Nonintrusive	10	3.3	1.16	10	3.7	.82	10	3.8	1.03
Appealability	10	4.9	.32	10	4.4	.84	9	4.8	.44
Feasibility	10	3.4	1.07	10	4.0	1.05	10	4.1	.99
Computerization	10	3.3	1.16	10	3.8	.92	10	3.5	.85
Executability	10	3.8	.79	10	4.5	.53	10	4.0	.94
Concordance	10	4.3	1.06	10	4.5	.71	8	4.1	.83
Prioritization (high)	10	3.4	1.17	10	4.0	.67	9	4.1	1.05
Prioritization (consensus)	10	3.4	1.26	10	3.6	1.26	8	3.8	1.04
Affordability	10	2.8	1.14	10	2.8	.79	9	3.0	1.00

[a]n is the number of respondents. There were 10 respondents to the second round of rating attributes. Where $n < 10$, the attribute was rated not applicable by one or more respondents.

[b]Mean is the mean rating or score among those rating the attributes.

[c]SD is the standard deviation of the mean.

[d]Documents methods of development and cites literature.

[e]Documents how reliability was established.

11

Needs for Future Research and Capacity Building

Throughout this report we have identified issues that we cannot presently resolve because the knowledge base is weak or inconclusive. These topics include, but are not limited to, how to measure quality of care reliably and validly, how to apply such measures efficiently, how to address deficiencies in quality of care when they are discovered, and how to evaluate systematic approaches and innovations in quality assurance. The knowledge base is also inadequate about the efficacy and effectiveness of health care services and technologies, that is, about what works in the practice of medicine (Roper et al., 1988).

In debating a redirected quality assurance program for Medicare, we concluded that the nation's capacity to undertake such an effort is weak. The numbers of practitioners and clinicians trained in appropriate research methods are inadequate. Too few caregivers and administrators are trained in quality assessment and assurance methods. In short, the need for capacity building, especially education and training, in the quality-of-care field is appreciable.

These deficits in our present state of knowledge and quality assurance manpower mean that the credibility of quality measurement and improvement can be questioned. Addressing these problems through a coherent research strategy, expanded training, and other quality assurance activities should be seen as fundamental prerequisites for improving our ability to measure and change the performance of providers of health care for the elderly.

This chapter examines research needs and capacity building. Most of our attention is given to outlining a research agenda for quality review and assurance, in keeping with the congressional charge to evaluate current research on methodologies for measuring quality of care and to suggest areas of research needed for further progress. First, we advance a framework for setting priorities for research topics; we also review past and current research efforts in the quality-of-care area. Second, we discuss in more detail the research efforts we believe should be pursued. Third, because we are not persuaded that research by itself will stimulate and support the progress that is needed (at least not in the timeframe contemplated), we discuss aspects of capacity building that we believe deserve high priority attention.

RESEARCH NEEDS

Overview

Research in quality-of-care measurement and quality assurance is our main concern. We do not address fields such as biomedical research or technology assessment, both of which have an indirect role in the information base for quality assurance, or research into the organization and financing of health care, access to care, or continuity of care. These aspects of health care delivery can strongly influence the quality of health care, but solutions to access and continuity problems are likely to lie outside the purview of quality measurement and assurance programs. A federal quality assurance program and its national, population-based databanks offer an unparalleled opportunity to track and document problems of access to care, fragmentation of care, and underuse of services.

We also do not survey the field of health services research, which is closely related to research in quality assurance. Two important links between these fields should be noted. First, the formal research methods and approaches for health services research are those most likely to be used in much of the research that will be called for later in this chapter. Second, much of the existing theory, tools and methods, and investigators in the quality assurance field come out of the health services research community.

A decade ago an Institute of Medicine (IOM) study committee stated that the "need for more knowledge about health services in the United States is becoming increasingly apparent to health care professionals, government officials, and the public" (IOM, 1979, p. 1). More recently Reinhardt (1989, p. 5) noted that "the development and implementation of a sustained, multidisciplinary research agenda is the only way that we will attract the best minds to this field [of health services research] and build a knowledge base over the next decade that will be useful for health professionals, consumers, payers, and policy makers." Substituting "quality of care" for "health services" yields equally true observations.

Berwick (1989) has proposed a broad conceptual framework on which a quality-related research agenda for the next decade might be built. One pillar is that of efficacy, or knowing what works, and includes an emphasis on technology assessment.[1] The second pillar is appropriateness, or using what works, and includes practice guidelines and standards. Execution of care, or doing well what works is the third pillar, and purpose of care, or clarifying the values and objectives of health care, is the fourth. According to Eddy (1984, p.75), "uncertainty, biases, errors, and differences of opinions, motives, and values weaken every link in the chain..." of efficacy, appropriateness, and execution. Brook and Lohr (1985) argued that greater returns from health services research would be realized when work on efficacy, effectiveness, variations in population-based rates of use, and quality of care were integrated into an operational model for policy, planning, and evaluation. Our view of a research agenda for quality review and assurance reflects this integrative or boundary-crossing approach; although we identify key topics, we believe that efforts along a broad, multidimensional, and multidisciplinary front will be required.

The research community must have orderly ideas about how to set research priorities. For broad quality-of-care issues, Lohr et al. (1988) advanced the following criteria for priority setting in research: (1) the history and persistence of the problem; (2) the likely utility, persuasiveness, and generalizability of the research; (3) the probability of obtaining data and results in a timely way; (4) the ease and cost of acquiring clinically valid data; and (5) the tradeoffs with other appealing allocations of research dollars. Within the dozen or so broad topics discussed later in this chapter, which we conclude deserve significant attention and investigation, are many competing subjects and problems. Congress and public- and private-sector funding agencies could apply such criteria in selecting topics of highest priority.

Current Knowledge Base on Quality of Care

The literature on quality of care and quality measurement is immense. Since World War II in particular, much work has been done on assessing quality of care, rather less on assuring quality of care.[2] For instance, a bibliography by Williamson (1977) listed about 3,500 publications in this field.

In the subsequent decade, that body of work has grown exponentially. At least one peer-reviewed journal, *Quality Review Bulletin* (QRB), is oriented exclusively to quality measurement and assurance. Also, the first issue of *Quality Assurance in Health Care*, the official journal of the International Society for Quality Assurance in Health Care (based in Stockholm, Sweden) has just appeared (Jessee et al., 1989). The nursing literature on quality assurance is also very extensive (Lang and Kraegel, 1989). Several publications, such as the *Journal of Quality Assurance* and the *Journal of*

Nursing Quality Assurance, are devoted to operational and management aspects of quality of care. Despite these targeted publications, this quality assurance work tends to be scattered over a wide array of clinical, management, evaluation, and health services research publications. Thus, tracking the knowledge base is a very difficult task.

In the spring of 1988, two leading journals published special issues on quality of care (*Health Affairs,* 1988; *Inquiry,* 1988). Several subjects have become especially topical: (1) measurement of patient outcomes and health status; (2) the impact of Medicare's Prospective Payment System (PPS) and other financing schemes on quality of care (Heinen et al., 1988; ProPAC, 1989; PPRC, 1989); (3) the extraordinary and unexplained variations in population-based rates of use of services across like geographic areas (Chassin et al., 1986; Schroeder, 1987; Brook et al., 1989); and (4) appropriateness of diagnostic and therapeutic procedures and ways to feed information on utilization back to clinicians in those geographic areas.[3]

Several federal agencies support work in quality assessment and assurance. The National Center for Health Services Research (NCHSR) has funded quality assessment studies for two decades (Brook and Lohr, 1985; Komaroff, 1985). NCHSR has also supported work in many related areas, such as patient and provider relations (Becker, 1985; Inui and Carter, 1985), health information systems (Pryor et al., 1985; Steinwachs, 1985), and clinical decision making (Doubilet and McNeil, 1985). With the new Agency for Health Care Policy and Research (AHCPR), especially its Medical Treatment Effectiveness Program, these efforts can be expected to grow.

The Health Care Financing Administration (HCFA) Office of Research and Demonstrations (ORD) supports nearly 300 research, evaluation, and demonstration projects on many health services and health policy topics relating to Medicare and Medicaid (ORD, 1988). The major focus is the relationship of Medicare program expenditures to reimbursement, coverage, eligibility, and management, but some studies examine the impact of the Medicare program on beneficiary health status, access to services, and use of services. As of 1988, for instance, HCFA was sponsoring about two dozen projects related directly or indirectly to quality of care (ORD, 1988), and the agency had proposed an "effectiveness initiative" to study and document the effectiveness of medical interventions of particular concern to the Medicare program (Roper and Hackbarth, 1988; Roper et al., 1988; IOM, 1989). HCFA's Health Standards and Quality Bureau (HSQB) and the Peer Review Organizations (PROs) are embarking on pilot projects related to assessing quality of care delivered to Medicare enrollees. HSQB also oversees the development of a Uniform Needs Assessment Instrument for evaluating the needs of Medicare patients for posthospital care. Finally, the American Medical Review Research Center (AMRRC, a PRO membership organization) is conducting a small area variations study that will compare utilization and outcomes across geographic areas and feed practice-pattern information back to physicians in those areas.

The private sector also supports work related to quality assessment, quality assurance, and patient health status. One case in point is the Robert Wood Johnson Foundation (1989), which is initiating a large-scale effort in hospital quality assurance. Other foundations, such as The John A. Hartford Foundation and the Pew Memorial Trust, support studies relating to utilization management and appropriateness of invasive procedures. The Henry J. Kaiser Family Foundation has funded work on functional health outcomes and health status measurement (Tarlov et al., 1989). In addition, major business coalitions are beginning to devote considerable attention to quality assessment and quality improvement; one instance is the work of the Midwest Business Group on Health (MGBH, 1989).

Gaps in the Current Research Base

This array of work and investment in quality-of-care studies is useful, but many gaps and deficiencies remain. Most quality assessment research has been narrowly focused on evaluating the level of quality of care for specific diagnoses, groups of patients, or types of institutions. Although perhaps only a small number of diagnoses or procedures may make up most of the issues in quality of care, past work tends not to be easily generalizable to other diagnoses, patient populations, or institutions.

Research into quality assurance and improvement is sparse. Very little is known about how to change the habits, practice styles, and standard operating procedures of physicians, nurses, and other caregivers, of institutions such as hospitals or prepaid group practices, or of health care organizations such as home health agencies. This gap is particularly significant for the quality assurance and continuous improvement models described in Chapter 2.

Little is known about the links between the process of care and the outcomes of care. In the absence of reliable and valid information about these relationships, reliable and valid measurements of quality of care are more difficult to construct; hence, changes in medical, nursing, and institutional practices are even more difficult to bring about.

The "art of care" deserves more attention. Little information is available on important aspects of the patient-provider relationship, on the role of patient values and expectations in achieving good outcomes, or on effective communication styles. Similarly, although the literature on patient satisfaction is growing (Cleary and McNeil, 1988), our understanding of how best to gather and to use information from patients, family members, and consumers in quality measurement and assurance efforts is only at a formative stage (Davies and Ware, 1988; Kaplan and Ware, 1989).

A related void in the knowledge base concerns data and data bases, although investigators are becoming more proficient at using some administrative data banks for research purposes (Roos, 1989). Among the questions deserving further study are the following: how best to gather quality-related information; how to validate the accuracy of data elements in patient management or insurance claims systems; and how to transmit, store, share, and link data and data files, yet protect patient and provider confidentiality and privacy. Finally, we know relatively little about how most effectively to feed back quality-related information to practitioners and institutional providers.

These lacunae in the knowledge base for quality measurement and assurance might be characterized as falling into one of three stages. They are (1) basic research (e.g., on measuring patient outcomes and on efficacy and effectiveness of health care interventions), (2) applied research (e.g., on translating the results of basic research into information and tools that can be employed in quality assurance programs), and (3) diffusion (e.g., the actual incorporation of such information and tools into real-life programs and the evaluation of those programs). The remainder of this section discusses key topics identified (somewhat arbitrarily) in these stages (Table 11.1), which we believe deserve high priority attention and funding.

Priorities for Basic Research

Table 11.1 illustrates the three basic stages of the research process into which we have categorized topics or areas of need for additional research. This table does not give an exhaustive account of research subjects, and some topics are discussed more fully than others in the following sections.

Variations, Effectiveness, and Appropriateness of Medical Care Interventions

The quality of care for Medicare beneficiaries can differ considerably from one area to area, beneficiary to beneficiary, doctor to doctor, and hospital to hospital. The appreciable variation in the use of services across areas or organizations is worrisome; nevertheless, we do not know from the literature on variations in care whether some people are getting too little care and others too much, because appropriateness cannot be inferred from low or high rates of use. Thus, it will be necessary to continue to study population-based variations in use of services and to document whether and how differences in rates correspond to differences in appropriateness.

The research community recognizes that many medical services are of little or no benefit to patients; some pose a substantial risk to patients (PPRC, 1989). Bunker (1988) contended that perhaps only 20 percent of what physicians do every day has been shown to be of clear value by well-designed clinical studies.

TABLE 11.1 Topics and Stages of Research in Quality Assessment and Assurance

Basic Research	Applied Research	Diffusion
Variations, effectiveness and appropriateness		
Process of care measures		
Technical measures		
Art of care measures		
Outcomes, health status, and quality of life		
Continuous improvement models		
	Linking process and outcome	
	Practice guidelines	
	Effectiveness of quality assurance interventions	
	Setting-specific issues	
	hospitals	
	ambulatory care	
	home health care	
	health maintenance organizations	
	Effect of organization and financing on quality assurance	
	Rural health care	
		Data systems and hardware
		Data sharing
		Data feedback and disclosure
		Program evaluation

Decisions to provide services are influenced by many factors including the organization of practice, reimbursement incentives, and availability of resources. Physicians often do not have enough information to predict whether a particular service or procedure will benefit the patient. Wennberg (1984), for instance, attributed much of the variation in the use of services to physician uncertainty.

Part of the reason for poor understanding of variations and appropriateness is the lack of broadly accepted information on effectiveness of services. Effectiveness, defined by PPRC (1989) as the probability of benefit to a given individual from a medical procedure applied to a given medical problem, relates to the value of resource use—that is, the combination of quality and cost. According to Roper and Hackbarth (1988), the goal of effectiveness research is to assure that any given patient receives the maximum benefit in improved health for any given level of health care expenditure. Appropriateness relates the procedures recommended for a given patient to the current knowledge of effectiveness. Knowledge about effective and appropriate medical care can be increased through clinical and health services research, including clinical trials, epidemiological studies, analysis of cost effectiveness, and assessment of techniques to influence clinical decision making.

Process-of-Care Measures

Technical aspects of care. Process-of-care measures have long been the yardsticks against which to measure quality of care. Properly evaluating the technical process of care requires the use of explicit criteria. Much needs to be done in the area of developing adequate process measures. This topic may be more an issue of application than of basic research; for instance, ways need to be found to make good criteria sets, which may be developed for research or program evaluation purposes, more easily accessible to quality assurance professionals.

Process criteria typically contain statements about diagnosis- or problem-specific elements of care that practitioners agree are relevant, important, and measurable. For instance, criteria sets may ask whether the right problems were identified and diagnosed, whether the correct diagnostic steps were taken, whether the appropriate treatments were recommended or delivered, and whether those treatments were correctly administered in a timely fashion. Developing criteria sets that are reliable, valid, and parsimonious with respect to data-collection requirements is a very difficult task, and existing criteria sets vary widely in these respects. Very few meet the standards of clarity, validity, reliability, flexibility, and clinical adaptability discussed in Chapter 10.

Art-of-care measures. The art of care is both extremely important and difficult to measure. This interpersonal dimension includes the practitioners' responsiveness to patient needs, ability to elicit information about patient preferences for treatment alternatives and generally their caring attitude. These aspects resist quantification, but they influence outcomes of care, often in the form of patient satisfaction. A substantial research effort is needed to establish the reliability, validity, and generalizability of the concepts and methods for measuring the art of care. These include the use of videotapes, written transcripts, and audiotapes in research settings and interviews, questionnaires, and self-report measures in ordinary practice settings.

A better understanding of the interpersonal and communication aspects of the care process implies a need to appreciate which factors can erode the sense of trust implied by the phrase the "doctor-patient relationship." Some attention should be given to the pressures on physicians that may undermine their relationship with patients. These include malpractice concerns and intrusive utilization management. Also important is the extent to which patients and their families appreciate the effect of such forces and pressures on practitioners.

Outcomes, Health Status, and Quality of Life

The importance of using patient outcomes in quality-of-care measurement is unquestioned. Measuring outcomes is a very complex task, and the need continues for research into the development of valid, reliable, and practical outcome measures. Research in this area should be viewed more broadly than merely the assessment of clinical or physiologic end results. It should include assessments of several dimensions of health and health-related quality of life as well as patient satisfaction.

Four basic facets of outcomes research warrant further examination (Lohr, 1988). The first is the link between process of care and outcomes, which is discussed below with respect to applied research. Second is the assessment of medical technologies in ways that will provide useful information about process of care; it underscores the need to strengthen the relationship between technology assessment and quality assessment (Brook, 1988; Greenfield, 1988; Mosteller and Falotico-Taylor, 1989).

A third facet of outcomes research calls for better ways to adjust outcome measures for severity of illness. Although HCFA has sponsored a large body of work in this area (ORD, 1988), severity adjustment remains a major area of contention; without agreed-on adjustors for severity (or risk), outcome measurement in quality assurance will always be open to criticism. Related to this is the need to improve the reliability and validity of outcomes as ways to screen for potentially poor quality care. Mortality statistics in which severity or expected patient outcomes are not well controlled, for example, can be very misleading.

Fourth and most critical is the need to expand and improve measures of health status and functional outcomes measures. Several good instruments exist. More are needed, for different settings of care for the elderly generally and for particular subgroups such as the very old or very frail. Although consensus about the appropriate domains of health status and quality of life to measure is considerable, this field is constantly evolving, and new concepts and measures (e.g., social and role functioning, and vitality) are continually being proposed, developed, and tested. Other conceptual problems center on how health status scales should be scored to yield summary information for quality assessment and assurance uses and whether health status scales can and should be aggregated into more global indexes. Steady support for research in this area is critical if the field is to avoid a confusing proliferation of measures whose similarities or differences are not apparent to or understandable by clinicians or quality assurance professionals.

The practical strengths and limitations of existing health status measures should be studied. Important problems involve length and complexity of questionnaires and obstacles to administration such as illiteracy, blindness, deafness, and language barriers. Methodologic studies should answer questions such as: What are the best ways to collect information directly from patients? How can medical record or insurance claims data be linked with those outcomes? How much information can be obtained from self-reports, especially by telephone? How can information be obtained from frail geriatric patients, especially those in long-term-care institutions? Is it possible to use "representative" patients (akin to Nielsen raters for television)?

Continuous Improvement Models

Research funding for continuous improvement should be directed to several different questions. First is to understand better the ways in which health care organizations can most effectively undertake the shift to the continuous improvement model. The move to implement this model is complex and time-consuming; knowing what strategies make it more feasible throughout an organization would be an important question to answer. A second issue concerns how to demonstrate to external customers (i.e., to patients, payers, and the community) the "value added" by fully implementing the continuous improvement approach. Third is the need to explore how health care is different from other industries (manufacturing, utilities, or other service industries such as education) and what that implies for the application of the continuous improvement model. Fourth, health care gives licenses for people to do things to other people (for good or for harm), which is not the same as a license to manufacture a car or to produce electricity. Therefore, there will always be a need for regulatory procedures, but how to achieve a blending of regulatory approaches with the internal, organization-based continuous improvement approaches is a difficult question warranting direct study.

Priorities in Applied Research

Linking Process and Outcomes

We have emphasized the need for basic research to develop and document good process and outcome measures because quality assessment and assurance will always need both types of measures. Establishing a causal link between process and outcome is also crucial. To understand the links (or lack thereof) between process of care and outcome requires that one develop complex models that encompass a full range of health outcomes, take into account different clinical approaches to the same clinical problems, and permit comparisons of process and outcome across different organizational settings and payment structures. The link between process and outcome must embody principles of patient values and preferences. Although these issues might be thought to be a matter of basic research, we discuss them here because well documented process-outcomes links are crucial to applied quality assurance.

Two major points for operational programs should be underscored. First, in quality assessment, making the appropriate choice of quality measures (e.g., process measures for physician office-based care or outcomes for long-term care) is critical. This task is facilitated when the relationships between processes of care and expected results for patients are reasonably well understood. Second, in quality assurance, the aim is to understand enough about problems in performance to know what to fix; outcome measures lacking a strong tie to process do not provide adequate guides to an operational quality assurance program.

Quality-of-care measures must encompass patient values and preferences. We know little about patient attitudes toward, expectations for, and preferences about health and health care or about how they might differ according to the patient's sociodemographic characteristics or health status. We know less about how to build such concepts into measures of quality of care, and whether they should be reflected in measures of technical or interpersonal care, in outcome measures, or both.

Practice Guidelines

Practice guidelines give recommendations about the appropriateness of medical interventions and are thought to contribute to better patient management.[4] As discussed above, relevant basic research in the realms of efficacy, effectiveness, and appropriateness will provide the intellectual and clinical base for clinical standards and guidelines. AHCPR, which has a direct congressional assignment concerning practice guidelines, may have a major role in this area.

Significant issues lie in the areas of applications and diffusion, particularly mechanisms for developing, testing, and promulgating such guidelines. Methods of consensus development, use of expert panels, and group judgment techniques must all be examined because they remain the primary mechanisms for practice guidelines development. Many questions can be raised, including: How should panels be assembled and conducted? What is the role of literature reviews and data, and how should information be conveyed to such panels? When do we conclude that consensus has been reached? Alternatively, when do we decide that irreconcilable differences among experts preclude the development of a guideline and instead point to the need for further clinical research?

Equally compelling questions can be raised about the dissemination and use of practice guidelines in everyday practice. For instance, what mechanisms work best for alerting the practicing community to the existence of such guidelines? How should clinicians in one specialty be informed about the existence of guidelines of interest to them that have been developed by a different specialty group? How can any practitioner be persuaded of the validity of guidelines that depart from his or her own long-established patterns of behavior and preferences?

Effectiveness of Quality Assurance Interventions

We may know more about modifying patient behavior than we do about changing professional and organizational behavior. Donabedian (1989) suggests that unique characteristics of the medical profession may promote or hinder quality assurance. These include a tension between autonomy in medical practice and accountability for its quality, mistrust of externally imposed quality review efforts, and a general unfamiliarity with quality assurance purposes and methods.

What, then, works best to change professional behavior? Educational interventions are often regarded as the preferred method for changing behavior. Some studies show continuing medical education (CME) to be effective, but other studies do not. Thus, a link between quality monitoring and CME must be created.

Komaroff (1985) called for continued research into the effectiveness of various interventions including education, medical audit with feedback, administrative restrictions, and positive and negative incentives. His priorities for research topics, which are as important today as they were then, included: (1) innovative corrective action plans involving various approaches to CME, such as refresher and mini-residencies, and satisfactory completion of specialty-based self-study programs and tests; (2) expanded consultation arrangements (including the use of telecommunications); (3) various mentoring or proctoring arrangements; (4) positive incentives, such as recognition among peers, monetary rewards, and the publication of good performance results; and (5) negative incentives, such as intensified review of cases, restrictions on practice, monetary penalties, exclusion from payment programs (e.g., Medicare), and other professional or financial sanctions.

This type of research is also pertinent to diffusion. It should be tied to ongoing quality assurance activities, with collaboration between researchers and quality assurance professionals. The cooperative efforts of PROs, AMRRC, and the research community in PRO pilot projects provide a useful model. The aims are to enhance the knowledge base and skills of clinicians and quality assurance staff and to speed the diffusion of successful new approaches to quality review and assurance. This will be especially important in fostering internal quality assurance programs based on the principles of continuous quality improvement.

Setting-Specific Research

One concept that has motivated the recommendations of this committee is that quality assurance and improvement within health care organizations should be encouraged and supported. In line with the above recommendation that the effectiveness of quality measurement and assurance be studied in real-life programs, we believe that some setting-specific issues warrant attention as well.[5]

Hospitals. In the past, health services and clinical studies have emphasized the hospital setting, and the problems of sustaining successful quality assurance efforts in hospitals are reasonably well understood. The Robert Wood Johnson Foundation (1989) is supporting a major initiative to improve the quality of hospital care for institutions that are interested in quality but lack the resources or expertise to address the issue adequately, and the Agenda for Change of the Joint Commission on Accreditation of Healthcare Organizations represents a considerable research investment. We applaud these efforts and encourage additional work on continuous improvement models of various sorts.

Ambulatory care. Recognizing that research in ambulatory care is in its infancy, our agenda gives very high priority to the development, testing, and implementation of standardized methods of quality assessment for care rendered in ambulatory care settings, especially care delivered in physician offices. One part of this research effort should be targeted toward procedures that were formerly done in the inpatient settings and are now often provided in the ambulatory care setting. In addition, our earlier emphasis on the art of care requires that ways be developed to measure that domain reliably and validly.

Quality assurance is probably harder for office-based care than for any other setting. Our research agenda emphasizes studies of innovative organizational mechanisms by which office-based physicians can use outside organizational resources in practice-based quality assurance. Examples include medical-specialty-based practice evaluation programs and programs whereby hospital-based clinicians participate in quality assessment of office practice through cooperative agreements. Some of these innovative approaches were identified during the study's site visits (see Volume II, Chapter 6, for examples).

Home health care. High priority should be given to developing, testing, and implementing methods of quality assessment and assurance for care rendered in the home. Particular emphasis should be placed on efficient outcome-based quality assurance methods that agencies can use internally. Ways to secure information about intangibles such as patient abuse or neglect should be examined. Further, the application of the Uniform Needs Assessment Instrument and similar functional assessment tools needs to be evaluated for hospital discharge and home health care planning. Other related issues are construction of a valid and reliable system for classifying home visits and the development and testing of measures of case-mix and severity of illness to determine the intensity of care needed by patients.

Medicare's home health benefit needs evaluation. In particular, some work could assess: (1) the impact of the "homebound" provisions on the use, continuity, and quality of home health care; (2) the impact of current requirements for care planning on use, continuity, and quality of care, with particular emphasis on the value and effect of requiring physicians to act as gatekeepers for changes in care plans; and (3) the economic and quality-of-care implications of physician referrals to physician-owned and hospital-based home health agencies.

Health maintenance organizations (HMOs). Prepaid group practices of all types offer a rich opportunity for research into quality assessment and assurance issues for several reasons. The most important is the opportunity to look at defined populations and, using that base, study quality-of-care factors that might predict enrollment into or disenrollment from such plans. In addition, HMOs tend to have much more advanced programs of quality assurance than do fee-for-service plans (with the exception of some large, nationally known multispecialty groups). These programs typically do not distinguish the elderly from the other age groups covered by the HMO; this suggests that research into factors that enhance or detract from the quality of care for all groups could pay considerable dividends.

HMOs and competitive medical plans (CMPs) eligible for Medicare risk-contract reimbursement have to meet certain federal conditions, which typically concern structural aspects of the plans more than process or outcomes of care. Research into the links between those structural components and process and outcome measures would be useful for external regulatory programs.

Hornbrook and Berki (1985) identified research priorities within the HMO industry. They included (1) the extent to which variations between prepaid group practices and fee-for-service settings arise from differences in resource availability, practice patterns, or management approaches; (2) the effect of duration of enrollment on the use and cost of health services and health status; and (3) the impact of membership in HMOs for special populations such as the elderly, the disabled, or the terminally ill. These questions, although only tangentially related to quality measurement and assurance, continue to warrant further investigation.

Rural Health Care

Several organizations (such as HCFA, the Robert Wood Johnson Foundation, the American Hospital Association, and the W.K. Kellogg Foundation) currently support research on the delivery of health care in rural areas, but additional work on assessing and improving the quality of care delivered to one of the nation's most vulnerable populations is justified. Congress has emphasized the need for studies on (1) the future of rural hospitals, (2) long-term health care for the rural elderly, (3) hospital care for the rural poor and uninsured, and (4) alternative delivery systems and managed care in rural areas. Among the questions that might be addressed are the following: What socioeconomic and demographic factors most affect access to health care services, use of services, and quality of care received by residents of rural areas, especially the elderly? What is the impact of a sole provider rural hospital on pricing, costs, and quality of health care services in rural areas?

In addition, we believe that research support should be directed at developing and testing specialized external quality review and assurance programs for small rural hospitals (or networks) that cannot undertake their own internal programs. We also endorse the development, testing, and dissemination of methods to extend the resources of rural health-care providers through such mechanisms as telecommunication for consultation, continuing medical education, and remedial education.

Effect of Organization and Financing on Quality Assurance Activities

Understanding the generalizability (or external validity) of quality assessment and assurance methods is important because such approaches are generally intended to be universal in their application. Organizational and financing arrangements influence the quality of care provided and limit the generalizability of quality assessment and assurance methods (Donabedian, 1989). These arrangements and their effects should be studied for the lessons to be learned about applying various assessment and assurance techniques to different settings and payment arrangements. As discussed in Chapters 8 and 9, controls over recruitment and staffing, equipment and material resources, and direct supervision of professional work may well be correlated with higher quality (Donabedian, 1989). One important topic for investigation, therefore, is the effects of structural characteristics, incentives (financial or other), and leadership styles on quality.

Priorities for Diffusion

Data Systems and Hardware

Efforts to improve the Medicare data bases will continue; one objective is to enhance their usefulness for quality measurement and quality assurance. Several problems should be addressed, including: (1) their content (e.g., only crude outcome measures are available); (2) the extensiveness and detail of information on diagnosis and services rendered; and (3) the reliability and validity of coded data (especially on diagnosis and procedures). Related to these problems are issues of key quality-related data missing because the services are not covered (e.g., prescription medications). A recent IOM project has identified limitations to the use of the Medicare files for effectiveness research (IOM, 1989; IOM, forthcoming), and the same drawbacks apply for quality assurance. The steps needed to overcome these problems do not, strictly speaking, lie in the realm of research; rather they need to be taken to enhance the possibility of doing quality-related research, and quality measurement and assurance, with insurance claims and administrative data.

Mechanisms are needed by which ambulatory claims data from the Medicare/Medicaid Decision Support Systems (see Appendix B of Chapter 4) can be used to screen for potential quality-of-care problems warranting more in-depth review or monitoring. Use of the Uniform Clinical Data Set in quality-of-care review (Chapter 6) should be evaluated further. Also, the addition of any health status measure to the Medicare insurance claims or other billing forms must be rigorously evaluated.

Outside the realm of the Medicare claims data files lie medical records and clinical information systems. Health care data systems are evolving: from informal (often idiosyncratic), manual systems for recording patient information, to personal computers for storing or analyzing small amounts of information, to mainframe systems for manipulating large files of clinical, administrative, and billing information. Further development and refinement of these systems and better empirical work in how to use them in quality review and assurance programs are needed.

Among the questions to be addressed is how to promote greater uniformity and standardization among systems maintained by different providers and programs. Using mainframe systems, personal and laptop computers (such as computer-assisted telephone interviewing and computer-assisted personal interviewing), and electronic record technologies should be studied in all facets of the quality assurance loop—data collection and analysis, provider feedback, and education. Another topic is how to build more patient-reported information, for example, on health status, into such systems. The final question is how to develop personal-computer-based algorithms for quality review.

Data Sharing

The multiplicity of external review activities we have observed throughout this study results in unacceptable duplication of effort, appreciable waste of resources, and considerable frustration on the part of providers. To minimize this duplication, some research funds should be devoted to developing ways that quality-related data can be shared in a timely manner among review entities. This would explicitly include examining the extent to which data collected by practitioners or institutional providers for an external agency or group (such as a state-mandated data commission or the Joint Commission) might substitute for data that the Medicare quality assurance program would otherwise require or collect. Interested parties will have to agree on specifications for standard clinical data sets for all settings in which Medicare beneficiaries receive care. Requirements concerning psychosocial and other health status profiles should be a part of those specifications.

Data Feedback and Disclosure

Two major issues arise with respect to the diffusion of quality-related information: feedback to practitioners and providers, and disclosure of information to the public. At the core of quality assurance is the need to make data available to providers in a steady stream to support their own activities and to serve as benchmarks for more detailed data analysis, while balancing the needs of privacy, confidentiality, and due process. The quality assurance field has little in the way of a conceptual framework and theory of feedback at present, and even less in terms of effective feedback mechanisms in place. Considerable attention should be given to this gap.

Some research funds should be invested in understanding how best to make quality-related information useful to, and available to, patient and consumer groups and the public at large. Although the release of hospital-specific mortality rate data has established the principle of the public's right to such information, it is not clear that the approach taken has been of particular use to either the provider or the patient community. Care must be taken to present data in ways that are useful to the intended audiences, rather than in ways that may anger, intimidate, or frighten them.

The release of provider-specific quality-related data also raises difficult problems concerning privacy, confidentiality, and due process issues. Individual rights and protection must be balanced with society's need for more and better aggregate information about medical practice and patient outcomes. The IOM examined these questions with respect to the Professional Standards Review Organization program some years ago (IOM, 1981) and they warrant reviewing in the context of our proposed Medicare quality assurance program.

Evaluation

Program evaluation and evaluation research are major disciplines in their own right. The principles and tools developed in those fields have not been systematically applied to the evaluation of quality assurance programs. We believe that research efforts relating to evaluation should be directed at three major questions.

First, how should the government evaluate the impact of the Medicare quality assurance programs on quality of care for the elderly? Evaluation criteria grounded in cost containment and cost savings do not seem appropriate for a quality assurance emphasis; criteria are needed that will reflect an effect (or lack of it) on quality of care. Second, what techniques could be used by a federal program (especially one that moves away from strict contracting toward grants, cooperative agreements, or other hybrid financing mechanisms) to evaluate its local agents? Third, what techniques would best let external quality assurance evaluators reduce intrusive external review for providers and practitioner groups when that is warranted by good performance and increase review for poor performance? Related to this is how to identify exemplary performers who might warrant special recognition or additional relief from external review.

CAPACITY BUILDING

We are not convinced that research by itself can accomplish improvements in quality measurement and assurance techniques needed for progress in this field. The capacity for conducting successful quality assurance programs calls for more than methods; it requires well-motivated and well-trained personnel. Thus we emphasize the need for investments in the training and development of professionals in the field of quality assurance and assessment. Because ultimately quality assurance cannot proceed without an appreciation of its purposes, methods, strengths, and limitations by the patient population, we also comment briefly on issues relating to patient education.

Professional Education

Capacity building can be viewed as having both short- and long-term components. In the short run, concepts and methods of quality assurance must be introduced to health care professionals already practicing in the health care field, and technical assistance must be provided to them. The aim is to train established professionals to assume responsibility for and to take leadership roles in quality assurance.

Methods to achieve these goals can take several forms. CME courses and in-service training programs can be used to introduce the need for, and the concepts and methods of, quality assessment and assurance. Curricula may be developed and implemented by quality assurance associations, such as the National Association for Quality Assurance Professionals (NAQAP) or the Joint Commission and by professional associations such as the Association of American Medical Colleges, the Association of Schools of Public Health, the Council of Medical Specialty Societies, the American Nurses Association and National League for Nursing, and similar organizations.

Quality assurance should be seen as a viable career path for physicians and other clinical professionals in much the same way as clinical administration has become a career path for some practitioners. For instance, NAQAP offers certification for professionals in quality assurance based on a written examination. However, practicing physicians must always be involved in quality assurance. Thus, the notion of developing career opportunities for practitioners does not imply that quality assurance can or should be delegated to a cadre of "specialists" in quality assurance.

Longer-range capacity building involves education and training in the concepts and tools of quality assurance as part of undergraduate and graduate professional training. Although we recognize that medical, nursing, and other training programs are already heavily burdened with teaching basic subject matters and skills as well as staying abreast of new areas of knowledge, we believe that the professionalism of health professionals requires a greater investment in the quality-of-care field.

Closely allied to the need for more health professionals trained in and committed to quality assurance is the need for better-trained researchers, especially those who will be in the forefront of research into quality measurement and assurance like that advocated in this chapter. Health professionals and researchers must gain proficiency in areas such as study design and statistics, clinical epidemiology, decision analysis, health law, information processing, and the like.

Patient Education

Informed consumers capable of asking questions and evaluating information about quality of care and quality assurance programs must be an integral part of the quality assurance process. By emphasizing desired patient outcomes in our quality-of-care definition, we are also emphasizing that informed patients who can participate effectively in decision making about their care are critical to good quality care.

The federal government should fund, sponsor, or produce printed and audio-visual materials for distribution to Medicare beneficiaries. These could take the form of newsletters, brochures, television programs, tapes, and the like. Such products should explain the Medicare program's interest in quality of care and how the program seeks to review and assure the quality of the care that it covers. These materials should also stress the importance of responsible, knowledgeable beneficiaries.

These communications should be geared to a range of educational, income, and cultural backgrounds. They should be simply written and include a steady stream of findings from research about the effectiveness of medical treatments. They should be augmented by an 800 number telephone line, by which Medicare beneficiaries or their representatives could gain leads to appropriate sources of information about the risks and benefits of care and about qualified providers of care. Because such information must be presented in a useable manner, the identification of practical dissemination techniques that will reach and be responsive to the public is crucial.

Continuous Improvement

Capacity building and training for continuous improvement have these same needs, particularly to develop the relevant curricula for graduate medical, nursing, and administrative education. Continuous improvement has three special foci as well: customer knowledge, the focus on processes, and statistical thinking. First, we know very little about what patients, employees, health care professionals, payers, and others need and want to know about quality of care, and even less about how the continuous improvement models (or indeed any quality assurance program) can satisfy those needs and wants. What might be called market research on these topics would be useful. Second, the process focus calls for attention to many repeated actions over time; in health care this can include repetitive steps in taking histories and physicals, ordering, processing, or reporting laboratory tests;

prescribing and dispensing medications; maintaining adequate medical records; and producing and sending bills. We need to develop better ways to help people understand the repetitive content of what they do so that they can recognize and correct inefficient aspects of these processes. Third, actions that continue over time are measurable and testable with statistical tools, but people are often apprehensive of learning and applying methods or instruments with even a simple mathematical basis. The issue is tied to problems of "enumeracy" in the society as a whole, but for implementing the continuous improvement model it means that some attention has to be given to training all members of the health care organization in the use of the basic tools of quality control.

FUNDING ISSUES

This chapter has focused on research priorities and capacity building. Meeting these needs would not be carried out solely by our proposed Medicare quality assurance program. Indeed, in some cases this would clearly be neither desirable nor practical.

Rather we expect that, of the work to be funded by the federal government, several agencies must be involved. Within HCFA, ORD would probably have a major role, although funding for pilot projects (like those now being conducted by the PROs) might continue to come through HSQB. The field of health services research has the most direct links to research on quality assessment and assurance, so we would expect AHCPR to have the major role in funding extramural research projects of the type recommended earlier in this chapter.

The efforts of major private sector groups will contribute greatly to these goals. Major foundations and groups within the business community have begun to invest in important projects. We hope that our research agenda will prove helpful to these parties as well.

With respect to capacity building, we note that elements of the DHHS Public Health Service other than AHCPR, most particularly those concerned with education and training of health professionals, will be significant. Again, the role of the private sector, including especially the major professional and educational associations, will be critical to the future success of these efforts.

SUMMARY

This chapter has discussed research needs and capacity building. We categorized research priorities, somewhat arbitrarily, into one of three stages: basic research, applied research, and diffusion. Priorities for basic research included the following topics: (1) variations, effectiveness, and appropriateness of medical care interventions; (2) process-of-care measures for both the technical aspects of care and the art of care; (3) outcomes, health status, and quality of life; and (4) continuous improvement models. Priorities in applied research included: (1) linking process and outcomes; (2) practice guidelines; (3) effectiveness of quality assurance interventions; (4) various setting-specific issues (relating to hospitals, ambulatory care, home health care, and HMOs); (5) rural health care; and (6) the effects of organizational and financing arrangements on quality of care and quality assurance. Finally, with respect to diffusion, we identified the following areas as warranting continued work and investigation: (1) data systems and hardware; (2) data sharing; (3) data feedback and disclosure; and (4) program evaluation.

Improvements in quality assurance and assessment call for much greater investment in the training of professionals in these fields. Capacity building must also include the patient, because informed patients are an integral part of successful quality assurance.

NOTES

1. Berwick does not explicitly distinguish efficacy (what works in ideal or controlled trial settings) from effectiveness (what works in the day-to-day practice of medicine) (OTA, 1978; Brook and Lohr, 1985), but his conceptualization can be understood to accommodate that distinction.
2. Chapters 8 and 9 of this volume discuss issues relating to quality-of-care measurement and quality assurance. Chapter 6 of Volume II describes different approaches to preventing, detecting, and correcting quality of care problems; it includes an extensive bibliography on these topics and a number of exhibits.
3. These types of issues are often subsumed under rubrics such as outcomes research and effectiveness research, both of which were receiving considerable support at the federal level and in the Congress as this study was being conducted. Several bills were introduced into the House of Representatives and the Senate during 1989 to strengthen the role of the Department of Health and Human Services (DHHS), and more particularly the Public Health Service, in research of this sort. The titles of the bills (e.g., "The Medical Care Quality Research and Improvement Act"; "The Patient Outcomes Research Act") make clear their intent. Among the steps contemplated was the creation of a new agency on health care research and policy. In addition, agency budgets would be increased for research into patient outcomes and the effectiveness of health care technologies and practices, the development of practice guidelines, and the appointment of various national advisory councils. These initiatives were still being debated as this report was being prepared. In December 1989, Title IX of the Omnibus Budget Reconciliation Act of 1989 (P.L. 101-239) terminated the National Center for Health Services Research and replaced it with the Agency for Health Care Policy and Research, a larger research organization in the Public Health Service. This move is seen as a significant expansion of the relevant research capacity of the DHHS.

4. Chapter 10 discussed the important characteristics of technology- and procedure-specific appropriateness guidelines and their uses both as an educational
tool for clinicians and as a mechanism for controlling the use of inappropriate
and unnecessary services.

5. As explained earlier in this report, we did not include nursing home care in this
study, but defining quality of care for the elderly broadly means that nursing
home care cannot be overlooked. The nursing home setting provides unique
opportunities for research into the quality and continuity of care for a relatively
stable population and for particular groups of patients, such as the very old or
those with chronic, disabling diseases.

The IOM made a series of recommendations to Congress about necessary
changes within the industry to improve quality of care (IOM, 1986). We concur
with research recommendations advanced by that commission. First were factors that affect demand for nursing home care: the rate and direction of change
in health status at advanced ages (which affects survival and the risk of institutionalization), increases in the availability of alternative long-term care services,
and the influence of PPS or other cost containment measures on the supply of,
demand for, and availability of nursing home beds. Second, that IOM committee argued that more work was needed to develop minimum nursing staff requirements (with respect to qualification and training) based on case-mix and to
compare the effectiveness of different staffing patterns, types of staff, and training requirements. Finally, that IOM report recommended a study on the costs
and benefits of single-occupancy versus multiple-occupancy rooms on the quality of life of nursing home residents. We would supplement these efforts with
work on outcomes of care, particularly measures that relate actual to expected
outcomes.

REFERENCES

Becker, M.H. Patient Adherence to Prescribed Therapies. *Medical Care* 23:539-
555, 1985.

Berwick, D.M. Health Services Research and Quality of Care: Assignments for the
1990s. *Medical Care* 27:763-771, 1989.

Brook, R.H. Quality Assessment and Technology Assessment: Critical Linkages.
Pp. 21-28 in *Quality of Care and Technology Assessment.* Lohr, K.N. and
Rettig, R.A., eds. Report of a Forum of the Council on Health Care Technol-
ogy. Washington, D.C.: National Academy Press, 1988.

Brook, R.H. and Lohr, K.N. Efficacy, Effectiveness, Variations, and Quality: Boundary-Crossing Research. *Medical Care* 23:710-722, 1985.

Brook, R.H., Kamberg, C.J., Mayer-Oakes, A., et al. *Appropriateness of Acute
Medical Care for the Elderly.* R-3717-AARP. Santa Monica, Calif.: The
RAND Corporation, 1989.

Bunker, J.P. Is Efficacy the Gold Standard for Quality Assessment? *Inquiry* 25:51-
58, 1988.

Chassin, M.R., Brook, R.H., Park, R.E., et al. Variations in the Use of Medical and
Surgical Services by the Medicare Population. *New England Journal of Medicine* 314:285-290, 1986.

Cleary, P.D. and McNeil, B.J. Patient Satisfaction as an Indicator of Quality Care. *Inquiry* 25:25-36, 1988.

Davies, A.R. and Ware, J.E. Involving Consumers in Quality Assessment. *Health Affairs* 7:33-48, Spring 1988.

Donabedian, A. Reflections on the Effectiveness of Quality Assurance. Paper prepared for the Institute of Medicine Study to Design a Strategy for Quality Review and Assurance in Medicare, 1989.

Doubilet, P. and McNeil, B.J. Clinical Decisionmaking. *Medical Care* 23:648-662, 1985.

Eddy, D. Variations in Physician Practice: The Role of Uncertainty. *Health Affairs* 3:74-89, Summer 1984.

Greenfield, S. The Challenges and Opportunities that Quality Assurance Raises for Technology Assessment. Pp. 134-141 in *Quality of Care and Technology Assessment*. Lohr, K.N. and Rettig, R.A., eds. Report of a Forum of the Council on Health Care Technology. Washington, D.C.: National Academy Press, 1988.

Health Affairs 7:1-113, Spring 1988. (Special Issue. The Pursuit of Quality.)

Heinen, L., Gorski, J.A., and Roe, W. Quality of Care Research and Projects in Progress. *Health Affairs* 7:145-150, Spring 1988.

Hornbrook, M.C. and Berki, S.E. Practice Mode and Payment Method: Effects on Use, Costs, Quality, and Access. *Medical Care* 23:484-511, 1985.

Inquiry 25:1-192, Spring 1988. (Special Issue. The Challenge of Quality.)

Inui, T.S. and Carter, W.B. Problems and Projects for Health Services Research on Provider-Patient Communication. *Medical Care* 23:521-538, 1985.

IOM (Institute of Medicine). *Health Services Research*. A Report of a Study. Washington, D.C.: National Academy Press, 1979.

IOM. *Access to Medical Review Data*. A Report of a Study. Washington, D.C.: National Academy Press, 1981.

IOM. *Improving the Quality of Nursing Homes*. Washington, D.C.: National Academy Press, 1986.

IOM. *Effectiveness Initiative: Setting Priorities for Clinical Conditions*. A Report of a Study. Washington, D.C.: National Academy Press, 1989.

IOM. *Effectiveness and Outcomes of Health Care*. Report of a Conference. Washington, D.C.: National Academy Press (forthcoming).

Jessee, W.F., Reerink, E., Reizenstein, P., et al. Quality Assurance in Health Care. Editorial. *Quality Assurance in Health Care* 1:1, 1989.

Kaplan, S.H. and Ware, J.E. The Patient's Role in Health Care and Quality Assessment. Pp. 25-68 in *Providing Quality Care: The Challenge to Clinicians*. Goldfield, N. and Nash, D., eds. Philadelphia, Pa.: American College of Physicians, 1989.

Komaroff, A.L. Quality Assurance in 1984. *Medical Care* 23:723-734, 1985.

Lang, N. and Kraegel, J. Quality of Health Care for Older People in America. Paper prepared for the Institute of Medicine Study to Design a Strategy for Quality Review and Assurance in Medicare, 1989.

Lohr, K.N. Outcome Measurement: Concepts and Questions. *Inquiry* 25:37-50, 1988.

Lohr, K.N., Yordy, K.D., and Thier, S.O. Current Issues in Quality of Care. *Health Affairs* 7:5-18, Spring 1988.

MBGH (Midwest Business Group on Health). *Value-Managed Health Care Purchasing: An Employers Guidebook Series.* Volume I: Project Conclusions; Volume II: Health Care Quality Assessment; Volume III: Purchasing System Evaluations; Volume IV: Site Specific Results on Health Care Purchasing. Chicago, Ill.: MBGH, 1989.

Mosteller, F. and Falotico-Taylor, J., eds. *Quality of Life and Technology Assessment.* Monograph of the Council on Health Care Technology. Washington, D.C.: National Academy Press, 1989.

ORD (Office of Research and Demonstrations). *Status Report, Research and Demonstrations in Health Care Financing.* Baltimore, Md.: Health Care Financing Administration, January 1988.

OTA (Office of Technology Assessment). *Assessing the Efficacy and Safety of Medical Technologies.* OTA-H-75. Washington, D.C.: U.S. Government Printing Office, 1978.

PPRC (Physician Payment Review Commission). *Annual Report to Congress.* Washington, D.C.: Physician Payment Review Commission, 1989.

ProPAC (Prospective Payment Assessment Commission). *Medicare Prospective Payment and the American Health Care System: Report to the Congress.* Washington, D.C.: Prospective Payment Assessment Commission, 1989.

Pryor, D.B., Califf, R.M., Harrell, F.E., et al. Clinical Data Bases: Accomplishments and Unrealized Potential. *Medical Care* 23:623-647, 1985.

Reinhardt, U. Statement of the Association for Health Services Research on the Medical Care Quality Research and Improvement Act (H.R. 1692). May 1989.

The Robert Wood Johnson Foundation. Call For Proposals: Improving the Quality of Hospital Care. Princeton, N.J.: The Foundation, May 1989.

Roos, L.L. Nonexperimental Data Systems in Surgery. *International Journal of Technology Assessment in Health Care* 5:341-356, 1989.

Roper, W.L. and Hackbarth, G.M. HCFA's Agenda for Promoting High-Quality Care. *Health Affairs* 7:91-98, Spring 1988.

Roper, W.L., Winkenwerder, W., Hackbarth, G.M., et al. Effectiveness in Health Care. An Initiative to Evaluate and Improve Medical Practice. *New England Journal of Medicine* 319:1197-1202, 1988.

Schroeder, S.A. Strategies for Reducing Medical Costs by Changing Physician Behavior: Efficacy and Impact on Quality of Care. *International Journal of Technology Assessment in Health Care* 3:39-50, 1987.

Steinwachs, D.M. Management Information Systems: New Challenges to Meet Changing Needs. *Medical Care* 23:607-622, 1985.

Tarlov, A.R., Ware, J.E., Greenfield, S., et al. The Medical Outcomes Study: An Application of Methods for Monitoring the Results of Medical Care. *Journal of the American Medical Association* 262:928-943, 1989.

Wennberg, J.E. Dealing with Medical Practice Variations: A Proposal for Action. *Health Affairs* 3:7-32, Summer 1984.

Williamson, J.W. *Improving Medical Practice and Health Care: A Bibliographic Guide to Information Management in Quality Assurance and Continuing Education.* Cambridge, Mass.: Ballinger Publishing Co., 1977.

12

Recommendations and a Strategy for Quality Review and Assurance in Medicare

This final chapter summarizes the Institute of Medicine (IOM) committee's main findings and conclusions and outlines our vision of an "ideal" quality assurance system. It states our explicit recommendations for a strategy and structure for a reformulated quality assurance system for Medicare, based on our findings and conclusions and in response to the congressional charges for this study. It describes in some detail how we think such a system might work, recognizing that many organizational and operational features of the system would not be completed until well into implementation. Finally, a section on implementation strategy briefly discusses tasks to be undertaken in three phases.

The committee debated many issues over the course of this project. On some issues it reached broad consensus, as reflected in our findings and conclusions. On others the committee was more divided on a stance to take, chiefly because of conflicting or insufficient evidence. Still other positions were arrived at only after weighing concrete findings against more intangible considerations of organizational, financial, or political factors.

Many approaches to a strategy for quality assurance in Medicare were considered in reaching our decisions and recommendations (some of which are briefly noted below). This chapter does not, however, give a rigorous organizational, financial, or political evaluation of different strategies that might be considered. We do not explicitly discuss the pros and cons or the benefits and side effects of the recommendations we have made or of possible alternative options. Our recommendations about a long-term strategy for Medicare quality assurance are explicated, although little solid evidence about risks or benefits of an as-yet untested strategy to be followed over a decade could be marshalled at this time. The decade-long implementation strategy we recommend is intended to provide information about the advantages and disadvantages of a new system so that its realization can be in some ways self-correcting.

FINDINGS AND CONCLUSIONS

The nation is generally perceived to have a solid, admirable base of good quality health care, and the elderly are usually satisfied with the quality of care they personally receive. Contrasting with this positive perception of the overall quality of care in the nation is a large body of literature that documents areas of deficiencies in all parts of the health sector. Some of these relate to overuse of unnecessary and inappropriate services, some to underuse of needed services, and some to inadequate technical skills, poor interpersonal care, or faulty judgment in the delivery of appropriate services.

The committee concluded that significant problems exist in quality of care and in our present approaches to quality assurance. The problems are sufficient to justify a major redirection for quality assurance in this country and, in particular, a more comprehensive strategy for quality assurance in Medicare.

Our major findings and conclusions include the following:

* A quality assurance program should be guided by a clear definition of quality of care.
* No single approach or conceptual framework to quality assurance is likely to suit all purposes.
* Regarding the elderly,
    —the elderly population continues to grow, both in absolute numbers and as a proportion of the entire population,
    —the average number of years lived after age 65 continues to increase, and
    —an increasing number of people in this population live with chronic illness and disabling conditions.
* Regarding Medicare and the elderly,
    —health care costs continue to rise,
    —pressures for cost containment increase, and
    —use of sites of care other than inpatient (i.e., outpatient and long-term-care facilities and home settings) continues to expand.
* Near universal coverage of the elderly population by the Medicare program gives them better access to health care than any other age group; nevertheless, gaps in coverage and financial barriers do exist and adversely affect quality.
* Regarding the burden of poor quality,
    —evidence of overuse of health services is substantial,

—underuse is hard to detect under existing surveillance systems, but we suspect it is considerable, and

—numerous examples of poor performance have been documented by health professionals in health services research studies.

- Different approaches to quality assurance may be necessary

  —for different sites of care (e.g., hospital, home care, or ambulatory settings) and

  —for different organizational structures such as health maintenance organizations (HMOs) and fee-for-service practices.

- Quality-of-care criteria sets

  —can be classified into three main groups, namely appropriateness (or clinical practice) guidelines, patient management and evaluation criteria, and case-finding screens, and

  —vary considerably in internal and external validity.

- Criteria for evaluating quality-of-care criteria sets

  —can be defined in terms of about two dozen substantive (or structural) attributes and implementation (or process) attributes,

  —differ by type of criteria set, and

  —can be grouped into larger clusters of substantive attributes (scientific grounding, latitude for clinical and patient judgment, design, and efficiency) and implementation attributes (implementation, ease of use, appealability, and dynamism).

- Currently available methods of quality assurance

  —suggest that a small number of outliers account for a large number of serious quality problems,

  —are inadequate in coping successfully with outlier providers,

  —tend to focus on single events and single settings,

  —may not identify underuse and overuse of services,

  —are constrained (sometimes in counterproductive ways) by regulatory and legal systems, and

  —are of questionable value in improving average provider behavior.

- The Utilization and Quality Review Peer Review Organizations (PROs) constitute a potentially valuable infrastructure for quality assurance. Nevertheless, it is the perception of the committee that PROs

  —give primary attention to utilization rather than quality,

  —focus on outliers rather than the average provider,

  —concentrate on inpatient care,

  —impose excessive burdens on providers,

  —do not use positive incentives to alter performance,

  —are perceived as adversarial and punitive,

  —use a sanctioning process that is largely ineffective,

  —are rendered relatively inflexible by program funding arrangements,

  —use methods that are redundant with other public and internal quality assurance programs, and

—have not been evaluated with respect to their effect on quality.

• Mechanisms for ensuring that hospitals meet the Medicare Conditions of Participation

—are generally sound in terms of the concept of "deemed status", but

—warrant strengthening in several aspects, especially the survey and certification procedures for hospitals that are not accredited.

• The present structure does not have the capacity to achieve a comprehensive and maximally effective quality assurance system. Required research and capacity building include

—basic methodological research,

—applications research,

—research on methods of diffusion,

—training of professionals in research skills, quality assurance, and continuous improvement, and

—methods to improve patient decision making.

Model of Quality Assurance for Medicare

Based on these findings and conclusions, the committee proposes a quality assurance system that: focuses on the health care decision making and health outcomes of Medicare beneficiaries, enhances professional responsibility and capacity for improving care, uses clinical practice as a source of information to improve quality of care, and can be shown to improve the health of the elderly population. This ideal system stands in sharp contrast to the existing quality assurance system; the latter relies too heavily on provider-oriented process measures, regulation, and external monitoring, contributes little new knowledge to improve the quality of care, and has not been evaluated in terms of impact on the health of the elderly. We believe that any future quality assurance program requires a better balance than exists today between regulation and professionalism, provider orientation and patient orientation, and process of care and outcomes.

Our proposed program for quality review and assurance aims to alter the mix of elements that make up such a program. We propose to shift the emphasis from current directions or tasks to ones that more fully reflect our vision of a quality assurance program (Table 12.1).

The current PRO program is inclined toward reaction, external inspection, and regulation. We suggest that the future Medicare quality assurance program be more proactive in data collection and feedback and that it actively foster professionalism and internal quality improvement. The present system heavily emphasizes providers and the process of care. We suggest that in the future it give more attention to patient and consumer concerns and decision making and that it adopt an aggressive outcomes orientation.

The present approach relies on monitoring information and on data collected for other purposes (such as billing), and it does little constructive

TABLE 12.1   Shifts in Emphasis for a Quality Assurance
Program for Medicare

Current Emphases	Future Emphases

Regulation
  Inspection
  External monitoring
	Professionalism
	  Improvement
	  Internal programs

Provider and process
  orientation
	Patient/consumer and outcomes
	  orientation

Mostly nonclinical information
  with no feedback
	Develop and use new knowledge
	  from clinical practice and
	  return information to providers
	  to improve decision making

Individual providers and
  incidents of care
	Systems of care and
	  episodes of care

Hospital focus	Broader focus on all settings of care

Little public accountability
  or program evaluation
	Greater public accountability and
	  program evaluation

feedback to providers. We propose a program that generates new knowledge from clinical practice and that returns that information to providers in a timely way that improves clinical decision making.

Although any quality assurance program must be concerned with individual providers and specific incidents of care, as is presently the case, we believe that the future program must place stronger emphasis on systems of care, the joint production of services by many different providers, and continuity and episodes of care. The Medicare peer review programs have traditionally focused on hospital inpatient care and have been able to do little or nothing with ambulatory, office-based care or care in other nonhospital settings. We thus see a need for a major thrust toward quality assurance in all major settings in which the elderly receive care. Quality assurance in those settings is important in its own right, but it also is necessary if patient outcomes and episodes of care are to become significant components of this new program.

A major deficiency of the present program, in our view, is the lack of evaluation and public oversight. It is virtually impossible to know what the nation is getting for the Medicare resources presently devoted to the peer review program or to know which parts of that program are successful and which are not. In our reformulation, therefore, we place considerable emphasis on public accountability, so that policymakers and the nation more generally can know what impact the program is having and can express their views about program goals and directions. Finally, in addition to these points, we note that the present program is not grounded in a firm conceptualization or definition of quality of care. We strongly believe the future program of quality assurance in Medicare should direct its activities on the basis of a clear understanding and acceptance of a definition of the concept of quality of care.

Alternative Options Debated by the Committee

The committee discussed several options for Medicare quality assurance at one point or another during its deliberations. Mostly these centered on what to do, or not do, with the existing PRO program. One clear option was to keep the PRO program more or less intact and simply recommend marginal changes (such as strengthening the sanctioning process and improving generic screens) in line with suggestions that have been made by other investigative or advisory bodies. This option was judged not responsive to the congressional charge ("to design a strategy") and in any case not sufficient to the task of creating a long-term strategy for quality assurance for the entire Medicare program. A variant on that option was to reduce the PRO program severely to a simple regulatory mechanism that would concentrate on outlier providers and practitioners, leaving to the private sector and professional organizations and associations all efforts at detecting less egregious but perhaps more prevalent quality problems and all quality assurance and improvement responsibilities. This seemed to lead to an artificial split in responsibilities and to make the PRO program even less appealing to the provider community than it is now, and it certainly would not enable the federal government to argue that it was doing all in its power to ensure that the elderly receive high quality care.

Another variant was to keep the PRO program more or less intact but to eliminate its regulatory or sanctioning powers and strengthen its educational powers. This was viewed as an unattractive option for at least two reasons. First, it undercut the vision of a comprehensive quality assurance program that the committee believed important. Second, the sanctioning powers of the PROs have value in terms of the leverage they provide the PROs in insisting that deficient practitioners and providers undertake corrective actions, including educational ones; removing that leverage threatened to make the PROs very ineffectual.

A completely opposite tack was to recommend that the PRO program be immediately terminated and replaced with something very different—for instance, a technical assistance program to aid the provider community in developing and maintaining their own quality assurance efforts, or a program that worked through other existing efforts such as those of state health departments or the Joint Commission for Accreditation of Healthcare Organizations. This option was considered to be neither practically nor politically feasible, particularly because even less evidence is available on the likely success of those alternatives than on the success of the current PRO program.

Other Key Questions

Other major splits developed as the committee moved through its deliberations. First, should the committee embrace the precepts of continuous quality improvement? Proponents argued strenuously for giving this new model a central place in the new Medicare quality assurance program. Others were more skeptical, believing that although the continuous improvement systems and their underlying philosophy and practical tools are attractive, the evidence of their success in dealing with clinical problems or in applications beyond the hospital setting provides an insufficient base for a major federal initiative.

Second, to what extent should patient outcomes be the main variables for judging quality of care? Many, if not all, members of the committee agreed that, in principle, good outcomes are the ultimate criteria for judging the quality of health care rendered. Many also recognized, however, that outcome measurement and outcomes management have severe technical drawbacks. They therefore argued that a focus on process-of-care measurement will always have to be part of any quality assurance, or continuous improvement, program.

A third disagreement centered on how much a quality assurance program should involve itself with cost containment and utilization control or can afford to do so without fatally undermining its quality assurance goals. In other words, to what extent should the PRO program, or its successor, be assigned responsibilities for utilization review and management tasks whose chief aim appears to be to control use of services? Should these tasks, such as prior authorization of procedures, be assigned elsewhere, for instance to Medicare fiscal intermediaries (FIs) or carriers?

The committee never completely settled on a single answer to these questions. In all cases (to embrace continuous improvement models, to base a new program exclusively on outcomes, or to move utilization management out of the quality assurance program), the committee opted for middle positions: support for continuous improvement for organizations that can successfully mount such efforts but retain a more traditional approach to quality review and assurance for the federal effort; emphasize both outcomes and process of care indefinitely; and retain only those utilization review activities that have a clear clinical or peer review component and serve an unequivocal quality-of-care purpose. The committee's basic position was that evidence accumulated through the lengthy implementation period for its recommended program should be used to help resolve these or other conflicts.

In summary, our conclusions and ultimately our vision of a Medicare quality assurance effort should be understood as reflecting our best collective judgment about an achievable strategy to pursue to ensure high quality care for Medicare beneficiaries in the face of many uncertainties about the organization and financing of health care in the 1990s. Although our recommendations may seem either too radical or not venturesome enough for some readers, we believe that they represent an appropriate synthesis of the evidence and experience to date and that they will provide a practical starting point and implementation strategy for the future. Our intermediate position on adopting the continuous improvement model as a guiding philosophy for quality assurance in Medicare is a case in point.

RECOMMENDATIONS

Our findings and our vision of a quality assurance system for Medicare have led us to 10 major recommendations. This section presents those recommendations, which are summarized in Table 12.2.

Medicare Mission and Quality Assurance

RECOMMENDATION NO. 1. **Congress should expand the mission of Medicare to include an explicit responsibility for assuring the quality of care for Medicare enrollees, where quality of care is defined as the degree to which health services for individuals and populations increase the likelihood of desired health outcomes and are consistent with current professional knowledge.**

Successful quality assurance resembles quality health care: both have elements of science and art. Effective implementation of a quality assurance program may depend on advanced assessment instruments and sophisticated data banks and on the motivation and commitment of the participants, but more is needed than tools and good intentions. Such a program must be directed to serve a health care mission important to both individuals and to society collectively.

A program of quality assurance should correspond conceptually and respond practically to an accepted definition of quality of care. For this report we have adopted the definition set forth in Chapter 1 and stated above. A quality assurance program responsive to desired health outcomes and attentive both to individuals and populations calls for a markedly stronger and broader mission statement than appears in the legislation that presently

TABLE 12.2 Summary of the Recommendations for a Strategy for Quality Review and Assurance in Medicare

RECOMMENDATION NO. 1. Congress should expand the mission of Medicare to include an explicit responsibility for assuring the quality of care for Medicare enrollees, where quality of care is defined as the degree to which health services for individuals and populations increase the likelihood of desired health outcomes and are consistent with current professional knowledge.

RECOMMENDATION NO. 2. Congress should adopt the following three goals for the quality assurance activities of the Medicare program:
1. Continuously improve the quality of health care for Medicare enrollees, where quality is as defined in our first recommendation;
2. Strengthen the ability of health care organizations and practitioners to assess and improve their performance; and
3. Identify system and policy barriers to achieving quality of care and generate options to overcome such barriers.

RECOMMENDATION NO. 3. Congress should restructure the Utilization and Quality Control Peer Review Organization (PRO) program, rename it the Medicare Program to Assure Quality (MPAQ), and redefine its functions.

RECOMMENDATION NO. 4. Congress should establish a Quality Program Advisory Commission (QualPAC) to oversee activities of the MPAQ and to report to Congress on these activities.

RECOMMENDATION NO. 5. Congress should establish within the Department of Health and Human Services a National Council on Medicare Quality Assurance to assist in the implementation, operation, and evaluation of the MPAQ.

RECOMMENDATION NO. 6. Congress should direct the Secretary of the Department of Health and Human Services (DHHS) to report to Congress, no less frequently than every two years, on the quality of care for Medicare beneficiaries and on the effectiveness of MPAQ in meeting the goals outlined in recommendation no. 2.

RECOMMENDATION NO. 7. Congress should direct the Secretary of DHHS to initiate a program to make the Medicare Conditions of Participation consistent with and supportive of the overall federal quality assurance effort.

RECOMMENDATION NO. 8. Congress should direct the Secretary of DHHS to support, expand, and improve research in and the knowledge base on efficacy, effectiveness, and outcomes of care and to support a systematic effort to develop clinical practice guidelines and standards of care.

RECOMMENDATION NO. 9. Congress should direct the Secretary of DHHS to establish and fund educational activities designed to enhance the nation's capacity to improve the quality of care it receives.

RECOMMENDATION NO. 10. Congress should authorize and appropriate such funds as are needed to implement these recommendations.

guides the Medicare quality assurance effort.[1] We believe a more explicit commitment to quality is needed to counter the perception by providers and beneficiaries that monitoring efforts in the Medicare program are primarily concerned with cost containment.

The Medicare program has a major responsibility to support quality assurance efforts that will not only address the technical components of health care but also respond to gaps in services, access problems, resource constraints, and ethical dilemmas that affect the quality of care. It must be alert to problems for both the users of Medicare services and the populations eligible to be served by Medicare who may not currently be receiving services.

The committee took the position, after much deliberation, intentionally to exclude resource constraints from the definition of quality. It did so in the belief that the quality assurance program would then be able to identify situations in the health care system where quality is being threatened because resource constraints have been tightened or could be improved if additional resources were available. That is, an effective monitoring system should be able to distinguish between quality and cost problems. This distinction recognizes that, in the future, some forms of explicit rationing of health care may be necessary, and we urge that quality-of-care concerns be taken into account when making such rationing decisions. The Medicare program may not be the sole responsible agent to resolve these issues, but its quality assurance program can assist in bringing the issues into the appropriate arenas for debate.

By focusing on health services, desired health outcomes, and levels of professional knowledge, our definition of quality calls for broad action by provider organizations and by the Medicare program in data collection, analysis, feedback, and dissemination. Clearly this implies a considerably expanded and richer conceptualization of the outcomes about which data will be acquired than has been evident heretofore in any (external or internal) quality assurance efforts. It also implies greater attention to the scientific knowledge base, to health care technology assessment, and to the actual processes of everyday practice. It requires that better use be made of what is known about the effectiveness of health care services and about the links between process and outcome. Finally, by highlighting the need for attention to both individuals and populations, we underscore the importance of requiring the Medicare program as a whole (and those vehicles used by it to serve defined populations, such as the risk-contract HMOs) to take responsibility for understanding the health outcomes of the populations for which they are accountable, not just for the persons actually served.

Quality Assurance Goals of the Medicare Program

RECOMMENDATION No. 2. Congress should adopt the following three goals for the quality assurance activities of the Medicare program:

• **Continuously improve the quality of health care for Medicare enrollees, where quality is as defined in our first recommendation;**
• **Strengthen the ability of health care organizations and practitioners to assess and improve their performance; and**
• **Identify system and policy barriers to achieving quality of care and generate options to overcome such barriers.**

We will recommend below an ongoing evaluation of the quality assurance program and its impact. These are the goals for which that program should be held accountable: improved health, enhanced capabilities of providers in quality assurance, and better understanding of broad system obstacles to high quality of care. These goals are at once more explicit and more comprehensive than the status quo.

Medicare Program to Assure Quality (MPAQ)

RECOMMENDATION No. 3. **Congress should restructure the PRO program, rename it the Medicare Program to Assure Quality (MPAQ), and redefine its functions.**

To discharge the responsibilities implied by earlier recommendations, Medicare will need a revised and expanded quality assurance program at the federal level. To underscore this shift, the focus and responsibility of this new program should be deliberately changed to quality of care and away from utilization or cost control. In addition, Congress should authorize the Secretary of the Department of Health and Human Services (DHHS) to support local entities in the performance of the MPAQ activities. We refer to these local entities as Medicare Quality Review Organizations (MQROs).

Our proposed program is described more fully later in this chapter (see sections on responsibilities and tasks of the MPAQ and the MQROs). Briefly, the MPAQ would be responsible for the planning and administration of the quality assurance program for Medicare: (1) to engage in long- and short-term program planning for MQROs (e.g., to define the program guidelines for the MQROs, to review applications and make awards to MQROs, and to provide or arrange for technical assistance to MQROs); (2) to monitor and evaluate MQRO operations and performance; and (3) to aggregate, analyze, and report quality-of-care data.

MQROs would have several primary responsibilities: (1) to obtain information on patient and population-based outcomes and practitioner and provider processes of care; (2) to analyze these data, making appropriate adjustments for case mix, patient characteristics, and other pertinent information by various types of providers; (3) to use these data to assess practitioner or provider performance; (4) to feed such information back to the internal quality assurance programs of practitioners and providers (as well as report it to the MPAQ); and (5) to carry out quality interventions and technical assistance to internal, organization-based quality assurance programs.

This information will serve important monitoring functions. MQROs must be able to identify providers at both ends of a "quality distribution" if they are to direct needed corrective action and to spotlight and reward exemplary performance. They should, however, be perceived by all providers and institutions as a source of objective, valid, comparable information that will facilitate priority-setting for and evaluation of internal quality assurance activities. To serve this public good function, MQROs, with guidance from MPAQ and outside help from technical assistance contractors, must devise reliable, valid, and sensitive methods for analyzing and disseminating data.

We expect that in many instances MQROs would be (or be similar to) the organizations with which the Health Care Financing Administration (HCFA) presently contracts through the PRO program. We do not believe that these entities must be statewide organizations. Instead, they might operate at substate, state, or multistate levels, depending on what configuration appeared to best suit the practicalities of data collection, analysis, and feedback, geography, and population.

MQRO activities should not be regarded as simply expanded PRO tasks, and not all that the PROs currently do should be part of the MQRO agenda. Rather, MQRO responsibilities will be redirected in line with the emphases shown in Table 12.1 to give a far more central role to data collection, analysis, and dissemination and to fostering internal quality assurance programs.

Public Accountability and Evaluation

RECOMMENDATION No. 4. Congress should establish a Quality Program Advisory Commission (QualPAC) to oversee activities of the MPAQ and to report to Congress on these activities.

RECOMMENDATION No. 5. Congress should establish within DHHS a National Council on Medicare Quality Assurance to assist in the implementation, operation, and evaluation of the MPAQ.

RECOMMENDATION No. 6. Congress should direct the Secretary of DHHS to report to Congress, no less frequently than every two years, on the quality of care for Medicare beneficiaries and on the effectiveness of MPAQ in meeting the goals outlined in recommendation no. 2.

We believe that the MPAQ and the impact it has should be rigorously evaluated. It needs to be accountable for public monies expended in this

TABLE 12.3 Relationships and Responsibilities of Main Constituents of the Medicare Program to Assure Quality

Government Agencies	Organizations	Primary Responsibilities
Congress of the United States	Quality Program Advisory Commission (QualPAC)	Advise Congress on strategies for quality assurance in Medicare and report on issues relating to quality of care for the elderly.
Department of Health and Human Services (DHHS)	National Council on Medicare Quality Assurance	Advise the Secretary of DHHS, the HCFA Administrator, and others on all aspects of MPAQ implementation, strategy, program planning, and operations.
	Technical Advisory Panel (TAP)	Advise the Secretary of DHHS, the HCFA Administrator, and others on public oversight and regular, formal evaluation of the MPAQ.
Health Care Financing Administration (HCFA)	Medicare Program to Assure Quality (MPAQ)	Long-and short-term program planning (MPAQ) (e.g., of MQRO activities). Monitoring and evaluation of MQRO operations and performance. Aggregation, analysis, and reporting of quality-of-care data.
	Medicare Quality Review Organizations (MQROs)	To obtain, analyze, use, and feedback quality-related process and patient outcome data to internal quality assurance programs of practitioners, agencies, and facilities providing care to the elderly. Report information to MPAQ. Initiate quality interventions and sanctions as needed.
	Technical Assistance Contractors	To give expert assistance in methods of quality assessment and assurance to MQROs and to internal quality assurance programs.

effort, and it needs to guard against the inclination of some organizations to work only on "easy" quality-of-care problems. Moreover, the MPAQ may find itself directly or indirectly affecting the Medicare program. This brings it foursquare into the public policy arena, where more extensive accountability and oversight enter the picture.

Thus, in addition to the MPAQ and its MQROs, we have recommended that two other entities—QualPAC and a National Council on Medicare Quality Assurance—be created to form a comprehensive structure to promote, coordinate, and supervise quality review and assurance activities at the national level. Furthermore, we call for a periodic report to Congress that describes the state of quality of care for Medicare beneficiaries and the impact of the MPAQ on quality of care. Because of the importance of these evaluation activities, we also suggest that the Secretary of DHHS establish a Technical Advisory Panel (TAP) to assist in the evaluation efforts. Table 12.3 summarizes the organizational relationships and responsibilities we have in mind.

These two organizations, which are described in more detail below, have four major purposes

- To bring a greater degree of public and scientific oversight and input into the quality assurance program;
- To provide a way for both the MPAQ and the MQROs to avail themselves of the most advanced techniques available through the private sector;
- To provide a basis by which the program itself can be more effectively evaluated; and
- To assist in program management and operations.

Congressional Commission: QualPAC

The QualPAC would have several main responsibilities. It should provide advice to the Congress on strategies and methods for improving quality of care for Medicare beneficiaries and on areas where quality improvement is needed. It should conduct studies and analyses as needed to form the basis for policy and programmatic recommendations related to MPAQ. A third responsibility would be to analyze aggregate and person-based national data from many sources, including the National Center for Health Statistics, to identify quality problems, such as access, at a population level. It should also integrate existing and new research findings to augment our knowledge about and methods for quality assessment and assurance. Finally, it should serve as a forum for all major interested parties to have a voice in the planning and evaluation of MPAQ activities.

QualPAC would be composed of appropriately qualified representatives of the public who are not officers or employees of the United States government and are representative of professions and entities concerned with or affected by activities relating to the MPAQ. It might, for instance, comprise:

- Individuals distinguished in providing health care (including at least one with experience in geriatrics);
- Experts in the field of quality review and assurance;
- Persons knowledgeable in the fields of insurance, health economics, law, ethics, and related areas;
- Persons distinguished in research, demonstration projects and evaluations with respect to health care and public programs; and
- Representatives of the elderly, consumers, labor and business.

Finally, we suggest that QualPAC could be established and run in much the same way as other Commissions set up since the advent of the Medicare Prospective Payment System (PPS), such as the Prospective Payment Assessment Commission (ProPAC) and the Physician Payment Review Commission (PPRC). QualPAC staff and resources should be comparable to those provided for the other Commissions. We advise that QualPAC be funded separately from the MPAQ at levels sufficient to enable it to carry out its duties.

Executive Branch Advisory Bodies: National Council and TAP

The National Council on Medicare Quality Assurance would have a pivotal role in achieving a constructive integration of MPAQ with quality-of-care management and research in the nation's health care system. It would be responsible for advising the Secretary of DHHS, the Administrator of HCFA, and the Director of the Health Standards and Quality Bureau (HSQB) on all aspects of MPAQ strategy, program planning, and operations. For instance, it could provide oversight for intramural research, for MQRO evaluation, and for the many decisions that will have to be made as the MPAQ is implemented.

To accomplish these objectives, the National Council must comprise representatives of top management and leadership of health care delivery institutions and systems, medical specialties, research institutions, and consumer organizations. The Secretary of DHHS would set the criteria for membership and operations of the National Council. The MPAQ would provide staff support.

We suggest that systematic evaluations of the MPAQ be conducted by an agency other than the one responsible for operating it; that is, formal MPAQ evaluations should be conducted outside HSQB (and perhaps outside HCFA). We further suggest that these evaluations be mounted at the outset of the program. To provide public oversight and strong evaluation expertise to this effort, we propose that the Secretary of DHHS empanel a second executive branch body, a TAP, to advise on MPAQ program evaluation, including the preparation of the periodic evaluation report. The Secretary would set the criteria for TAP membership (which we believe should include a majority of experts from outside the government), define its operational characteristics, direct the production of the periodic impact report to Congress, and determine which agency in the Department would conduct the MPAQ evaluation.

We suggest two other organizational and financing features for these bodies. The first concerns membership. Cross-representation of members would be valuable; thus, chairpersons or other persons delegated by the chair of each body might be ex officio members of one of the other two entities. The second concerns funding. For QualPAC, we suggest authorizations and appropriations independent of those for MPAQ, because the QualPAC would be accountable directly to the Congress. The other two advisory groups could be financed out of MPAQ annual appropriations.

Finally, we do not mean by this to preclude special reviews by other executive branch agencies, such as the Office of Inspector General (OIG). Furthermore, it is probable that congressional arms, such as the General Accounting Office (GAO) or the Congressional Budget Office (CBO), might continue to be asked to investigate particular aspects of the MPAQ. Nevertheless, we do not view these agencies as appropriate entities for ongoing evaluation of MPAQ. Moreover, in addition to the reports from the Secretary of DHHS, we have implicitly invested in the QualPAC the responsibility of periodic evaluation reports directly to Congress about the progress and impact of the MPAQ.

Hospital Conditions of Participation

RECOMMENDATION No. 7. **Congress should direct the Secretary of DHHS to initiate a program to make the Medicare Conditions of Participation consistent with and supportive of the overall federal quality assurance effort.**

We have emphasized throughout this report the use of process-of-care information and especially patient outcomes data in evaluating quality of care. Nevertheless, all conceptual frameworks of quality assurance emphasize the importance of the capacity of an organization to render high-quality care—essentially a structural measure. Indirectly, such capacity is measured through mechanisms such as accreditation. In the case of the hospital sector and Medicare, this translates into deemed status for those facilities accredited through the Joint Commission for Accreditation of Healthcare Organizations and certification through state survey and certification agencies for those not so accredited.

In Chapter 5 and in Volume II, Chapter 7, we discuss several problems with the current HCFA program for survey and certification of hospitals and for delegating certification of unaccredited hospitals to state agencies, and we propose several actions for HCFA to take to address those problems.

Four steps deserve attention. First, HCFA should update the Conditions of Participation, and their related standards and elements, within the next two years and periodically thereafter (no more infrequently, say, than every three years). The revised conditions should require hospitals to use up-to-date quality assurance procedures and to adopt any structural or process standards that are shown to be related to quality of patient care.

Second, HCFA should continue to support the concept of deemed status for hospitals. The agency should encourage the Joint Commission in its efforts to develop a state-of-the-art quality assurance program and to disclose information to the agency about conditionally accredited and nonaccredited hospitals in a timely fashion. HCFA should also maintain contact with Joint Commission activities to ensure that the Joint Commission's accreditation program remains consistent with the intentions of the emerging MPAQ.

Third, HCFA should increase the capacity of the survey and certification system to encourage and enforce compliance with the conditions (i.e., for those hospitals not meeting them by virtue of deemed status), specifically (1) to specify the size and composition of state survey teams; (2) to use survey procedures and instruments that focus more on patients and less on medical records; (3) to develop explicit national decision rules for determining compliance and taking enforcement actions; (4) to adopt intermediate sanctions, such as fines or temporary bans on Medicare admissions, that better match the severity of the quality problem; and (5) to increase the number of federal inspectors to evaluate state agency performance (through validation surveys) and to inspect hospital facilities.

Finally, HCFA should improve the coordination of federal quality assurance efforts by developing criteria and procedures for referring cases involving serious quality problems between the MQROs and the Office of Survey and Certification.

Research and Capacity Building

RECOMMENDATION NO. 8. Congress should direct the Secretary of DHHS to support, expand, and improve research in and the knowledge base on efficacy, effectiveness, and outcomes of care and to support a systematic effort to develop clinical practice guidelines and standards of care.

RECOMMENDATION NO. 9. Congress should direct the Secretary of DHHS to establish and fund educational activities designed to enhance the nation's capacity to improve the quality of care it receives.

We applaud the recent attention and support that Congress and DHHS have given to effectiveness and outcomes research and to efforts to stimulate the development of clinical practice guidelines. We endorse expanded funding for all these efforts. DHHS should also undertake broad efforts to improve coordination of data systems and data collection activities within the Department.

Financial, technical, and other support for research and special projects is also needed in the following areas:

• quality assessment and assurance methods, including continuous improvement models, technical and art-of-care process measures, and outcomes, health status, and quality of life measures;
• links between process of care and patient outcomes;
• efficient data collection and analysis methods appropriate to both process of care and outcomes;
• effectiveness of quality assurance interventions;
• effect of setting of care, organizational factors, and financing on quality of care and quality assurance;
• population-based variations in use of services;
• rural health care;
• data systems and hardware;
• methods of data sharing, feedback, and disclosure; and
• improved methods of program evaluation.

We define capacity building as activities that will enhance the ability of professionals and patients to assess and to improve quality of care. Chapter 11 discussed the research and capacity building efforts that we believe would contribute most to the quality assurance mission of Medicare. With respect to the latter, three steps warrant priority attention:

• Training health care professionals in the research skills needed to conduct a broad range of quality-related studies;
• Educating current and future health care professionals in applied quality assurance and continuous improvement concepts and techniques; and
• Educating patients and consumers about how best they can contribute to evaluating and improving the care they receive and participate in decision making about their health care.

Funding

RECOMMENDATION NO. 10. **Congress should authorize and appropriate such funds as are needed to implement these recommendations.**

The MPAQ must be adequately funded from the start, if it is to be successfully implemented and operated. Annual funding levels for the

Medicare peer review programs have barely reached one-half of 1 percent of Medicare expenditures over the past decade; PRO budgets, at about $300 million per year, are closer to 0.3 percent of expenditures. We concluded that this level of support, given the many different and complex assignments Congress has given the PRO program, seemed insufficient to the task, although greater efficiency can probably be attained.

The new MPAQ entails a considerably expanded data collection, analysis, evaluation, and technical assistance effort, all aimed at improving quality of care. In addition, we assume that Congress and HCFA will continue to expect the MPAQ to do much of what the PRO program does now in the quality assurance area, even as the latter turns over to other agencies emphases on cost and utilization control and other peripheral duties. Regardless of possible efficiency gains or other developments that might otherwise occur in the PRO program, however, we conclude that an increase in the MPAQ budget over present PRO levels is necessary.

We have not specified a target amount for several reasons. First, implementation of this proposed program will take a long time, and many details will emerge only as the program progresses. Moreover, internal and external quality assurance efforts have an element of joint production, and not all the activities envisioned in this proposed plan may involve new costs. Nevertheless, a reasonable estimate of the costs of this program might be that, eventually, they will reach as much as double the investments in the present PRO program, but it should be recognized that this is an order-of-magnitude estimate, not a detailed point estimate.

Such sums should be used for all MPAQ administrative, operational, and evaluation activities. These would include (but not be limited to) all data collection, analysis, and feedback activities related to quality review and assurance as well as any activities related to utilization review or management that clearly serve primarily a quality-improvement goal. Funding would cover whatever research in quality review and assurance methods and approaches is sponsored by the MPAQ. These would include pilot projects and experimental efforts at the MQRO or individual provider level, such as initiating a program of awards for exemplary performance. Finally, it would include evaluations of the impact of MPAQ on patient outcomes and quality of care.

This recommendation is potentially costly. We have concluded, however, that an underfunded quality assurance program, as we judge the PSRO and later the PRO programs to have been, cannot discharge its responsibilities effectively and is thus wasteful of the funds it is provided. It earns little respect from the provider community, and it cannot demonstrate any meaningful impact on either quality of care or the health of the beneficiary population.

The program we are proposing is intended to overcome some of those pitfalls. Its aims are to provide a considerably enhanced body of knowledge about the health and well-being of the elderly and current medical practice and to improve the mechanics of quality review and assurance in all major settings of care. Furthermore, we have built into our proposals a rigorous evaluation component, so that society can know what it is getting for its investment. In our view, the MPAQ simply will not be able to accomplish its objectives with funding that remains at historical levels, and we thus advocate an appreciable increase in support.

ORGANIZATIONAL AND OPERATIONAL FEATURES OF THE MEDICARE PROGRAM TO ASSURE QUALITY

This report responds to a congressional charge to design a strategy for quality review and assurance in Medicare. We have three aims. The first is to have in place a fully functioning program by the year 2000. The second is to have many of its parts operating well before that time. The third is to create a system that can grow and mature well into the next century, when health care needs, health care delivery systems and financing mechanisms, and social realities may be vastly different from those we encounter today. Achieving these aims will require patience, the commitment of considerable public and private resources, and appreciable good will among all those who have a stake in the success of the Medicare program and of quality assurance more generally. Although the approach we outline is a substantial undertaking, we believe the benefits of a sensitive, well structured quality assurance program for Medicare beneficiaries is worth the effort.

Starting Points

The conceptual foundation of the MPAQ approach is the classic triad of structure, process, and outcome. We also draw on five constructs of the continuous improvement model: (1) to differentiate external quality monitoring from internal quality improvement and assurance efforts; (2) to emphasize increased use by internal programs of data on outcomes, systems, and processes of care; (3) to reward providers that implement successful internal quality improvement programs; (4) to focus on a broad range of "customer" outcomes that include those of patients, practitioners, and the broader community; and (5) to foster cooperative communication and negotiation between many different pairs of parties in the health care delivery setting.

The practical starting point for the MPAQ is the existing Medicare program and the private, local organizations that presently do (or could) carry out the current PRO agenda. We emphasize transition, not starting over, and we believe that many elements of the PRO program—those that foster quality improvement—can and should be retained. Our decision to recommend steady transition from the present PRO program to the MPAQ reflects our judgment that an abrupt end to or shift from a complex existing program with historical ties to earlier Medicare peer review efforts is neither desirable nor feasible. At the same time, we have renamed the program to emphasize the substantial changes in concept and function that we have recommended.

Structure

The Federal and Local Levels

Our model of quality assurance has three levels. The first level is that of the federal program, the MPAQ. It might also embrace other organizations that operate nationally and that might be considered complementary to this effort, such as the accreditation programs of the Joint Commission or the National League of Nursing. The middle level is that of local or regional entities, the MQROs. As we have stated previously, MQROs would have a considerable data collection, analysis, and feedback function. The functions and activities of both these levels are described more fully below. The third level is one based on internal, organization-based quality assurance and continuous quality improvement models.

The Internal Organization Level

We have given considerable recognition to the emerging concepts of continuous quality improvement and organization-based, internal quality assurance efforts, because self-review and self-regulation remain the hallmark of the healing professions. We do not prescribe the approach to quality assurance that such institutions, agencies, or practices might take because that, in our view, should be left to the discretion of providers. We comment here on what we expect they would do, recognizing that we have proposed an external program intended to detect and correct problems that internal quality improvement efforts miss.

Some internal quality assurance programs may pursue traditional quality assurance efforts. Others may implement advanced continuous quality improvement models. Still others may experiment with novel review and assurance activities tailored to their particular needs and circumstances. The MQROs should encourage and assist the development of all such efforts, for instance, by sending provider-specific information back to internal organization-based programs in a constructive and timely manner. Although we expect internal programs to use outcome data for their own purposes, as is basic to continuous improvement models, we also expect them to emphasize the actual systems and processes of care as a means of knowing where to act when problems arise or where to improve care more generally.

Internal programs should document their quality-assurance procedures and results. Although the choice of specific approaches to solve quality problems would be left to individual providers or institutions, they should be able to document that their surveillance systems identify and attempt to solve important quality problems.

For instance, providers might institute programs designed to monitor and correct overuse of inappropriate and unnecessary services, to identify problems with underuse of services (including poor access to care across an episode of care as well as inappropriately low use of specific types of services), and to examine the process of care for poor performance. Because of our emphasis on patient-provider decision making, we also hope that providers would give more attention to educating their professional and support staffs in this area, and to informing patients about health and quality-of-care issues and about the choices they can make concerning their own health care. Education for professionals should include feedback of new knowledge from clinical practice data to inform their ongoing clinical decisions.

If internal programs cannot document their quality assurance procedures and impact, or if the results of the external MQRO monitoring suggest that these activities are not being done well, then the MQRO will have to become more actively involved. Such MQRO interventions might involve abstracting process-of-care information on-site, consulting in the planning of quality assurance activities, imposing corrective actions of the sort now available to PROs, and pursuing new intervention strategies developed during the implementation of the MPAQ.

Operational Overview of the Proposed Model

An Emphasis on Outcomes

A central theme of our recommendations and the proposed program for quality assurance in Medicare is a greater emphasis on the outcomes of care. Attention to outcomes offers several advantages. It allows monitoring of the system while leaving the providers unconstrained to undertake their own quality improvement efforts. It calls for systematic data collection that can be used to inform workers in the health care field about how process components are related to specific outcomes. It fosters looking across time and appreciating the temporal and service links within episodes of care. It emphasizes those aspects of care that are most relevant to patients and to society.

The evolution of an outcome-based quality assurance program will require several steps. Objective and reproducible outcomes must be defined, these outcomes must be adjusted for patient-specific risk factors, and the role of specific processes of care in producing these outcomes must be evaluated. Generally, outcomes should be related to specific patient conditions, diagnoses, and problems. Because the knowledge, skills, and systems are not yet available to put this program in place for a broad set of conditions and care settings, it will necessarily have to develop incrementally.

Operationally, we picture a local or regional unit, not unlike the current PROs, that would be responsible for collecting systematic information on patient outcomes and care. We begin with hospitals and inpatient care, because such facilities address some of the larger problems in medicine. We would immediately include other forms of care that substitute for inpatient hospital care, such as ambulatory surgery. We would then extend this approach to other forms and settings of care—nursing home, home care, and ambulatory care—as quickly as feasible, allowing for more technical development in these areas.

Systematic information on patients' outcomes would be collected across a number of dimensions. The MPAQ and MQROs must choose outcomes that are easily and reproducibly defined, are feasible to obtain, and are important to Medicare beneficiaries. These outcomes could include mortality and medical complications, relevant physiologic measures, functional outcomes (such as patients' mental and emotional status), physical capabilities (such as the ability to walk or climb stairs), activities of daily living (such as bathing, dressing, feeding, and toileting), placement of the patient at home or in a long-term-care facility, and patients' and families' satisfaction with care.

A very difficult aspect of outcome-directed quality assurance efforts will be to adjust outcomes for the risk factors present in the population being studied. This will be necessary to ensure that comparisons of the outcomes of patients who are treated by different physicians, groups, and hospitals or who are covered by different plans are appropriate.

The choice of the initial conditions to be studied must reflect the availability of information about known risk factors. For example, few data are available that predict the mortality, morbidity, loss of function, development of confusion, or discharge site of elderly patients admitted to a hospital with pneumonia. For patients with a hip fracture, by contrast, numerous authorities agree that mental status, functional status before the fracture, associated medical conditions, age, sex, and race affect both the mortality and recovery of function. Thus, a study of patients with hip fractures can adjust for risk factors more effectively than a study of elderly patients hospitalized for pneumonia.

Effective outcome studies must ensure that information on all relevant risk factors is identified and collected at the time that care is provided (e.g., at hospital admission for patients with fractured hips). When needed information is difficult to obtain from retrospective medical chart review (such as the patients's mental status and function before the fracture), it must be obtained prospectively.

The adjustment of outcome for these risk factors will require analytical expertise. This expertise must be available to the MQRO for the system to have scientific credibility and to be effective.

Studying outcomes, however, does not yield a complete picture of quality of care. In addition to risk adjustment, the appropriateness with which patients are selected to receive a particular health intervention must also be taken into account. For example, particular hospitals or surgical teams may have extremely low risk-adjusted operative morbidity and mortality if they select for surgery patients who are very healthy and do not need the operation under study.

Adjusted, comparative information would be returned to the appropriate providers. Those providers whose performance is significantly poorer than the mean would be asked to examine their activities carefully, to identify the specific systems or processes of care that may have contributed to these results, and to make appropriate corrections. Follow-up studies should be performed in appropriate time frames to assess the impact of these corrections. Failure to improve would result in closer monitoring and potentially more stringent actions, including public disclosure of their status. We emphasize the need for creative responses by MQROs to the wide range of situations they will encounter in monitoring the quality of care rendered in so many different and new settings.

Aggregate information would also be shared with provider groups to serve as a basis for better understanding of effective patient management interventions. This information would form part of a national data base to be used to improve clinical decision making.

The size of this undertaking means that not all discharges could be monitored for outcomes. At least some conditions would be studied nationally for periods of time to acquire adequate comparative data. In other cases, regional needs (perhaps based in part on variations in performance) might be used as the basis for selecting conditions to include in the outcomes agenda.

Importance of Process of Care

This attention to outcomes is not intended to slight the importance of process-of-care measurement. Process measures have strengths missing in an outcome focus. These areas include the lack of sensitivity of outcome measures for detecting certain rare but catastrophic events. Process-of-care measurements also reflect the need to use process measures as proxies for outcomes for patients with complex medical conditions where the many variables that influence outcome of care cannot be controlled. Further, the long lead time required for some adverse outcomes is such that process surrogates are needed. Many small processes are what make up the health care that produces the outcomes of interest and are thus the critical element of the continuous improvement models.

Much of the process evaluation in our program is expected to be carried out by the providers themselves. Related activities, such as the development of clinical standards and criteria for appropriateness, will be best done by national groups informed by data generated by this quality assurance program. For instance, the increased interest and research in effectiveness and outcomes of care should enrich the literature in the near future. The MPAQ or MQROs should encourage, stimulate, and participate in this work as much as possible.

It will be very difficult for the MQRO or any external agency to identify (let alone respond to) the aspects of the process of care mainly responsible for good or poor outcomes. That is best done by the internal quality assurance departments of these institutions, organizations, or provider groups. For example, the MQRO would report to a hospital on the results of patients with fractured hips treated at that institution. The quality assurance department of this hospital would be responsible for studying all aspects of care, from pre-operative assessment, surgical technique, post-surgical care, inpatient rehabilitation, discharge planning, and rehabilitation in a nursing home or home health care, to determine which aspect of this care was responsible for any problems with care.

Continuity and Quality Assessment

The emphasis on care beyond a single setting or facility is a new direction in quality assurance. It is essential if ultimate outcomes are to be understood and affected. Superb inpatient care followed by poor posthospital care, for instance, cannot be acceptable. Each care provider and institution is part of a system of care. Each must recognize a responsibility to ensure that the continuum of the process of care brings a good outcome for the patient.

Potential Problems and Limitations

It is appropriate to acknowledge real or potential drawbacks with this model. First, this design is ambitious and far-reaching. It will be more difficult to develop in the ambulatory and home care setting than in the institutional one.

Second, even though important progress has been made for inpatient hospital care, the data and methods to implement such a system today are inadequate or not easily transferable from other research applications. For instance, ways to collect appropriate outcome data efficiently, to adjust properly for risk and severity of illness, and to create distributions of providers by outcomes all need further development. It is this dearth of off-the-shelf methods applicable to a broad-scope quality assurance program that necessitates the 10-year implementation strategy we describe later in this chapter (and the research agenda offered in Chapter 11). The evolution of this model will require an extensive research and development phase, moving from such hospital-based conditions as fractured hips to outpatient conditions such as hypertension and congestive heart failure.

Third, any quality assurance system has the potential for "gaming" by providers; a program as invested in promoting internal quality improvement efforts as this one is more at risk for such gaming. For instance, patients may receive procedures or other services they do not need; their functioning after the service might be very good on occasion, skewing the overall outcome scores upward without taking the overuse of services into account. Relying on self-review, delegated review, and self-regulation are problematic approaches, and they deserve careful study.

Fourth, we have emphasized transition from a complex, poorly received program that currently relies on local organizations of varying effectiveness and reputation, rather than an abrupt shift to something completely new, because of the potential value of the expertise and inter-organizational relationships that already exist. Some critics may view this decision as the equivalent of pouring new wine into old wineskins, and that may prove to be true. We assume, however, that existing physician-based organizations can turn successfully to this new strategy more readily than completely new organizations can be invented.

Fifth, there is little experience to draw on to evaluate a program as complex and ambitious as this one. The program therefore runs a considerable risk of seeming to be ineffective, inefficient, and wasteful of society's dollars. The issues of gaming and lack of evaluation experience in particular point to a need for public oversight and rigorous evaluation and prompt us to recommend the expanded evaluation components described earlier.

Priority-Setting for MPAQ Resources

One charge to this committee was to develop criteria that could be used to set priorities in the allocation of resources, both funds and personnel, in reviewing and assuring quality of care. Resource needs can be expected to increase as the action plan for MPAQ is implemented. We propose that the following general criteria be considered in establishing the priorities for allocating resources for the Medicare quality assurance effort.

- The allocation of resources should reflect a balance between short-term and long-term goals.
- High priority should be given to strengthening the capacity of those assessing health care in two areas, detecting and correcting quality problems, as well as in continuously improving quality of care.
- Efforts to improve knowledge about and the performance of "change agents"—those persons, tools, and programs that make happen what has been identified as desirable or necessary if quality of care is to be improved—must be given early attention.
- Evaluation of all levels of MPAQ and MQROs must be given high priority from the start of the program.
- Resources should follow the need and the opportunity for impact. Rigid national formulae and regulations for reviewing care should be relaxed in favor of local decision making about the types of quality problems, the settings of care, and the systems of care that warrant most attention.
- Activities that support the infrastructure of the MPAQ and the MQROs should receive adequate and long-term sustaining resources. These include data collection, analysis, and feedback mechanisms.
- Adequate funding should be made available for the technical assistance aspects of the proposed program.

RESPONSIBILITIES AND TASKS OF THE MPAQ

PPS and Cost Containment

The MPAQ may continue in the short run to have Medicare program responsibilities beyond the quality assurance effort, because many functions now administered through the PRO program are related to the PPS reimbursement structure of Medicare. Although the committee has identified the lack of clarity in the mission of Medicare as a major issue, we also acknowledge some advantage in consolidating functions such as utilization review within the same operating program. We concluded that the MPAQ should have flexibility in determining to what extent the current non-quality-related review activities should be administered by its local MQROs, presumably retaining those that require clinical data expertise.

The issue of where utilization review should be conducted is a particularly difficult one. Many experts have the strong opinion that utilization review and quality assurance should be separated, so that no stigma of "cost containment" attaches to the organization chiefly responsible for quality assessment and assurance. Nevertheless, utilization review has always had a place in the quality assurance armamentarium. In some cases it may be virtually indistinguishable from quality assurance, as in the cases of prior authorization procedures that clearly forestall an unnecessary and potentially risky procedure or retrospective review efforts that identify poor medication-prescribing patterns.

The basic question is whether these activities should be split between two entities so as to avoid the conflict between cost control and quality assurance, or at a minimum whether the review function and payment decisions (or retrospective denials) functions should be separated. That is, should the nation incur the costs of a "double" review effort so as to preserve a desirable dividing line between cost containment and quality assurance? Should all prospective or retrospective utilization review be assigned to other entities, such as Medicare FIs or carriers? We conclude that those utilization review activities for which clinical (or peer) judgment is paramount, as well as those that clearly serve a quality-assurance role, should remain with the MPAQ (and the MQROs). Continued monitoring is needed, of course, to ensure an appropriate balance between a focus on overuse and a focus on underuse and poor performance in the overall process.

Program Planning For MQROs

Reconsideration of PRO Functions

The continued usefulness of several aspects of the present PRO program can be questioned (see Chapter 6 and Volume II, Chapter 8). In the fee-for-service sector, these review activities include several PPS-related activities such as diagnosis-related group (DRG) validation and physician attestation, day and cost outlier review, Medicare code editor review, and invasive procedure review. For the prepaid group practice sector, aspects of the PRO program warranting reconsideration include the three-level (limited, basic, and intensified) approach for reviewing risk-contract HMOs and competitive medical plans (CMPs) and the procedures for records and case selection.

Other issues should be considered in the early planning for MPAQ. One group of questions concerns quality measurement techniques to prevent and detect problems: (1) the reliability, validity, sensitivity, specificity, and feasibility of hospital generic screens; (2) the pending generic screens for nonhospital settings; and (3) the computerized screening algorithms for the Uniform Clinical Data Set (UCDS).

Another group of questions centers on the functions assigned to PROs, FIs, and carriers—in particular, the appropriate delegation of responsibility for utilization review whose chief aim is that of utilization or cost control rather than quality assessment. Questions related more to quality assurance include the following: (1) current approaches to corrective action and sanction options; (2) denials for substandard quality of care; and (3) consumer outreach and education that could be more efficiently accomplished on a national basis.

Cutting across all these issues are three broad problems: (1) the administrative procedures used by HCFA for funding and oversight of the MPAQ; (2) HCFA's survey and certification capability as it relates to Medicare Conditions of Participation; and (3) sharing data with voluntary accreditation groups, state boards of licensure, accreditation, and certification, and the National Practitioner Data Bank. As to sharing data, we urge that specific attention be given to how the data to be collected by hospitals for the Joint Commission (as part of its hospital-based Agenda for Change and clinical indicators projects) can be coordinated with or mapped to the data required by certain state data commissions and thence to data required for this quality assurance program. Much of this information is likely to be duplicative; at least for the hospital sector, we believe that it could be collected only once and put to multiple purposes.

Concerning the parts of the PRO program to retain or to phase out, a thorough review of current PRO program elements—in the context of our proposed MPAQ—is needed. We suggest that at an early stage HCFA should review, with the assistance of the National Council, the third PRO Scope of Work (SOW) and related contract modifications to determine what elements need to be deleted, modified, or expanded and what new elements must be added to facilitate a timely and efficient transition to MPAQ. Because of the singular importance of Congress in assigning tasks to the PRO (and now MPAQ) program, this review might be coordinated with the first meeting of the QualPAC, so that explicit advice to Congress about needed changes (additions or repeal) in existing legislation can be made. No changes to the third SOW should be made until that review is completed, except as necessary to conform to congressional legislation that may be enacted in the meantime and to enable existing PROs to conduct or finish certain pilot projects already underway in the areas of post-acute review, ambulatory care review, and small area analysis.

For assistance with this program review, the advice of QualPAC and the other Medicare commissions might be sought. This might be accomplished, for instance, through joint meetings. The agendas might include: (1) determining whether some of the activities related to PPS (e.g., DRG validation, monitoring of hospital notices of denials, and similar tasks) or to cost containment (e.g., prior authorization of services) are still needed, and (2) deciding whether the MPAQ and MQROs remain the proper sites for those activities.

MQRO Funding

Program planning depends heavily on the financing mechanism selected for MQROs. The contracting strategy for the PROs has become over-specified and rigid; it is not conducive to the long-term goals of this program. We advise that the MPAQ use a grant or cooperative agreement mechanism in preference to the current contracting approach.

In establishing program plans for MQROs, the MPAQ will need either to streamline its Request for Proposal/SOW efforts or to establish mechanisms by which it can design and publish grant or cooperative agreement solicitations. Some hybrid funding mechanisms might be developed, for instance with data collection per se being a contracted operation and innovative quality assurance efforts a cooperative agreement operation. In any case, the MPAQ should allow ample time for response from potential awardees (e.g., a minimum of 60 days).

The MPAQ should consider establishing standing review panels for evaluation of proposals. Such review panels might include individuals from outside HSQB, outside HCFA, and perhaps outside the federal government to ensure adequate representation of appropriate interested parties. For instance, the agencies or offices charged with the responsibility of outcomes and effectiveness research might be represented.

Clinical Conditions

As described more fully in the section on MQROs, we envision a considerably expanded data acquisition effort aimed at outcomes of care, use of services, and processes of care. With respect to the first, outcomes information should be related to important patient conditions and problems. In keeping with our desire to introduce more innovation and flexibility into the quality assurance effort, we do not believe that the national MPAQ should mandate all the patient conditions on which outcomes and other information should be collected. Rather, we propose a two-pronged approach: some "national" conditions on which all MQROs would collect and report data and some "MQRO-specific" (state-, locality-, or region-specific) conditions selected by the MQROs. Among those suggested later in this chapter, for instance, are major cardiovascular, pulmonary, and cerebrovascular conditions and surgical procedures common in the elderly population.

The MPAQ should establish and announce the criteria by which all conditions would be selected and choose a set, or sets, of national conditions according to those criteria. A crucial selection criterion might be high likelihood of quality-of-care problems. The MQROs should be expected to justify their choices of local conditions against the same criteria, and the MPAQ should have the right to disapprove MQRO choices.

In work for HCFA relating to the Effectiveness Initiative, the IOM used the following criteria in recommending key patient conditions for effectiveness and outcomes research: (1) high prevalence of the illness in the elderly population or in particular subgroups of the elderly; (2) burden of the illness on the elderly; (3) substantial variation in per-person use of services or in the outcomes of care for the condition (i.e., variation beyond that explained by differences in patient characteristics, severity of illness, or health resources in a geographic area); (4) relatively high costs to the Medicare program of reimbursing for condition-related diagnostic and therapeutic services; (5) existence of alternative strategies for managing the care of patients with the condition that are in dispute or reflect professional and clinical uncertainty; and (6) reasonable availability of data. The criteria for selecting conditions for quality review (e.g., in HMO ambulatory care) are also discussed in Chapter 6, Volume II. These or similar criteria might be used or adapted for the MPAQ effort.

Technical Assistance

MQROs will not necessarily have all the data collection, analysis, and reporting capabilities envisioned by this strategy, especially in the beginning. Thus, technical assistance will need to be available to them. High-priority areas for such aid would include: (1) identifying local patient conditions for outcomes follow-up; (2) developing ways (e.g., computer hardware, software, and criteria) to gather, analyze, and interpret data; (3) refining methods for timely feedback of constructive, comparative information; and (4) designing procedures and policies for triggering more intensive review of individual provider institutions.

Comprehensive assistance of this sort probably cannot be rendered directly by MPAQ personnel or by staff of DHHS regional offices. Thus, we suggest that one or more technical assistance contractors be engaged for this purpose (Table 12.3). Their principal job would be to provide standardized, state-of-the-art assistance to MQROs in all aspects of outcome and process-of-care measurements. In addition, these technical assistance bodies would undertake a major educational effort to assist the MQROs in assimilating in a timely fashion findings and products from the research community.

MQRO Evaluation

MQRO evaluation will probably require two components. First, we support continuation of multi-year funding for MQROs, but interim (e.g., annual) evaluation of progress and performance will be needed. Second, we have placed considerable emphasis on outcomes of care. Because MQROs will not be able to show instantaneous success, we believe that short-term progress and performance elements should also be built into the evaluation design.

A major task for the MPAQ at the outset will be to establish clear criteria by which MQRO performance will be evaluated. We advocate heavy emphasis on documentation of impact on quality of care and on the success with which MQROs foster the development of internal quality-assurance efforts by providers. Because one aim of our proposed program is to encourage diversity, objective evaluation of the MQROs using uniform "scales" cannot be the sole assessment technique. More implicit criteria, such as site visits by expert peer panels analogous to major grant reviews, may be more appropriate.

The evaluation criteria must place greatest emphasis on quality of care and performance and less emphasis on cost savings and on meeting specifications of financing instruments (such as precise numbers or timing of completed reviews). The MPAQ should seek assistance with the evaluation plan for MQROs from the National Council.

We do not minimize the legitimate concerns of the legislative and executive branches about the costs of the Medicare program. We have concluded, however, that evaluating the MPAQ and MQROs on the basis of how well they monitor the implementation of PPS or other radical changes in Medicare financing, or on how much money they save, would seriously distort the quality assessment and assurance goals of the program. Tracking the implications and actual effects of quality improvement on expenditures and costs remains an important component of program evaluation, but we are advocating a deliberate shift in the evaluation criteria of MPAQ away from dollar savings and toward quality improvement.

Special Factors Relating to the Elderly

Many ideas generated by this study are transferable or generalizable to other public sector programs such as Medicaid and to the private sector; we hope that will happen. Nevertheless, from the point of view of quality of care, the elderly are a special and often vulnerable group. Complex chronic health states, frailty, inability to gain access to needed care, isolation, and similar factors all have significant implications for undermining the quality of their health care. We believe, therefore, that the MPAQ should mount specific efforts to clarify what factors must be taken into account in designing and operating a quality assurance program that will meet the special needs of the elderly.

Public Oversight and Administrative Rulemaking

Our proposal calls for the MPAQ to be sensitive to several major issues: the burden of harm of poor quality; the effect of organization and financing on quality of care; the state of scientific knowledge; adversarial, punitive, and burdensome quality assurance activities; methods, tools, and interventions; clarity of goals; and resource availability. That agenda, plus the need for public input and oversight of a program as ambitious as this one, require that QualPAC and the National Council be kept informed of program plans.

More importantly, a formal advise-and-consent relationship needs to be established between either QualPAC or the National Council (or both) and the MPAQ for all major program decisions and regulations.

We also advise that formal public notice and rulemaking steps should be followed in MPAQ program planning. Guidance for this can be found in the rules of the Administrative Procedure Act and in recent recommendations of the Administrative Conference of the United States relating to the PRO program (as discussed in Chapter 6).

Data Analysis and Reporting

Because we give the MQROs the main responsibility for data collection, analysis, and use, that aspect of this strategy is described in the next section. Certain data, however, will be reported to the national MPAQ. These data should be designed to provide an "epidemiology" of quality-of-care problems for the Medicare population as a whole (which implies that the size of the MQRO areas should be large enough to develop reasonable estimates). Although the major source of information for the MPAQ will be data collected through the MQROs, we do not mean to constrain the MPAQ to just those data. For instance, it might be appropriate for the MPAQ to contract with the National Center for Health Statistics for population-based surveys that would supplement MQRO data.

One premise of our proposed model is that the MPAQ exemplify activities and performance expected of MQROs. Hence, the MPAQ should report on patterns of high use of apparently inappropriate or unnecessary care. It should identify health problems or geographic areas in which beneficiaries appear to be receiving too little care. This underuse may arise from Medicare benefit, coverage, and reimbursement policies, its own or others' utilization management and prior authorization efforts, or independent provider decision making. It should also support analyses intended to clarify the types of technical and interpersonal care problems that most frequently arise across the country. Analyses in all three areas would give explicit attention to beneficiary characteristics, such as degree of frailty, geographic area, income, race, and ethnicity.

Information on this epidemiology of quality problems will be disseminated in four ways: to DHHS officials, to QualPAC, to the provider community, and to the public. The level of aggregation of the information would differ, in accordance with existing rules of confidentiality and privacy and in accordance with the uses to which the information would be put.

RESPONSIBILITIES AND TASKS OF THE MQROs

Overall, our program attempts to reinforce the belief that quality assurance belongs primarily in the province of the professional and the provider organization and only secondarily (or in the face of failure of the professional or the organization) in the province of the external review agent. To this end, we have designed an oversight function for the MQROs that rests heavily on data collection, analysis, and feedback. We emphasize, however, that our strategy assumes a long developmental period in which several operational options might be tested. Details in the remainder of this section are intended to illustrate possible options.

General Points

Four Assumptions

First, different types of efforts will be needed for hospital episodes (including post-acute care), for physician office-based care, and for other services such as home care. Second, we see the data collection and analyses efforts taking place in "cycles," for instance, three-month follow-up periods for hospital care. Third, we believe that fee-for-service and prepaid group practice review should be made as alike as possible, and thus we make no major distinctions here about how such review, data collection, or analysis should proceed. Prepaid group practice settings and some large multispecialty clinics lead the typical fee-for-service office-based setting in ambulatory care review. The MPAQ might therefore apply techniques from the private sector group practice experience to the fee-for-service arena, rather than develop completely independent ambulatory care review systems de novo. Fourth, we expect that some form of peer review will always be needed, regardless of how successfully MPAQ moves to outcome measurement or how effective provider-based continuous quality improvement programs become. The criticisms of the PROs' peer review capabilities (discussed in Chapter 6), however, will have to be satisfactorily resolved.

Types of Data

Information collected and used by both the external program (MPAQ and the MQROs) and internal quality assurance programs should include structure, process, and outcome variables. We expect these to be defined in part to reflect the unique health care needs of the elderly.

Structural variables. We view structural data as less important than either process or outcome data. Their main use is to reflect the organization's capacity to deliver high-quality care, documented through its own quality-improvement systems or reflected in information about licensing, certification, and accreditation. Structural information will, however, always have a place in quality assurance. Therefore, we suggest that the MPAQ have a more decisive role in setting Medicare Conditions of Participation and in determining whether provider organizations have met those conditions. One condition should be that the organization has a viable internal quality assurance program that can document solutions to important quality problems. Information from MQROs should contribute to those determinations.

Process-of-care information. For quality assurance purposes, information on the process of care is central. It is required for: (1) documenting continuity of care across settings and among providers; (2) detecting and verifying problems of overuse of services; (3) identifying populations having difficulty gaining access to care or otherwise facing problems of underuse of services; and (4) pinpointing cases of obviously poor performance.

Process information may indicate the reasons for those problems, which can range from Medicare program policies and financial incentives, resource constraints, and cost-containment efforts, to deteriorating practitioner knowledge or technical skills. Examining the process of care will also be important for those providers identified as having poor outcomes. Presumably, by correcting processes of care they know to be deficient, they can improve those outcomes. Finally, process data point to inappropriate, unnecessary, and poor care, especially in situations in which outcomes are not a good measure (e.g., ambulatory care for acute ailments).

We have emphasized patient and clinician decision making in our conceptual model. Assessment of this activity clearly belongs more to the provider organization and its internal quality improvement program than to the federal Medicare program and the MQROs. The practical consequence of this is to place the bulk of the process measurement effort on the internal programs. An important aspect of this will be to ensure that such internal data collection serves as many purposes simultaneously as possible—that is, the needs of the organization and those of external quality assurance bodies.

There are instances, however, in which the MQROs might conduct their own process-of-care evaluations. The first instance is in serious cases of poor performance of those providers monitored chiefly by outcomes, at least (or especially) when such providers voluntarily seek such outside help and technical assistance. The second is in routine collection of process data for all providers, so that information on the process-outcome links can be expanded.

The third instance is when individuals or agencies file complaints about providers. Some quality assurance groups have found this a productive way to identify quality problems (especially those of poor technical or interpersonal practices). Furthermore, it helps to meet the MPAQ's responsibility to maintain constructive relationships with the patient community.

The fourth instance is in evaluating ambulatory care, such as that delivered in physician office-based practice, where process measures are presently the main assessment tool. For this last case in particular, the MQROs will need to develop special approaches. Process-of-care management is one area where the technical assistance function will be crucial.

Outcomes data. Both external and internal quality assurance efforts should involve a broad set of health status outcomes. In keeping with our focus on desired health outcomes, we suggest that all major domains of health status and quality of life, such as physical, mental, and social functioning and satisfaction with care (Chapter 2), should be included. Data should be sought from the four sources discussed below (under Sources of Data). It is in this realm that we see a greatly expanded need for obtaining data directly from enrollees (both users and nonusers of care) concerning expectations about care, preferences for outcomes, actual outcomes, and satisfaction.

To use patient outcomes in a quality assurance program, they must bear some demonstrable relationship to process of care. Such relationships, however, are not well documented in the clinical or quality-of-care literature. Although the volume of clinical data may be very large, most experts identify the process-outcome link as a very weak link indeed in the quality assurance chain. This may indicate that much of the poor care identified by process criteria is not accompanied by poor outcomes, at least in the short run, although such care still needs to be improved.

Use of services data. The MQROs will collect (or acquire from other public agencies or private sector bodies) information on population-based rates of use of services. These will be aggregated at the local level into profiles for categories of enrollees (e.g., the very old, those enrolled in capitated systems, or those residing in underserved areas) and for providers. MQROs will report data to the MPAQ, so that population-based rates of utilization can be aggregated and analyzed at the national level, in particular when categories of enrollees are too small in number to support significant analysis by a given MQRO.

Sources of Data

We see four main sources of information: (1) administrative data bases; (2) medical charts and similar records; (3) providers; and (4) Medicare enrollees. For instance, the administrative or insurance claims data banks will be a good (necessary, but not sufficient) source of information about use of services. Medical chart information will be gathered by the provider or the MQROs, or both, after care is rendered; in the future, such information might also be forwarded electronically when computerized medical records are widely available.

Information on patient outcomes will usually involve direct contact with physicians, patients, or proxies by questionnaire, telephone, or direct interview. It may also come from tracking administrative records for evidence of later use of services, institutionalization, or death.

Clinical information needed for case-adjustment might be taken from hospital discharge data sets mandated at the state level, the Joint Commission's clinical indicators, or the Medicare UCDS. The MPAQ might differ from the UCDS effort in two ways. First, the chart abstracting or data reporting would stop short of the very large number of elements now in the UCDS. Second, MPAQ would emphasize a different selection of cases. For instance, it might expand the random and the disease- or condition-specific case selection and reduce the emphasis on abstracting cases that PROs review for reasons only tangential to quality or outcomes.

Overview of Data Collection and Analysis

We foresee two parallel review efforts, defined mainly by setting of care. One major form of review focuses on services provided by hospitals, quasi-inpatient facilities, such as ambulatory surgery clinics, and institutions and agencies that render posthospital care. The other major form of review focuses on office-based ambulatory care. In what follows, the details should be taken as illustrative, not prescriptive.

Topics for Review: Conditions and Sentinel Events

In keeping with our focus on three categories of quality problems—poor technical care, overuse, and underuse—we suggest that MQROs might study several "tracers" or "conditions" per category. For instance, if nine review conditions were to be studied, three might be selected nationally and the remainder locally. More (or fewer) conditions might be studied in any review cycle, depending on the extent of the problems expected or the length of time needed for adequate outcomes data collection.

Conditions. Selection of tracers or conditions by a given MQRO would be based on input from local providers in accordance with priorities set by the MPAQ and the National Council. Guidance from QualPAC, on the basis of its analyses of national data, might also be sought. Among the types of conditions warranting systematic follow-up of outcomes of inpatient or surgical care are hip fracture and hip replacement, cerebrovascular diseases such as stroke, cardiovascular and pulmonary problems such as acute myocardial infarction, chronic obstructive pulmonary disease, and congestive heart failure, and cataract removal and lens implantation. Some MQROs might elect to study elective procedures widely subjected to prior authorization.

Among diagnoses that might be considered for ambulatory care review are highly prevalent chronic illnesses such as hypertension, arthritis, and heart disease. Other conditions are those that, with adequate ambulatory care, should not result in hospitalizations for their own complications. For example, appropriate care for diabetes should forestall hospitalization for diabetic ketoacidosis, although it would not necessarily be expected to forestall hospitalization for atherosclerotic complications.

Sentinel events. In addition to the nationally and locally defined conditions, sentinel events might serve as indicators of possible problems. Criteria to guide the selection of sentinel events include: (1) sensitivity to identifying problems of overuse, underuse, and poor technical care for Medicare enrollees; (2) appropriateness for the health care setting under review; and (3) expected burden of harm of each of the three types of problems for a given setting.

The MPAQ, with guidance from the National Council, could develop optional sentinel events from which MQROs might elect a minimum number. MQROs might also be able to propose local sentinel events as triggers for all providers in their jurisdiction. Complaints to MQROs might also serve as possible triggers. MQROs would be encouraged to work with institutional providers and specialty groups to conduct ad hoc studies to expand the knowledge base on the sensitivity, specificity, reliability, and validity of both sentinel events and outcome measures.

Hospital and Other Inpatient Episodes

In keeping with our concerns about coordination of care and a desired focus on episodes of care, we propose that the MQROs begin their oversight and monitoring with hospital and other quasi-inpatient episodes. By this we mean an index admission to a hospital or an ambulatory surgical clinic plus all post-discharge care rendered by home health agencies, nursing homes, and other facilities (e.g., the hospital or clinic). An example of how information on outcomes, process of care, and certain other variables (e.g., severity of illness) might be collected and analyzed follows.

Example. On a periodic basis, the MQRO would receive from hospitals, ambulatory surgical centers, home health agencies, and post-acute care nursing homes basic administrative data on all discharged Medicare patients who meet the condition-specific or sentinel-event criteria. Approximately three months after discharge, the MQRO would follow up by telephone or possibly by face-to-face interview; either all or specified samples of patients would be contacted. Special procedures would be adopted for review of care of patients who had died in the interim and for those who could not be located. (To the extent that providers could perform this function in a verifiable way, the MQRO could receive information from providers rather than collect it themselves.)

The interview would obtain three major types of outcomes data: (1) symptoms and general health status (i.e., functioning) before the health care encounter; (2) the same information at the time of the interview; and (3) satisfaction with the health care encounter. Included in this interview might be items intended to elicit patients' values or preferences for their levels of health status before and after the health care encounter.

At some point during that three-month period, the MQRO (or provider) would abstract the medical chart to obtain information on general health and functional status on admission and discharge, key indicators of severity, process-of-care measures, and the appropriateness of admission and of any procedures. Similar medical record data would also be collected for all patients not otherwise accounted for above (e.g., those who had been discharged dead or those lost to follow-up).

After this data collection process has been completed for, say, a 12-month period (e.g., four cycles of three months each), the MQRO would analyze the data. (Interim aggregation and analysis could be conducted, especially if the particular condition or sentinel event under study is a long-term review topic.) Specifically, the MQRO might use information from the telephone or personal interviews to construct an observed quality outcome score and information from chart review to develop an expected quality outcome score. The MQRO might then develop an expected probability of a specific outcome for each reviewed patient; from these scores, condition- or event-specific observed-to-expected ratios or profiles could be calculated for providers. Ultimately, the MQRO might be able to aggregate profiles for a given provider into global performance profiles.

Home Health Care

We recommend that MQROs monitor the care rendered by home health agencies to all elderly clients, not just to those who become home health care recipients after discharge from a hospital or ambulatory surgical clinic. Data collection and analysis could mimic procedures given in the hospital example above (e.g., health and functional status, satisfaction, indicators of severity, and process measures when home health care is started and periodically thereafter). Because there is so little experience in this area, however, we believe that a significant pilot-testing effort will be needed.

This is an area where outcomes—health status and satisfaction—are particularly important. Several groups are working on various outcome measures for home health care, and the Uniform Needs Assessment Instrument may be useful in this enterprise (see Volume II, Chapter 6 for more discussion). Thus, we would expect the MQRO effort to draw heavily on the experiences and instruments now in various stages of development and testing.

Ambulatory Care

Both overuse and underuse of services are of concern in the physician-office setting. In addition, this setting has its share of technical and interpersonal problems. To tackle all these problems requires both provider-oriented and patient-oriented information, which implies that information should be obtained from physicians, office charts, and patients.

We know far less about methods for reviewing the quality of care in the ambulatory setting than those for inpatient care. In the coming years, information from PRO pilot projects, HMO experiences, and research and demonstration studies focusing on outcomes management in ambulatory care should help to close that gap. In addition, some existing assessment methods might now be used to monitor overuse and underuse of outpatient surgery. Thus, within a few years we believe that MQROs will be in a better position to expand their oversight and monitoring responsibilities to the physician's office. Some illustrative steps are suggested below.

Example. Medical record information might be abstracted on-site (in cycles of perhaps once or twice a year). In later years, chart-based information might be available electronically from the physician's office. Both outcome and process-of-care measures would be relevant. Generic health measures, such as functioning and well-being, would be emphasized given the high prevalence of chronic conditions among the elderly seeking office-based care; health status assessment surveys might be completed on-site with a lap-top computer.

To address our concerns with technical and interpersonal skills, process measures need to be developed that reflect clinical issues, patient participation in decision making, adherence to agreed-on regimens, and satisfaction. Some of these data would be obtained through patient interviews, perhaps scheduled to correspond to the cycles for medical record abstraction. The selection of process measures must take into account the complexity of care frequently received by the elderly. Less emphasis would be placed on specific actions or interventions and more emphasis on processes that relate to primary and secondary disease prevention, counseling, continuity and coordination of care, pain reduction and other quality-of-life dimensions, reinforcement of dignity and independent functioning, and "interactive" issues such as multiple medications, diet, and nutrition.

Self-administered practitioner questionnaires (for, e.g., physicians or nurse practitioners) might be used for periodic data collection on practice patterns. Data might include many of the same elements that previous studies have indicated to be relevant to outcome. Among these are referral and consultant patterns, preventive care and patient education programs, access to facilities and to technologies such as x-ray and laboratory services, satisfaction with one's practice, and the availability and use of community-based nonmedical support services.

Medicare Part B (Supplementary Medical Insurance) files may also provide data to the MQROs for use in developing profiles of ambulatory services utilization by community or population subgroups. Such data might identify indicators for more intensive data collection efforts. Coverage of outpatient prescription drugs would mean that "Part C" files would also be a valuable source of quality information. For instance, models already exist to use drug tracers to identify potential complications or interactions of medications.[2]

To the extent that data collection focuses on an episode of care, the analysis provides a better understanding of the quality of the ambulatory care. As advances are made in the knowledge base on the link between process and outcome in the ambulatory setting and as ambulatory management information systems improve, the major target of analysis might be patient-physician decision making, using criteria mapping and algorithms that include patient preferences. MQROs should work closely with the health care community in interpreting such data, in particular for solo practitioners or small groups for whom the MQROs' analyses may be a major source of information for improving performance in physicians' offices.

Overview of Feedback, Data Reporting, and Data Sharing

Feedback

Feedback and data reporting have three primary dimensions: information made available to internal quality assurance programs and practitioners, to the public, and to policymakers. Although making data available in a timely way to the latter audiences (data reporting) is an important goal, we believe that designing effective mechanisms for giving information back to practitioners and provider institutions (feedback) is central to our proposed quality assurance program. Thus, we advise that the MPAQ give considerable attention at the outset to testing various options for provider feedback.

Example. The MPAQ, through the MQROs, should plan and test models for feedback of patient outcome and process-of-care data to practitioners and providers. These models should yield reliable, valid information on individuals or institutions that permits comparisons with peer groups; the information should be timely; and it should be presented in an easy-to-interpret manner. Because feedback is so important to an efficient and effective quality assurance program, we believe that such models should be developed and tested according to rigorous scientific standards. Implementation of all feedback and data-reporting mechanisms for the entire MPAQ program might, in fact, be delayed until such testing has occurred and until the QualPAC has had an opportunity to review and comment.

Data Reporting and Public Disclosure

A major principle of the MPAQ is that reliable, valid, and useful data ought to be available to or placed in the public domain. A corollary is that misleading information and poorly presented data are harmful to providers and, ultimately, to the public. We take the position that forestalling the latter takes precedence over accomplishing the former.

Example. Each MQRO might release selected information on providers to the public, initially perhaps on only a few procedures or outcomes. Eventually, they might well release information that gives distributions or rankings of providers.

We have specified neither the criteria for release of performance information to the public nor the procedures for MQROs to follow. Much depends on the technology of quality measurement and assurance methods— the reliability and validity of outcome measures, for instance, and the adequacy of case-mix and severity adjustors. The credibility and usefulness of these data must be thoroughly established. Moreover, providers must be given the opportunity and the necessary time to review and act creatively and responsibly on such information before its release.

The MPAQ should develop procedures and timeframes to be followed by MQROs before the public release of information. The advice of the QualPAC and the National Council should be sought in this effort. Such procedures might specify different timetables depending on whether the ratings or rankings are positive or negative. "Good news" (i.e., for those providers determined to be exemplary) might be released fairly quickly, whereas "bad news" (i.e., for poor quality providers) might be held to give them a reasonable amount of time to undertake changes to improve performance.

Example. The MPAQ might set in place a mechanism for regularly disseminating aggregate analyses on, say, the use of services by beneficiary groups to policymakers, legislators, and the public. This might include the mandated impact report delivered biennially to Congress, but many other options might be considered, including routine publication of utilization data in a manner similar to the *Vital and Health Statistics* series of the National Center of Health Statistics. Such reports should address both overuse and underuse of services as national data on quality problems become available. The information should be presented in a format that provides state-level analyses when possible. Because a separate DHHS agency has been charged with the development and promulgation of practice guidelines, the MPAQ might also make its information available as necessary to that agency.

Data Sharing

Related to data reporting and feedback is data sharing, which attempts to make use of the range of public- and private-sector quality review and improvement efforts in ways that minimize duplicative data collection and reporting. Any program as obviously data-intensive as this one risks duplicating the data collection, analysis, and reporting efforts of internal programs themselves and of other external efforts, particularly those of the accrediting bodies and state agencies.

We propose that considerable efforts be made to enable these groups to share quality-related information so that duplication of effort and waste of resources can be minimized. This explicitly includes sharing information and experiences across MQROs, between major units of HCFA and within HSQB (e.g., between the Office of Research and Demonstrations and HSQB, and between the offices in HSQB responsible for MQROs and those responsible for survey and certification), between HCFA and the Joint Commission, and between HCFA (or the MQROs) and state agencies. The laws and regulations governing release of peer review and other quality-related data (e.g., those from state-mandated data commissions and those collected under the auspices of the Health Care Quality Improvement Act) appear to be unclear, possibly contradictory, or open to interpretation. Thus, we believe that a careful review of the relevant statutes, regulations, and case law is needed.

Public Disclosure Versus Confidentiality and Privacy

The issues of protecting raw data, certain research data, peer-review deliberations, and the like from disclosure via the Freedom of Information Act are extremely complex. Despite our support for the principle of public disclosure, we believe that this subject deserves full examination at a national level, perhaps by QualPAC or an outside institution.

Overview of Quality Interventions

Performance Profiles

MQROs might aggregate outcome and process-of-care data into performance indicators or profiles for individual providers for feedback and data reporting. The example we used earlier was observed-to-expected ratios for outcomes measures, but many other possibilities exist. The structure, content, scoring, and interpretation of such profiles should be thoroughly tested and reviewed by QualPAC, the National Council, and the technical assistance contractors before final promulgation.

Quality Interventions

With respect to quality interventions, the MPAQ (and hence the MQROs) will be confronted with a dilemma. They must balance the need for predictable and equitable intervention strategies for all providers with an emphasis on local decision making, flexible response to different problems, and support for emerging internal quality improvement programs. This dilemma becomes especially acute when the main focus of a quality assurance program is on outcomes of care, and especially when outcomes attempt to take patient values and preferences into account.

Our basic position is that the MPAQ will need to articulate explicit bases or common factors for choosing among intervention options and then leave individual decisions to MQROs. In theory, our approach would not be very different from the PRO program's present quality intervention plan (Chapter 6). It gives broad authority for many different types of interventions—from notification of concern about a quality problem through mandated continuing medical education of many sorts, to intensified review, and finally to various legal and financial sanctions. Issues concerning the current PRO and OIG sanctioning process will need to be addressed, however.

In practice, not all the operational components of the PRO program (such as severity levels or weighted triggers for quality interventions) would necessarily be retained indefinitely. Other innovative interventions should be developed. Options for dealing with outlier providers should be strengthened (e.g., mandated consultations for certain clinical problems). More important are efforts to assist internal quality assurance programs to handle their own problems and to find ways to stimulate improvement across the broad spectrum of practitioners and providers.

In other words, MQROs would ultimately have a clear set of options (established through a rulemaking process) and clear directions on how to select among them. With our emphasis on local decision making and flexibility, we expect that different MQROs might well adopt different interventional and correctional approaches, but they would have to do so within well-defined guidelines.

In our view, innovative options for responding to quality problems have not been fully developed by any federal quality assurance program. Virtually no good strategies for working with quality distributions exist, certainly none that relate to health outcomes of the sort advocated in this proposed program or to organizations that are attempting to implement continuous quality improvement models. For that reason, we suggest that some demonstrations or quasi-experiments be conducted to explore the feasibility and effectiveness of various approaches that MQROs might take to quality interventions.

Example. In the event of poor scores on the performance profiles or a single egregious problem, one local MQRO might simply notify the provider, agency, or practice group to suggest some first-order responses. If these seem appropriate and later data indicate a satisfactory resolution, no further MQRO action would be needed. If no correction is evidenced, then the MQRO would intervene more directly, first by taking on many of the actions normally reserved to the internal quality mechanism and then by using stronger remedies (such as stiff sanctions) for uncorrected problems.

Example. A different MQRO might establish the policy of requiring all providers ranked in the lowest third of a quality distribution to adopt a six-month corrective action. This MQRO would evaluate those providers carefully at the end of that six-month period. It might also conduct a 100-percent concurrent review for all providers ranked in the lowest sixth of the quality distribution, using explicit process measures and instruments approved by MPAQ and the National Council.

Sanctions

We recognize the need for continuance of a sanctioning authority for MPAQ and MQROs. Sanctions (e.g., exclusions and monetary penalties) are a topic of considerable debate as this report is being prepared (Chapter 6). We have adopted no formal position on these issues except to note the conclusions in Chapter 6 that generally support the recommendations of the Administrative Conference of the United States. The many obstacles to broadening the options for sanctions, maintaining equity across types of providers, and otherwise strengthening this aspect of the MPAQ's and MQROs' response to intractable quality programs deserve a separate, in-depth examination, perhaps by QualPAC or another outside body.

IMPLEMENTATION STRATEGY AND PHASES

This section outlines proposed steps in a 10-year implementation strategy; the timeframe is fiscal year (FY) 1991 to FY 2000. We divide this strategy into three phases and identify basic tasks in those phases (Table 12.4). Many steps imply ongoing activities; when this is so, we identify the step at the time we would expect it to begin and do not necessarily follow it through the full implementation period. Special projects, studies, and activities begun in Phase II may well continue into Phase III. As with other parts of this chapter, details should be considered illustrative, not prescriptive.

Phase I: Years 1 and 2

Establish the MPAQ and its Adjuncts

Congress and DHHS should establish the MPAQ. Necessary steps include adopting Recommendation nos. 1 to 5, providing the appropriate authorizations and appropriations for the MPAQ and QualPAC, staffing QualPAC and the National Council, and detailed program planning for MQROs.

TABLE 12.4 Overview of Implementation Activities, by Phase

Phase	Activity
Phase I: Years 1 and 2	Establish MPAQ,[a] MQROs,[b] QualPAC,[c] and National Council for Medicare Quality Assurance
	Start program evaluation activities and appoint Technical Advisory Panel (TAP)
	Review existing PRO program features and Conditions of Participation
	Begin long-term research and capacity-building efforts
Phase II: Years 3 to 8	Design and test approaches for data collection, data analysis, and information dissemination
	Conduct special projects on
	Quality distributions
	Improve average level of performance and foster continuing improvement models
	Incentives for good and exemplary performance
	Responses to outliers
Phase III: Years 9 and 10	Move to full implementation based on outcomes of work in Phase II
	Continue public oversight, program evaluation, research, and capacity building

[a]Medicare Program to Assure Quality
[b]Medicare Quality Review Organizations
[c]Quality Program Advisory Commission

Steps to improve the public oversight and evaluation of the program should be initiated.

Evaluation

Planning for MPAQ evaluation activities should begin in Phase I. Congress or DHHS, or both, should articulate MPAQ goals in legislation or official policy (Recommendation no. 2), which would be used as the criteria against which the MPAQ should be evaluated. Fundamental changes in the organization or financing of health services for the elderly may have a significant impact on quality and should be included in the evaluation. If the office assigned the MPAQ evaluation responsibility calls on a TAP to assist in the planning, implementation, and documentation of periodic MPAQ evaluations, the TAP would be appointed in this phase.

We have advised that this evaluation component include a periodic report from the Secretary of DHHS to Congress on implementation of MPAQ and on the success of MPAQ in meeting its goals. Thus, planning for the first impact report to Congress should begin early in Phase I, and the first report should be delivered during Phase I (Recommendation no. 6). As a rule, we would expect this report to be related to the goals of the MPAQ. Because we are concerned about the dangers of premature evaluation, however, we suggest that the first such report cover only the progress of implementing MPAQ.

Other Activities

Several other program planning and implementation tasks would begin in Phase I. Among them are the review of current PRO program activities and the changes suggested with respect to hospital Conditions of Participation (Recommendation no. 7). The shift from contracting to a grant or cooperative agreement mechanism (or hybrid mechanisms) would start in this phase.

We have advocated strong support for research in the area of quality assessment and assurance and in related subjects. We have also argued for a much more forceful effort at capacity building. Work in this area should be started in this phase, although because we see it as needing to outlast the implementation of MPAQ, we discuss these topics more fully in the section on Phase III, below.

Phase II: Years 3 Through 8

The middle phase of implementation involves data collection, analysis, information dissemination, and special projects. These activities focus on the design, testing, and implementation of major components of the MPAQ model. We assume that these activities would be started in the second or third year of the MPAQ and generally would take anywhere from three to six years to complete. We assume further that the best of the approaches would then be incorporated into the full MPAQ in Phase III.

Data Collection

The importance to this Medicare quality assurance program (and to the Medicare program more broadly) of a greatly enhanced data base on use of services, patient outcomes, and the process of care is difficult to overstate. To create and maintain such an information base, only the foundations of which are in place, and to make it useful for assuring the quality of health care for the elderly over the long run is a massive undertaking. Because the development and testing of such a system is necessarily evolutionary and must be responsive to environmental and technical factors, putting this data collection effort in place can be expected to take the middle part of this 10-year strategy.

Design and implementation of the data-collection efforts would focus on use of services, processes of care, and patient outcomes, as discussed in earlier sections of this chapter. Detailed action plans for this work might be developed with the guidance (or advice and consent) of the National Council and QualPAC. Research or demonstration projects could be conducted as needed.

Data Analysis Capabilities

The data analysis capabilities for MPAQ exceed those available in contemporary quality assurance programs, both public and private. Thus, HCFA will need to begin early in this phase to expand and improve its internal data analysis capacity and, more importantly, the data-analysis capacity of the MQROs. Specific attention should be given to strengthening several key elements, especially analytic personnel and computer capability. The technical assistance effort—that is, using outside expert consultants on an advisory or contractual basis—would be implemented in Phase II.

Information Dissemination

Our proposed program calls for a sophisticated approach to feeding useful clinical practice and quality-related information back to practitioners and provider institutions of all types. Few good models of such feedback loops exist in contemporary quality assurance programs. Therefore, Phase II activities would include considerable efforts to design and test such models, which would be coordinated with the data collection and analysis projects.

Compared with research and demonstration projects concerning feedback to providers, we see less need for projects related to public release of information or to data sharing. These are as much policy issues as technical ones. Some formal, external studies of these issues might be undertaken during this phase, with a focus on their legal, regulatory, and policy ramifications.

Special Projects

Distinguishing providers on the basis of quality and outcomes. If MQROs are to be able to respond differently to providers according to their performance in rendering superior, acceptable, or only poor care, they have to be able to create "quality distributions" of providers. To overcome the conceptual, practical, and political difficulties implied by this aspect of the program, we recommend that DHHS sponsor or conduct a series of studies to test different methods of creating quality distributions for the major types of Medicare providers. Such analyses should be conducted by or with the assistance of outside experts in the appropriate research fields. The final choices as to what types of methods would eventually be used should not be made until the QualPAC has had the opportunity to review and comment.

Improving the average level of performance. Improving average performance (shifting the curve) is critical to the MPAQ; so is fostering better internal, organization-based quality assurance programs. Because this is such a new area, various research, demonstration, and pilot projects will be needed during Phase II. These studies might be (1) done through joint efforts of the MQROs and individual providers, (2) focused on geriatric-specific quality concerns, (3) be community-wide, and (4) involve several providers in either similar or different care settings. Existing PRO pilot projects could be absorbed into this program.

Incentives for good and exemplary performance. Early in Phase II, the MPAQ should study ways to identify and reward both good and exemplary (or superior) providers. Lowering the amount of intrusive external review to which good providers are subjected is the probable first step. Other incentives to be investigated might include publishing superior rankings, awarding special recognition for performance and innovation, selective contracting, and sharing information on exemplary providers with private third-party purchasers. No incentive plan would be put in place until the QualPAC has had an opportunity for review and comment.

Dealing with outliers. At some point, providers not meeting criteria for satisfactory performance on the quality indicators will have to be subjected to more intensive review and other quality interventions, as they are now.

A mechanism would also be devised for real-time intervention in the event of catastrophic malfeasance or poor performance. Special attention needs to be given to how the MPAQ and MQROs should respond to very poor performance because of the decentralized nature of this program.

Phase III: Years 9 and 10

Our goal is a functioning quality assurance program at the end of this 10-year period, one that can respond creatively to changing environmental circumstances. Some of these circumstances can be foreseen (even if their particulars cannot be specified), such as a larger and older elderly population and different Medicare payment systems. Others are a matter of speculation, such as the strength of the nation's economy.

Most of the reforms suggested for the first two phases of this implementation strategy are intended to provide a firm foundation for this program. They will take several years to implement fully; most should be completed by Phase III, so that they can be folded into a fully operational program over the last two years of the implementation strategy. In Phase III, we would expect to see a shift from demonstrations to implementation, continued improvement in quality of care and in the conduct of quality assurance, and a major reassessment to determine if the MPAQ is on target.

We discuss four other topics for Phase III—public oversight of the Medicare quality assurance effort, program evaluation, research, and capacity building—because of their very broad and long-range public policy implications. Although activities in these areas are expected to start in Phase I, we emphasize here the need for steady investment by DHHS because of the broad nature of the work and the larger policy implications for the Department.

Public Oversight

A consistent theme in this report has been engagement of patients and consumers in quality assurance. A corollary is that the public is entitled to have some voice about public monies spent on quality assurance programs and to bring quality-related problems to the policymakers' attention.

We have implicitly invested these responsibilities in QualPAC, but all facets of the Medicare program should be represented. Therefore, we suggest that efforts be coordinated among all the Medicare Commissions (especially ProPAC, PPRC, and QualPAC), to avoid duplication of effort and forestall major policy gaps. Among the issues that might be monitored is the likelihood and severity of quality problems confronting the MPAQ as reimbursement mechanisms and Medicare benefits change over the 1990s, but other issues may well arise.

To accomplish this coordination, Congress might direct that the Commissions meet jointly, say once every other year, in addition to or as part of their regularly scheduled meetings. This could be done as a single three-party meeting or as a series of meetings between the QualPAC and another Commission on a rotating basis. Other coordinating efforts, such as staff communications, should also be encouraged.

Evaluation of the MPAQ

We strongly emphasized rigorous program evaluation in this report. To this end, we suggested that HCFA devise and test various program evaluation activities in Phases I and II, including ways to assess the cost-effectiveness of a quality assurance program. This effort goes beyond evaluating the success of individual MQROs and focuses on the program itself, not on its agents.

By Phase III, a formal, operational program evaluation effort (outside the MPAQ) should be in place. Approximately 1 percent of the monies appropriated for the MPAQ program itself might be directed to this evaluation effort.

Research

Success for this proposed program depends heavily on adequate testing of many different models for data collection, analysis, and feedback. We expect that some of this will be done through MPAQ and the MQROs. A goodly portion would be done by other research and demonstration mechanisms available to HCFA and DHHS.

We wish to emphasize the need for continued, indeed expanded, research on certain other topics (as outlined in Chapter 11), even as we acknowledge the attention that Congress has very recently drawn to this area. Priorities for steady long-term research support that are not subsumed in the special projects and other efforts discussed specifically for MPAQ include at least the following areas: (1) variations, effectiveness, and appropriateness of clinical interventions; (2) practice guidelines and the mechanisms by which they can be developed, refined, disseminated, and updated; (3) measures of the technical and interpersonal aspects of the process of care; (4) measures of health status and health-related quality of life; (5) methods for changing provider and practitioner habits, behaviors, and performance including those related to continuous quality improvement; (6) data and information management systems; and (7) program evaluation.

Capacity Building: Supporting the Field of Quality Assurance

If quality assurance is to move forward forcefully, it will require a corps of professionals prepared to provide both technical skills and leadership.

At present we lack an adequate number of such professionals to staff a national set of organizations. An early priority must therefore be to establish training programs to prepare these health professionals. The educational programs would likely require a year of study and could be built on existing programs in epidemiology, health services research, and biostatistics.

Two approaches must be pursued. First, education for existing staffs and those senior professionals already in or about to enter this work will have to use techniques of intensive continuing education and technical assistance. Second, more organized programs of training with field experience will be needed to prepare a new cadre of health workers with the tools needed to collect and apply information based on outcomes in quality assurance. Attention to the tools employed in continuous quality improvement is warranted.

Resources will be needed to underwrite the curriculum development and to support the education of these professionals. Especially because many will be asked to forego more lucrative professional activities, support for the educational programs other than traditional tuition will be necessary. Ways to make quality assurance more of a profession with a clear career path should be developed. As with the research effort, this work must be carried on well after MPAQ implementation has ended.

SUMMARY

This chapter has presented our strategy for a quality review and assurance program for Medicare. The new program, which this strategy aims to have in place by the year 2000, is intended to respond to several major issues

- the burdens of harm of poor quality of care (poor personal performance, unnecessary and inappropriate services, and lack of needed and appropriate services);
- difficulties and incentives presented by the organization and financing of health care;
- the state of scientific knowledge;
- the problems of adversarial, punitive, and burdensome quality assurance activities;
- the federal role in quality assurance;
- the adequacy of quality review and assurance methods and tools;
- the tension between dealing with outliers and improving the average;
- the clarity of goals of a quality assurance program for Medicare; and
- the human and financial resources for quality assurance.

Our proposed program will evolve from the present Medicare PRO program but will have several different emphases. It will focus far more directly on quality assurance, it will cover all major settings of care, and it will emphasize both a wide range of patient outcomes and the process of care. It will also have a greatly expanded program evaluation component and greater public oversight and accountability. These new emphases present extraordinary challenges.

We advance 10 recommendations to support our proposed program. The first two change the mission of Medicare to include explicit goals for assuring the quality of care for Medicare enrollees, in accordance with this committee's definition of quality of care.

Three recommendations establish the MPAQ, MQROs, and two advisory bodies, namely the QualPAC for Congress and the National Council on Medicare Quality Assurance for the Secretary of DHHS. A related recommendation directs the Secretary of DHHS to report periodically to Congress on the quality of care for Medicare beneficiaries and the impact of the new MPAQ program on that care. Another recommendation calls for a program to improve both the accreditation and the certification procedures related to Medicare Conditions of Participation.

Two recommendations call for the Secretary of DHHS to support and expand research and educational activities designed to improve the nation's knowledge base and capacity for quality assurance. The final recommendation asks that Congress authorize and appropriate the necessary funds to implement all the preceding recommendations.

We also outline a strategy to implement the MPAQ over a 10-year span. Phase I would establish the MPAQ and its adjuncts, institute key program planning and evaluation activities, review PRO program activities, institute changes in hospital Conditions of Participation procedures at HCFA, and begin broad research and capacity building activities across the Department.

Phase II would focus on design, testing, and implementation of data collection, data analysis, and information dissemination mechanisms. It would also include special projects on four issues: distinguishing providers on the basis of quality and patient outcomes; improving the average level of performance; providing incentives for good and exemplary performance; and dealing with outliers.

In Phase III, tasks begun in Phases I and II would be completed and full implementation of the MPAQ would begin. In addition, four issues of special long-range concern would be addressed. Two of these involve the MPAQ directly, namely, public oversight and accountability and program evaluation. The third and fourth are research and capacity building, which encompass issues well beyond the implementation of the Medicare quality assurance program and hence involve policy issues for all of DHHS.

The MPAQ strategy outlined in this chapter is skeletal, yet very ambitious. We made our recommendations aware that the system of care in the next century will likely be very different from today's. The steps described were intended to show how the nation and the Medicare program might move from "here" to "there" over the next decade, to produce a quality assurance program responsive to that changing environment and whose principles will stand the tests of time and change.

We close by emphasizing the diversity of support for addressing the extraordinary challenges of quality assurance. The Medicare program has a responsibility to assure the quality of care for the elderly population; by no means does it have the sole responsibility. Patients, providers, and societal agents all must participate in this strategy for quality review and assurance if we are to meet these challenges. It is our hope and expectation that this strategy will accomplish a goal shared by all involved with medical care for the elderly—the improvement of quality for all.

NOTES

1. The act establishing the Professional Standards Review Organizations (P.L. 92-603) set out to promote effective, efficient, and economical delivery of health care services of "proper quality"; it uses terms such as "medically necessary," provides for the "exercise of reasonable limits of professional discretion," and refers specifically to "services for which payment may be made under the Social Security Act." The legislation creating the Peer Review Organization program (P.L. 97-248) does not materially change that focus; for instance, the duties and functions of PROs are to assure the quality of services for which payment may be made by Medicare and to eliminate unreasonable, unnecessary, and inappropriate care provided to Medicare beneficiaries.

2. Repeal of the Medicare Catastrophic Coverage Act eliminated the outpatient drug benefit and, by extension, development of the Part C medications files. The importance of medications data for comprehensive understanding of the quality of care rendered to the elderly remains as great as ever, however.

Acknowledgments

The contributions of many individuals and organizations to the committee's work deserve acknowledgment.

The committee expresses its deep appreciation to all individuals and groups who contributed to and testified for the study's public hearings and to those who gave generously of their time and knowledge during the study's site visits. Because of the very large number of persons and associations included in these groups, they are identified in materials contained in Volume II of this report. We also express our gratitude to the members of the elderly community and the practicing physicians who participated in the study's focus groups; their identities are confidential.

The committee thanks the authors of background papers prepared for this study which were used extensively by the staff and committee in their deliberations and in drafting this report. These experts include: Miriam Adams, Thomas Bubolz, Avedis Donabedian, Elliott Fisher, Catherine Hawes, Karen Josephson, Janet Kraegel, Norma Lang, Margaret O'Kane, Heather Palmer, Gail Povar, Evert Reerink, Leslie Roos, Noralou Roos, Laurence Rubenstein, Lisa Rubenstein, and Andrew Heath Smith. We thank Joann Richards of Mercy Hospital Systems for providing useful data and compilations on quality assurance and related activities collected through a recent hospital survey. We also extend our appreciation to the members of the criteria and standards expert panel: William A. Causey, Arthur J. Donovan, Leonard S. Driefus, David M. Eddy, Lesley Fishelman, Sheldon Greenfield, Robert J. Marder, Jane L. Neumann, Bruce Perry, and Ralph Schaffarzick. We are especially grateful to Paul Batalden, R. Heather Palmer, Henry Krakauer, Leslie Roos, Kenneth Wagstaff, and Harry S. Weeks for stimulating presentations to the committee.

The committee is particularly grateful to the members of the study's

Technical Advisory Panel (TAP) for their interest, support, and assistance throughout the project. The individuals and organizations on the TAP included: Jenean Erickson and Judith Brown, American Health Care Association; Deborah Bohr, American Hospital Association; Lynn Jensen and Jim Rodgers, American Medical Association; Carole Magoffin, American Medical Review Research Center; Norma Lang, American Nurses Association; Lawrence C. Morris, Blue Cross and Blue Shield Association; Margaret E. O'Kane, Group Health Association of America, Inc.; Jane Majcher, Health Insurance Association of America; James S. Roberts, Joint Commission on Accreditation of Healthcare Organizations; Frances Kay Cerjak and Francis Appel, National Association of Quality Assurance Professionals; Ruth Galten, National Association of Home Care; Richard E. Curtis and John Luehrs, National Governors Association; Jesse B. Barber, National Medical Association; and Lou Glasse, Older Women's League.

The contributions of the report's authors should be acknowledged. The study director, Kathleen N. Lohr, had primary responsibility for the entire report. In addition, chapters for which members of the project staff were specifically responsible were as follows: Chapters 1 and 2, Jo Harris-Wehling; Chapters 3 and 4, Allison Walker; Chapter 5, Michael McGeary and Jo Harris-Wehling; Chapter 6, Kathleen Lohr; Chapters 7, 8, and 9, Molla Donaldson; Chapter 10, Kathleen Lohr, Molla Donaldson, and Jay Bautz; Chapter 11, Kathleen Lohr and Allison Walker; and Chapter 12, Kathleen Lohr. We also acknowledge the valuable support of project consultants Elaine Elinsky and Jay Bautz and our subcontractor for the focus groups, Mathew Greenwald & Associates, Inc.

We are indebted to several members of the Institute of Medicine (IOM) professional staff. Marilyn Field provided considerable and timely assistance in the review and revision of several chapters of this report. The assistance and support throughout the study of Bradford Gray, formerly of the IOM and now at Yale University, was especially appreciated. Richard Rettig was particularly helpful in the early stages of planning and initiating the study. We also thank Alan Kaplan, an attorney and consultant in Washington, D.C., for assistance throughout the study and particularly with regard to the Medicare Peer Review Organization program, where he has many years of experience and great expertise.

The Study to Design a Strategy for Quality Review and Assurance in Medicare would not have been possible without the dedicated efforts of several members of the IOM staff, including H. Donald Tiller, Administrative Assistant; Dorothy Sheffield, Administrative Secretary; Lisa Chimento, Financial Specialist; and Thelma Cox, Denise Grady, and Theresa Nally, Project Secretaries. Wallace Waterfall provided much helpful editorial advice. In addition, the unflagging support and guidance of Karl Yordy, Director of the Division of Health Care Services, deserves special mention.

Finally, support for this study was provided by the U.S. Department of Health and Human Services, Health Care Financing Administration. We thank John Spiegel and Harvey Brook, of the Health Standards and Quality Bureau, for helpful responses to our inquiries and requests during the study. In addition, we particularly wish to acknowledge the considerable assistance and guidance of the government's project officer, Harry L. Savitt, of the Office of Research and Demonstrations.

Index

Index

A

AAAHC, *see* Accreditation Association for Ambulatory Health Care

ABA, *see* American Bar Association

ABMS, *see* American Board of Medical Specialties

Access
  barriers, 2, 24, 29, 31, 96, 110, 225-227, 258, 276, 369
  to care, 2, 52, 344, 346, 389, 402
  to information, 36, 37, 170, 248, 293, 350
  to PRO rules, 192
  public programs for improving, 34, 96, 256
  research needs, 344, 346, 381
  to services, 19, 29, 52, 79-80, 225, 288, 346
  underdiagnosis/undertreatment, 226-227
  underuse and, 23, 52, 225-226, 275, 284, 389
  utilization management and, 30, 111

Accountability, for quality of care, 20, 32, 36, 37, 241
  and autonomy, 290
  and continuous quality improvement, 62-64
  and oversight for PRO program, 193, 197, 372, 379-383, 420
  and prepaid practice, 193-195
  professional, 49, 244
  for public monies, 7, 52, 145

Accreditation, 53, 56, 267-269; *see also* Joint Commission on Accreditation of Healthcare Organizations

Accreditation Association for Ambulatory Health Care, 268

Accreditation Manual, 124, 267

Accreditation Council for Graduate Medical Education, 271

ACGME, *see* Accreditation Council for Graduate Medical Education

Activities of daily living, 83, 89-90, 91, 390

ADLs, *see* Activities of daily living

Administrative data sets, 274-276

Administrative Procedure Act, 148
Adverse patient occurrences, 281-283
    incidence, 214-215, 218
Agenda for Change, 56, 61, 125, 355,
    396; *see also* Joint Commission
    on Accreditation of Healthcare
    Organizations
AHA, *see* American Hospital Asso-
    ciation
Algorithms, clinical (patient care),
    178, 272-273, 278-279, 307,
    310, 322, 327, 395
AMA, *see* American Medical Asso-
    ciation
Ambulatory care
    certification, 268
    quality problems, 246-250
    research needed, 355
    review in, 142, 177, 194, 196-197,
        238, 256-257, 407-408
American Bar Association, 219
American Board of Medical Special-
    ties, 270, 271
American Hospital Association, 120,
    307
American Medical Association, 220,
    270, 271
American Medical Peer Review As-
    sociation, 182
American Medical Review Research
    Center, 179, 346, 355
AMPRA, *see* American Medical Peer
    Review Association
AMRRC, *see* American Medical
    Review Research Center
Appropriateness
    of care, 111, 159, 221-224, 316,
        391
    guidelines, 3, 272-273, 304-306,
        319-321, 325, 328, 370, 418;
        see also Practice guidelines
    research, 345, 353-354

Art of care, 25, 219, 350-351; *see
    also* Quality-of-care indicators/
    measures
Attributes
    of criteria sets, 311-319
    implementation, 316-319
    of medical profession, 289-292
    of QA methods, 49-50, 266-267
    substantive, 3, 311-316
Autopsy, 266, 286, 287

                          B

Beneficiary
    complaints, 170, 217-218, 252
    number of, 100
    relations, 169-170
Bi-cycle model, 62, 293; *see also*
    Quality assurance, models
Burden of harm
    differentiating among contributing
        factors, 209-210
    overuse and, 208, 210, 220-224
    of poor quality care, 27, 31-32
    quality problems and, 207
    sources of information about, 210-
        211
    of technical and interpersonal
        quality, 207-208, 209-210, 211-
        219
    underuse and, 209-210, 225-230

                          C

Capacity building, 3, 14-15, 360-363,
    384-385, 418-419
    and continuous improvement, 362-
        363
    patient education, 362
    professional education, 361-362
    research needs, 343
Career paths, 361

Carriers, 102, 374, 395; *see also* Medicare, claims processing
Case conferences, 228, 286-288
Case-finding
  complaints, 170, 217-218
  generic screens, 154-156, 160, 183-186, 228, 281-283, 307-388, 323
  see also Individual case methods
Case management, 219, 252
Case mix, 11, 12, 247, 259, 308, 356, 378, 409
Certification
  board, of health professionals, 53, 246, 266, 267, 269, 270-272, 278, 361
  Home Health Agencies, 82, 251, 252
  hospitals, 111, 120, 121-122, 128, 129, 130, 135, 371, 420
  physician attestation, 156
  preadmission, 140
  see also Licensure; Survey and Certification
CHAP, *see* Community Health Accreditation Program
Claims data, 54, 248, 249, 255; *see also* Medicare Statistical System
Clinical indicators, 132-133, 283-284, 308, 396
Clinical information systems, 243-244, 248-249
  research needs, 358
CME, *see* Continuing medical education
CMP, *see* Competitive medical plans
Coding
  accuracy, 242-243, 255, 275-276, 277, 279, 280, 281
  ambulatory, 249, 255
  ICD-9-CM, 242-243, 257, 275

Part B, 255-256
see also Common Procedural Terminology
Common Procedural Terminology, 257, 275; *see also* Coding
Community Health Accreditation Program, 252, 268
Competitive medical plans, 100-102
  research needed, 356-357
  review in, 173-177, 188, 193-195, 256-257
  see also Health maintenance organizations; Prepaid care
Complaints
  beneficiary, 170, 217-218, 252
  patient, 287-288, 288-289
Complication rates, medical, 266, 281; *see also* Quality-of-care indicators/measures
Computers, *see* Clinical information systems; Data
Conditions of Participation, 7-8, 111, 138, 396, 401-402
  enforcement, 129-131
  federal role, 131-132
  HCFA and, 8, 124-125, 128-131, 134-135
  history, 120-124
  inspection, 128-129
  quality assurance condition, 125-128
  recommendations, 383-384
  shift from capacity to performance standards, 124-125
Continuing Medical Education, 162, 270, 292-293, 354, 361; *see also* Physician education
Continuity of care, 13-14, 29-30, 392
Continuous quality improvement, 294, 374-375
  accountability, 58, 62-64
  applications, 61

capacity building and, 362-363
customers and suppliers, 46, 59-60
defined, 46
model assumptions and constructs, 58-61, 387-388
PDCA cycle, 59
research, 352, 362-363
see also Industrial quality control
Corrective actions/plans, 160-163, 216-217
Cost containment, 97, 111, 309, 360, 374, 394-395
CPT, see Common Procedural Terminology
Credentialling, 269
Criteria, quality assurance
development, 323-325
for allocation of resources, 393-394
for evaluation and management of care, 322-322
for successful quality assurance, 3, 49-52
mapping, 249
relationship among criteria sets, 308-309
sets, 277-279, 303-309, 310-319
and standards, 277-279
Customers, 58-60; see also Continuous quality improvement

D

Darling v. Charleston Community Hospital, 241
Data
bases, 243-244, 274-277, 281, 403-404, 415; see also Medicare Statistical System
collection and analysis, 178, 400, 404-408, 415

disclosure/reporting/dissemination/sharing, 15-16, 34, 170-171, 359-360, 408-410, 415-416
fee-for-service, 255-256
hospital, 243
prepaid care, 256-258
see also Claims data; Clinical information systems
Decertification, 129, 130, 131, 133, 181-182,
Decision making, 20-25, 56
patient, 22, 362, 385, 402, 407-408
physician, 22, 63, 207-208, 244, 278, 315, 327, 402, 408
and population-based outcomes, 36-37
Deemed status, 7-8, 111, 119, 134; see also Medicare Program to Assure Quality
Defining quality of care, 2, 4-5, 20-25, 375-377
Delegated review, 142-143, 179, 199; see also Professional Standards Review Organizations
Department of Health and Human Services, 1, 140
current responsibilities, 102, 119
evaluation of PRO program, 192-193
PRO contracting authority, 149
recommended responsibilities, 6-8, 14, 378, 379, 381-385, 413-414, 416, 420
regulatory and enforcement authority, 135, 163, 216-217
DHHS, see Department of Health and Human Services
Diagnosis-related groups, 97, 224, 228
definition, 108-109
validation, 156-159

Discharge
    planning, 223, 224, 156, 178, 184
    premature, 156, 223, 225, 227-
      228, 245
    review, 156
Disciplinary actions, 48, 215-216
DRGs, *see* Diagnosis-related groups

E

Education
    patient, 169, 362
    physician, 139, 162, 177, 292-293,
      361-362
Effectiveness/efficacy, 30
    medical care, 19, 23, 178
    of interventions, 289-297
    research, 348-350, 354-355
Elderly
    access to care, 2, 31-32, 79-80,
      93, 96, 230, 369, 399
    activity limitations, 89-90
    chronic illness and impairment, 2,
      88-89
    expenditures, 105-108
    federal role in support of, 84-85
    geographic distribution, 72-73
    health insurance, 75
    health status, 85-91
    income, 75-79
    life expectancy, 2, 85-86
    living arrangements, 73-75
    Medicare issues for, 2
    mental health, 90-91
    mortality, 86-88
    nursing home residents, 74-75, 81-
     82
    race and ethnicity, 71
    rate of population growth, 2, 69-
     71
    satisfaction with care, 1
    sex ratios, 71
    support ratios, 71
Elderly, use of services
    community-based services, 83-84
    home health care, 82-83
    hospital, 79
    long term care, 81-84
    nursing home, 81-82
    physician, 79-81
EMCROS, *see* Experimental Medi-
    cal Care Review Organizations
Enforcement, 128-131, 133-134, 253;
    see also Sanctions and sanc-
    tioning process
    DHHS authority, 135, 163, 216-
     217
    OIG authority, 145, 163-167, 189,
     200, 411
Episodes
    of care, 177, 239, 247-248, 405-
     406
    of illness, 239
Ethics, in health care
    autonomy, 23, 290
    beneficence, 25
    equity, 24
    fidelity, 25
    fiduciary relationship, 25
    nonmaleficence, 25
Evaluation of programs
    PRO, 180-182, 192-193, 260
    MPAQ, 379-383, 399-400, 414,
     417-418
    MQRO, 398-399
Exemplary performance, 16, 47, 323,
    416; *see also* Incentives
Expenditures
    by elderly for health care, 105-
     108
    health care, 28-29, 103-105
    Medicare, 28-29, 105-108
Experimental Medical Care Review
    Organizations, 139

F

Federation of State Licensing Boards, 215, 216
Fee-for-service, 3, 73, 254-256
  and accountability for care, 194-195
  alternatives to, 100-102, 112
  conflict of interest, 25, 48
  data, 255-256
  and medical records availability, 193
  and overuse, 140, 230
  prepaid system contrasted with, 254
  prevention of quality problems, 246, 255-257
  quality review in, 173, 175, 177, 182, 188, 194-195, 196, 254, 401
  types of problems, 256
Feedback, 408-409
  to clinicians, 254, 292-293, 359, 415-416
  loop, 15, 249
FI, see Fiscal intermediaries
Findings and conclusions, 2-4, 369-371
Fiscal intermediaries, 102, 138, 225, 374
FSLB, see Federation of State Licensing Boards
Funding
  for MPAQ, 9-10, 385-387
  for MQRO, 396-397
  for PRO program, 171-173
  for research, 363

G

GAO, see General Accounting Office
General Accounting Office, 145-146, 167, 183, 192-193, 212, 217, 383

Generic screens
  case-finding, 323
  characteristics, applications, and processes, 154-156, 160, 281-283
  limitations and problematic aspects of, 183-186, 282-283
  strengths, 282
  see also Adverse patient occurrences; Occurrence screens
Guidelines, 30
  appropriateness, 3, 272-273, 304-306, 319-321, 325, 328, 370, 418
  patient management, 272-273, 306-307, 322-323
  research, 353-354
  see also Generic screens; Practice guidelines

H

HCFA, see Health Care Financing Administration
HCQIA, see Health Care Quality Improvement Act
Health accounting, 62; see also Quality assurance models
Health Care Financing Administration
  Bureau of Policy Development (BPD), 121
  and Conditions of Participation, 8, 124-125, 128-131, 134-135
  Health Standards and Quality Bureau (HSQB), 120, 121, 128, 132, 140, 346, 363
  and HMO/CMP review, 177-182
  hospital-specific mortality rates, 35, 280, 308
  Office of Research and Demonstrations (ORD), 346, 351, 363
  procedures, 148, 192-193
  and PSROs, 143, 145
  research, 346

responsibility for Medicare program, 120
responsibility for quality, 34, 110
Health care personnel/professionals distribution
  manpower, 27-28, 58, 159, 343
  training, *see* Capacity building
  see also Physician
Health Care Quality Improvement Act, 148, 171, 410
Health maintenance organizations, 100-102
  accountability, 193-195
  data, 256-258
  quality review in, 173-177
  prevention of problems, 246, 256
  research needed, 356-357
  see also Competitive medical plans; Prepaid care
Health services research, 344
Health status assessment, 20, 26, 34, 57, 286, 406-407; *see also* Activities of daily living
  of the elderly, 85-91
  research needs, 351-352
HMOs, *see* Health maintenance organizations
Home health
  agencies, 82
  case management
  financing, 250-251
  homebound provisions, 82, 83, 356
  Medicare certification, 82, 251-252
  quality problems, 218-219, 250-254
  research needed, 356
  review in, 186-187, 406-407
  state licensure, 251-252
  visits per person, 82-83
  voluntary certification, 252
Hospitals
  adequacy of QA mechanisms, 3

  certification, 111, 120, 121-122, 128, 129, 130, 135, 371, 420
  data, 243
  discharge rate surveys, 79
  elderly use of care, 79
  mortality rates, 208, 280, 291; *see also* Quality-of-care indicators/measures
  nosocomial infections, 125, 154, 156, 184
  outcomes of care, small area analysis, 179
  readmissions, 161, 186, 227, 275
Hospital care, 79, 241-245

I

Incentives, 16, 47, 51, 293-294, 416
Individual case methods, 247, 286-289, 307-309
Industrial quality control, 58-61; *see also* Continuous quality improvement
Information management, *see* Clinical information systems; Data
Inspection, state
  Conditions of Participation, 128-129
  see also Certification; Licensure
Intermediaries, *see* Fiscal Intermediaries
Intervening care, 160, 187, 196; *see also* Medicare Peer Review Program; Readmission, to hospital

J

JCAHO, *see* Joint Commission on Accreditation of Healthcare Organizations
Joint Commission on Accreditation of Healthcare Organizations
  Agenda for Change, 56, 61, 125, 355, 396

decision rules, 129-130, 134
deemed status, 7-8, 111, 119, 134
see also Certification; Conditions of Participation; Decertification

L

Legislative charges to IOM, xii
Liability, 159, 211-215; *see also* Malpractice
Licensing, 162, 171, 269-270
Licensure, 251-252, 269-270; *see also* Certification
Life expectancy, 26, 85, 86
Long term care, 81-84, 91-93

M

Malpractice, 35-37, 211-215, 220; *see also* Liability)
Market forces and competition, 33, 35, 37, 220-221, 296
Medical records, 134, 141, 178, 191, 241-242, 255, 258, 318, 358-359
Medicare
  administration, 102
  claims processing, 102
  Conditions of Participation, 111
  data systems, *see* Medicare Statistical System
  deductibles and coinsurance, 104
  enrolled population, 100
  expenditures, 28-29, 105-108
  financing, 103
  HMO and CMP risk contracts, 100-102
  Hospital Insurance (Part A), 97
  legislation related to, 98
  Medicare Insured Groups, 102
  mission, 4-5, 96, 375-377
  prospective payment system, 79-80, 82-83, 107-109, 394-396
  quality assurance goals, 5, 110-111; *see also* Conditions of Participation; Medicare Peer Review Organizations; Utilization Management
  Supplementary Medical Insurance (Part B), 99
Medicare Peer Review Organizations (PROs)
  ambulatory review, 194, 256-257
  beneficiary complaints, 170
  beneficiary relations, 169-170
  contracts, 148-149
  data acquisition, sharing, and reporting, 170-171
  denials for substandard quality of care, 190-191
  DRG validation, 149, 156-159
  funding, 171-173
  generic screens, 154-155, 160, 183-186
  HMO and CMP review, 173-177, 193-195
  home health review, 186-187
  intervening care, 160
  interventions (QIP), 161-163
  Manual, 148
  nonhospital review, 159-160, 196-197
  organizational characteristics, 148
  outreach, 170
  oversight, 193, 197, 372, 379-383, 420
  physician review, 187
  preadmission and preprocedure review, 159
  PRO pilots, 179-180
  provider relations, 170
  quality interventions, 161-3
  required review activities, 149-160, 169-171
  review of rural care, 159, 188-189
  sanctions, 163-169, 189-190

scope of work, 154-156, 159
triggers (weighted), 162-163
waiver of liability, 159
Medicare Peer Review Organization
    Program
administration of program, 148
administrative procedures, 192
controversial aspects of, 182-195
costs, funding, 171-173
enabling legislation, 147-148
evaluation (program), 180-182,
    192-193, 260
peer review, 188-189
PROMPTS-2, 180
review of rural care, 159, 188-189
SuperPRO, 180-182
UCDS (Uniform Clinical Data
    Set), 177-179
Medicare Program to Assure Qual-
    ity, 1, 10-14, 378, 387-400
allocation of resources, 393-394
evaluation/public oversight, 379-
    383, 399-400, 414, 417-418
implementation strategy, 14-17,
    412-419
funding, 9-10, 385-387
operational overview, 12-14, 389-
    392
problems and limitations, 392-393
research, 418
responsibilities, 394-400
special projects, 416-417
structure, 388-389
Medicare Quality Review Organiza-
    tion, 378-379, 400-410
data, data collection, and analy-
    sis, 401-408, 415
evaluation, 398-399
feedback, data reporting, and data
    sharing, 408-410, 415-416
funding, 396-397
quality interventions, 410-412
reconsideration of PRO functions,
    395-396

review topics, 404-405
Medicare Statistical System (MSS),
    (M/MDSS), 117-118
Mental health, 90-91
MPAQ, see Medicare Program to
    Assure Quality
MQRO, see Medicare Quality Re-
    view Organization

N

NAQAP, see National Association of
    Quality Assurance Profession-
    als
National Association of Quality As-
    surance Professionals, 361
National Center for Health Services
    Research, 346
National Center for Health Statistics,
    69, 79, 90
National Committee on Quality As-
    surance, 268
National Council on Medicare Qual-
    ity Assurance, 379, 382-383
National League for Nursing, 252,
    268
National Practitioner Data Bank, 171,
    396
NCHS, see National Center for
    Health Statistics
NCHSR, see National Center for
    Health Services Research
NCQA, see National Committee on
    Quality Assurance
Net benefit, 4, 21, 22, 320
NLN, see National League for Nurs-
    ing
Nosocomial (hospital-acquired) in-
    fections, 125, 154, 156, 184
Notices of denial, 196; see also
    Medicare Peer Review Organi-
    zation Program
Nursing homes, 74-75, 81-82

O

OBRA, *see* Omnibus Budget Reconciliation acts

Occurrence screens, 307-308; *see also* Adverse patient occurrences; Generic screens

Office of Inspector General
    activity on interventions and sanctions, 167, 169, 217
    enforcement authority, 145, 163-167, 189, 200, 411
    evaluation of PRO program, 193
    procedures for recommending sanctions to, 166
    recommendations on penalties, 189-190
    recommended role of, 383

OIG, *see* Office of Inspector General

Omnibus Budget Reconciliation Act of 1986, 1, 148, 173, 180

Omnibus Budget Reconciliation Act of 1987, 102, 148, 149, 190, 252, 253

Omnibus Budget Reconciliation Act of 1989, 191

Organizational change, 294-295

Outcome measures, 266, 405
    in ambulatory care, 247, 406-407
    in Conditions of Participation, 128
    in data bases, 276, 358; *see also* Outcomes data
    distinguishing providers on basis of, 16
    in health status assessment, 284, 286
    for home health care, 253, 406
    limitations of, 13, 128, 132, 259, 276, 286, 358, 391, 402, 409
    in MPAQ, 12-13, 386, 389-391
    nonintrusive, 266
    OBRA requirements, 253

patient-provider decision-making process and, 36
    process links with, 6, 21, 51, 62, 54, 316, 348, 353, 357, 364, 377, 391-392
    research needs on, 273, 351, 353, 357, 383-384
    scales, 253
    severity adjustment, 351
    strengths of, 286
    in structure-process-outcome model, 53, 56-58

Outcomes
    art-of-care and, 350-351
    assessment, 247, 253, 266-267, 276, 277, 319, 405, 406
    and burden of harm, 207
    continuity of care and, 13-14
    of the elderly, 200
    in home health care, 218, 250-251, 253
    of hospital care, small area analysis, 179
    longitudinal, 196
    management, 74, 407
    physician certification and, 271-272
    population, 11, 196, 259
    provider-patient relationship and, 25
    research, 8, 327, 346-347, 397-398
    underuse and, 226
    volume of services and, 276-277
    see also Surgical mishaps

Outcomes data
    collection of, 390-391, 393, 397, 404-408, 415
    confidentiality, 360, 409
    from data bases, 273-275
    general points, 279-280
    hospital mortality rates, 280
    lack of, 58, 134, 135
    medical complications, 281

recommended scope of, 403
uses, 5, 7, 10, 12, 15, 247, 377,
  383, 387, 388-389
Outliers, 46-47, 141, 208, 416-417;
  see also Physician, performance
Outreach, 170
Overuse
  and burden of harm, 208-209, 210,
    220-224
  defined, 208
  fee-for-service and, 140, 230
  and underuse, 210

P

Patient
  complaints, 287-289
  compliance, 241
  decision making, 22, 362, 385,
    407-408
  education, 169, 362
  management guidelines, 272-273,
    306-307, 322-323
  privacy/confidentiality, 359-160
  records, 242; *see also* Medical
    records
  reports, 284-285
  satisfaction, 244, 284-285, 347,
    350-351
Patrick v. *Burget,* 245
PDCA cycle, 59
Peer review, 148, 154, 170, 188-189,
  198, 244
Performance
  exemplary, 16, 47, 323, 416
  profiles, 244, 410-411
  standards, 62, 124-125
Physician
  attestation, 140
  education, 139, 162, 177, 292-293,
    361-362; *see also* Continuing
    Medical Education
  manpower, 27-28

payment, 31, 99-100
performance, 16, 47, 141, 416-
  417; *see also* Outliers
Physician Payment Review Commission, 110-111, 187-188
Pilot projects, PRO, 179-180
Policies and procedures, 192, 241
Population-based measures, 36-37,
  63; *see also* Quality-of-care
  indicators/measures
Potentially compensable events, 213;
  see also Liability
PPRC, *see* Physician Payment Re-
  view Commission
PPS, *see* Prospective payment system
Practice guidelines, 272-273, 328
  research needs, 353-354;
  see also Guidelines
Practice variations, 222
  small area analysis, 222-223
Premature discharge, 156, 223, 225,
  227-228, 245
Prepaid care, 100-102, 194-195, 246,
  256-258; *see also* Competitive
  Medical Plans; Health maintenance organizations
Preventable deaths, 214
PROs, *see* Medicare Peer Review
  Organizations
Process measures of quality, 54-56,
  277-279, 350-351, 391-392,
  402-403
  linking process with outcomes,
    279-280, 353
  see also Quality-of-care indica-
    tors/measures
Professional Standards Review Organizations
  activities, 140-142
  costs, 143
  delegated review, 142-143
  impact, 146

National Council, 144
sanctions, 145-146
structure, 140
Professional incompetence, 215
Professionalism, 18, 32-33, 291
ProPAC, *see* Prospective Payment Assessment Commission
Prospective Payment Assessment Commission, 17, 29, 107, 109-110, 184, 227-228, 346, 382
Prospective payment system, 79-80, 82-83, 107-109, 227
and cost containment, 109, 394-396
PSROs, *see* Professional Standards Review Organizations
Public good, 34, 379
Public oversight
MPAQ, 399-400, 417-418
PRO, 193, 197, 372, 379-383, 420

Q

Quality assessment, defined, 45-46
Quality assurance
defined, 45
ideology, 296
international perspective, 61-62
leadership, 296
purpose of, 46-47
professional responsibility for, 32-33
public responsibility for, 33-34
Quality assurance, models
bi-cycle model, 62, 293
continuous improvement, 58-61
focus, 3
health accounting, 62
MPAQ, 371-373
structure/process/outcome, 53-58, 387
traditional and continuous improvement models compared, 62-64

Quality assurance, programs
criteria for judging success of, 49-52
external, 48-49
federal, *see* Conditions of Participation; Medicare Peer Review Organization Program
findings and conclusions, 2
internal, 47-49, 268, 388-389
Quality of care
criteria for review, *see* Criteria, quality assurance
definitions, 4-5, 20-25, 375-377
effect of organization and financing, 295-297
research needed, 357-358
Quality-of-care indicators/measures
complication rates, 281
mortality rates, 280
nosocomial infections, 125, 154, 156, 184
reliability and validity, 266-267, 311-314
retrospective methods, 221, 226, 277-279
structural measures, 53-54
volume of service, 276-277
see also Generic screens; Outcome measures; Population-based measures; Process measures of quality
Quality-of-care problems
in ambulatory care, 246-250
correcting, 244-245, 249-250, 253-254
detecting, 242-244, 247-249, 252-253
differentiating among problems, 209-210
in home health, 218-219, 250-254
interpersonal care, 208
overuse, 220-224
preventing, 241, 246, 251-252
technical care, 207-209, 211-219

underdiagnosis/undertreatment, 226-227, 228-229
underuse, 209, 225-230
see also Art of care
Quality interventions
    MQRO, 410-412, 416
    PRO, 161-163, 167-169
QualPAC, see Quality Program Advisory Commission
Quality Program Advisory Commission, 7, 379-382

R

Readmission, to hospital, 161, 186, 227, 275
Reappointment and privileging, 240, 241
Recommendations
    capacity for quality, enhancement of, 8-9, 384-385
    funding, 9-10, 385-387
    goals for Medicare quality assurance, 6, 377-378
    Medicare Conditions of Participation, 8-9, 383-384
    mission of Medicare, 5-6, 375-377
    National Council on Medicare Quality Assurance, 7, 379, 382
    PRO program restructuring, 6, 378-379
    public accountability and evaluation program, 6-7
    Quality Program Advisory Commission, 7, 379-381
    report on quality of care, 7, 379
    research into efficacy, effectiveness, and outcomes of care, 8-9, 384-385
Regulation, in medicine, 33
    Administrative Procedure Act, 148
    Code of Federal Regulations, 120
    PRO, 192, 147-148
    PSRO, 145-146

TEFRA, 101, 110, 147-148, 188
    see also Conditions of Participation
Reliability, 226-227, 311-314
Reminders, clinical, 244, 266, 273-274
Reports, patient, 284-285
Research
    access to care, 344, 346, 381
    ambulatory care, 355
    appropriateness, 345, 353-354
    capacity building, 343
    clinical information systems, 358
    CMPs, 356-357
    continuous quality improvement, 352, 362-363
    effectiveness, 348-350, 354-355
    funding, 363
    guidelines, 353-354
    HCFA, 346
    health services, 344
    health status assessment, 351-352
    HMOs, 356-357
    in home health, 356
    MPAQ, 418
    outcomes, 8, 327, 346-347, 397-398
    practice guidelines, 353-354
    practice variations, 222-223
    priorities for, 345
    rural care, 357
    severity of illness, 351
Resource allocation, 393-394
Resource constraints, 24, 377, 402
Retrospective review, 140-141, 162, 221, 277-279, 310
Rewards and penalties, 256, 266, 293; see also Incentives
Risk
    adjustment, 275, 277, 391; see also Severity of illness
    contracts, 100-102
    management, 35-37, 208, 241, 283; see also Liability; Malpractice

Rulemaking and public notice, 148, 192

Rural care, 27, 29, 99, 108, 135, 159
and peer review, 188-189
research needs, 357

S

Sanctions and sanctioning process, 145-146, 216-217, 412
PRO, 163-169, 189-190
recommendations to OIG, 169

Satisfaction, 1, 20, 21-22, 23
patient, 244, 284-285, 347, 350-351

Severity of illness
adjustment, 12, 243, 255, 280-281, 383, 405
research into, 351

Shifting the curve, 16, 47, 416; *see also* Physician, performance

Small area variations analysis, 179-180, 276, 222-223, 346-347; *see also* Pilot Projects; Practice variations

Statistical control (quality control), 58

Structural measure of quality, 53-54, 56-58, 268, 378

Study methods
criteria-setting panel, xiv
focus groups, xiv
public hearings, xiv
site visits, xiv

Suppliers, 35, 59-60; *see also* Continuous quality improvement; Customers

Surgical mishaps, 213

Survey and certification, 4, 7, 8, 14, 121, 124, 128, 129, 132-135, 180, 410; *see also* Conditions of Participation; Joint Commission on Accreditation of Healthcare Organizations

Surveys
of activity limitations in elderly, 90
of defensive medical practices, 220
health status assessment, 407
of home health quality problems, 218, 240
of hospital discharge rates, 79
measurement of quality through, 53, 56
patient satisfaction, 279, 284-285
of PRO impact, 182
recommended, 400
of underuse, 226

T

TAP, *see* Technical Advisory Panel

Tax Equity and Fiscal Responsibility Act, 101, 110, 147, 148, 188

Technical Advisory Panel, 382-383

Technical quality, 207-208, 211-219
defined, 207-208
and interpersonal care, 207-208, 211-219, 296, 353
see also Quality-of-care problems

TEFRA, *see* Tax Equity and Fiscal Responsibility Act

U

UCDS, *see* Uniform Clinical Data Set

Underdiagnosis and undertreatment, 226, 227, 228-230; *see also* Quality of care problems

Underuse, 225-230
access to care and, 23, 52, 225, 226, 275, 284, 389
and burden of harm, 209-210, 225-230
defined, 209
and outcomes, 226
and overuse, 210

surveys of, 226
see also Quality-of-care problems
Uniform Ambulatory Care Data Set, 248
Uniform Clinical Data Set, 177-179, 186, 395, 404
Uniform Needs Assessment, 180, 227, 346, 356, 406
Use of services; *see* Elderly, use of services; Overuse; Underuse
Utilities, 36, 57, 61, 352
Utilization management, 30-31, 36, 37, 111, 140-141, 374, 394-395
Utilization and Quality Control Peer Review Organizations Program, *see* Medicare Peer Review Organizations; Medicare Peer Review Organization Program

V

Validity/validation, 51, 316
of appropriateness guidelines, 319-320, 328
of DRGs, 156-159
of patient evaluation and management criteria, 328
of quality of care indicators/measures, 266-267, 311-314
Value purchasing, 36
Variations, 222-223
research, 348-350
small area, 179-180, 222-223, 276
Volume of services, 276-277